Download Your Included
Ebook With Supplemental Materials Today!

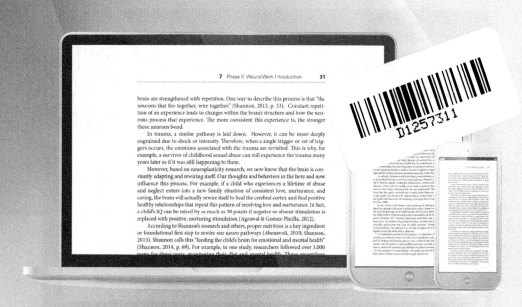

Your print purchase of *Guided Participation in Pediatric Nursing: Relationship-Based Teaching and Learning With Parents, Children, and Adolescents* **includes an ebook download** to the device of your choice— increasing accessibility, portability, and searchability!

Supplemental materials include:

- An outline of the guided participation processes and competencies
- Case studies that bring clarity to the process of guided participation
- Guided participation competence checklists for nurses and for parents
- Nutrition education for infants and Common Illness Guidelines for Families of Premature Babies
- Mom and Baby video

ental materials today at:
r the access code below:

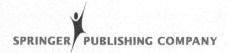

ACCESS YOUR ONLINE COURSE FOR GUIDED PARTICIPATION

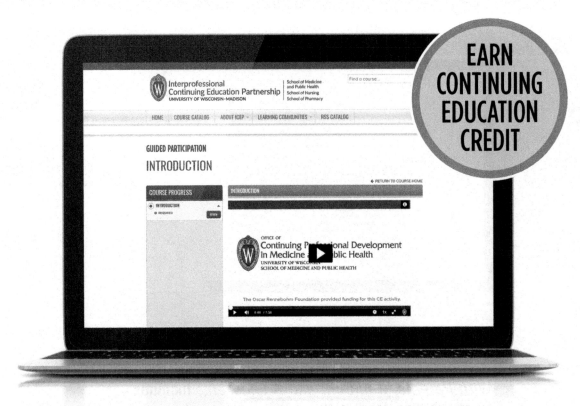

EARN CONTINUING EDUCATION CREDIT

Enhance your application of guided participation in your practice through this case-based online course. The course dives into principles, core concepts, and methods. Upon completion, you'll be equipped to initiate or expand guided participation in your practice.

START TODAY!*

Interprofessional Continuing Education Partnership
UNIVERSITY OF WISCONSIN–MADISON

School of Medicine and Public Health
School of Nursing
School of Pharmacy

JOINTLY ACCREDITED PROVIDER™
INTERPROFESSIONAL CONTINUING EDUCATION

ACCREDITATION STATEMENT
In support of improving patient care, the University of Wisconsin–Madison Interprofessional Continuing Education Partnership is accredited by the American Nurses Credentialing Center (ANCC), the Accreditation Council for Pharmacy Education (ACPE), and the Accreditation Council for Continuing Medical Education (ACCME), to provide continuing education for the healthcare team.

*This enduring activity is subject to periodic review and update.

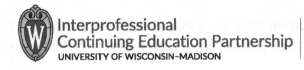

HTTPS://CE.ICEP.WISC.EDU/GUIDED-PARTICIPATION

The Oscar Rennebohm Foundation provided funding for this CE activity.

Guided Participation in Pediatric Nursing Practice

Karen F. Pridham, PhD, RN, FAAN, is professor emerita at University of Wisconsin School of Nursing. Her prolific career as nurse-researcher, scholar, and educator at the University of Wisconsin (UW)–Madison School of Nursing spans 40 years. Although retired from classroom teaching, she continues in an active program of research, while providing leadership in pediatric nursing to students and colleagues at the UW–Madison School of Nursing. She is responsible for a theory-based nursing intervention that has distinguished the UW–Madison School of Nursing as a leader in advancing the care of infants, children, and adolescents. Called guided participation, the approach offers nurses and other professionals strategies to assist mothers or parents with developmentally appropriate interventions for children experiencing healthcare challenges. It also tailors support for caregiving to parents' needs and goals. Dr. Pridham has published more than 70 peer-reviewed scholarly articles and has disseminated her research through posters and presentations regionally, nationally, and internationally. In 2010, she was one of the authors of a series of articles, "Furthering the Understanding of Parent–Child Relationships: A Nursing Scholarship Review Series," which won an award in the *Journal for Specialists in Pediatric Nursing*. She is the recipient of the coveted 2013 MNRS Lifetime Achievement award from the Midwest Nursing Research Society, and was inducted into the Sigma Theta Tau International Nurse Researcher Hall of Fame in 2015. Both awards recognize Dr. Pridham for her record of excellence in research and education and a distinguished career that has yielded outstanding accomplishments to advance the nursing profession.

Rana Limbo, PhD, RN, CPLC, FAAN, is senior consultant and associate director of Resolve Through Sharing® (RTS), Gundersen Medical Foundation, in La Crosse, Wisconsin. Dr. Limbo, a co-founder of the bereavement program RTS in 1981, has developed areas of expertise in relationship-based care, perinatal bereavement and perinatal palliative care, guided participation, and curriculum development. She is internationally recognized for her leadership, scholarship, and clinical expertise in bringing the domain of perinatal bereavement to the forefront of bereavement care. She is the author of numerous articles and book chapters, and co-author or co-editor of several books including *Meaningful Moments: Ritual and Reflection When a Child Dies* and *Conversations in Perinatal, Neonatal, and Pediatric Palliative Care*. Dr. Limbo worked with both Drs. Pridham (advisor) and Schroeder (same doctoral cohort) during her tenure as a doctoral student at UW–Madison in the 1990s. Her awards and recognitions include induction as a Fellow in the American Academy of Nursing; invited member of the International Work Group on Death, Dying, and Bereavement (IWG); two-term presidency of the Pregnancy Loss and Infant Death Alliance (PLIDA); AWHONN Excellence in Leadership award, 2017; and the *American Journal of Nursing* AJN Book of the Year award for *Perinatal and Pediatric Bereavement in Nursing and Other Health Professions* (2016). Her past and current research interests include miscarriage, guided participation, perinatal palliative care, feeding and growth of preterm infants, and caregiver suffering and grief.

Michele M. Schroeder, PhD, RN, CPNP, has been the pediatric clinical nurse specialist (CNS) at UnityPoint Health (UPH)–Meriter Hospital in Madison, Wisconsin since 2001, transitioning to family care in 2017. Previously, Dr. Schroeder provided leadership to nursing and to interdisciplinary care with the University of Wisconsin–Madison Interdisciplinary Pediatric Pulmonary Team and Training grant as a pediatric pulmonary CNS. She has also served as assistant professor/lead pediatric nurse practitioner of Child Health Option at Marquette University as well as senior research specialist at University of Wisconsin–Madison School of Nursing. She holds key nursing leadership positions at UPH–Meriter, and has responsibility for these programs: Journey to Excellence, Competencies, Professional Development and Education, and a DAISY award. Dr. Schroeder has authored numerous peer-reviewed publications. With guided participation as the foundation, her clinical, scholarly, and research interests include partnering with families in the care of their children, including learning to navigate systems of care (hospital, clinic, and community); development of working models of caregiving (parent and nurse); mentoring nursing and interdisciplinary colleagues in the care of children and their families; and fostering the development of professional nursing practice at individual and systems levels.

Guided Participation in Pediatric Nursing Practice

Relationship-Based Teaching and Learning With Parents, Children, and Adolescents

KAREN F. PRIDHAM, PhD, RN, FAAN
RANA LIMBO, PhD, RN, CPLC, FAAN
MICHELE M. SCHROEDER, PhD, RN, CPNP
Editors

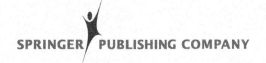

SPRINGER PUBLISHING COMPANY

Springer Publishing Company, LLC
11 West 42nd Street
New York, NY 10036
www.springerpub.com

Acquisitions Editor: Elizabeth Nieginski
Compositor: diacriTech, Chennai

ISBN: 978-0-8261-4043-2
ebook ISBN: 978-0-8261-4044-9
Supplemental Material ISBN: 978-0-8261-4032-6

Supplemental material for readers can be accessed at springerpub.com/pridham

18 19 20 21 22 / 5 4 3 2 1

The author and the publisher of this Work have made every effort to use sources believed to be reliable to provide information that is accurate and compatible with the standards generally accepted at the time of publication. Because medical science is continually advancing, our knowledge base continues to expand. Therefore, as new information becomes available, changes in procedures become necessary. We recommend that the reader always consult current research and specific institutional policies before performing any clinical procedure. The author and publisher shall not be liable for any special, consequential, or exemplary damages resulting, in whole or in part, from the readers' use of, or reliance on, the information contained in this book. The publisher has no responsibility for the persistence or accuracy of URLs for external or third-party Internet websites referred to in this publication and does not guarantee that any content on such websites is, or will remain, accurate or appropriate.

Library of Congress Cataloging-in-Publication Data
Names: Pridham, Karen F., editor. | Limbo, Rana K. (Rana Kristina), editor. |
    Schroeder, Michele M., editor.
Title: Guided participation in pediatric nursing practice :
    relationship-based teaching and learning with parents, children, and
    adolescents / [edited by] Karen F. Pridham, Rana Limbo, Michele M.
    Schroeder.
Description: New York, NY : Springer Publishing Company, LLC, [2018] |
    Includes bibliographical references.
Identifiers: LCCN 2018011529| ISBN 9780826140432 | ISBN 9780826140449 (e-book)
Subjects: | MESH: Health Education--methods | Pediatric Nursing--methods |
    Teaching | Professional-Family Relations | Parenting | Infant | Child |
    Adolescent
Classification: LCC RJ245 | NLM WY 159 | DDC 618.92/00231--dc23 LC record available at https://
lccn.loc.gov/2018011529

Contact us to receive discount rates on bulk purchases.
We can also customize our books to meet your needs.
For more information please contact: sales@springerpub.com

Printed in the United States of America.

To my mother, Mildred Frick, who helped me

learn and study guided participation ways, and to

my husband, Walter, and children, Bert and Ruth,

who traveled the paths with me.

To Paulette for her compassionate guidance

every day.

With much love to my parents, Charles and

Frances, whose daily example has taught me

more than they will ever know about living with

integrity, joy, and gratitude. Thanks for always

being there for me!

Contents

SECTION III

Guided Participation in Caring for Children With Acute and Chronic Conditions

SECTION IV

Guided Participation in Mental and Behavioral Health of Children and Families

Guided Participation in the Care of Children

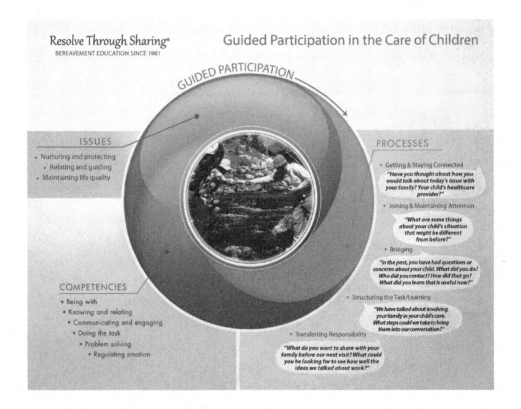

Many elements of guided participation (GP) are represented in this photo of a father assisting his daughter across slippery rocks in a mountainous stream. Both father (expert guide with years of hiking experience) and daughter (novice hiker with less experience) bring their own resourcefulness to the excursion. At the same time, each has a backpack, which could be filled to the brim with past experiences, worries and concerns, sense of responsibility, or numerous other things. The rocks are slick and the novice needs to cross the stream. Both may slip and get their boots wet, but the guide has more practice at righting himself. The guide brings the novice along, demonstrating a relationship that is strong, and showing the novice about how insecurities can be overcome. At the end, both have learned important elements of GP: skill does not guarantee success, but getting your boots wet strengthens problem solving. Finally, those clasped hands tell the story: "I'm here," "We're together," and "Human connectedness helps solve problems."

Rana Limbo

Contributors

Laura J. Ahola, MSN, RN, CNML, Nurse Manager, Pediatric Universal Care Unit, University of Wisconsin Health American Family Children's Hospital (AFCH), Madison, Wisconsin

Lori S. Anderson, PhD, RN, CPNP-PC, NCSN, Clinical Professor, Director for eSchoolCare (eSchoolCare.org), University of Wisconsin–Madison School of Nursing, Madison, Wisconsin

Janine M. Bamberger, MS, RDN, CD, Clinical Nutrition Manager, Children's Hospital of Wisconsin, Milwaukee, Wisconsin

Polly Belcher, BSN, RN, Retired Public Health Nurse, City of Milwaukee Health Department, Milwaukee, Wisconsin

Lisa F. Brown, PhD, RN, Associate Professor, School of Nursing, Virginia Commonwealth University, Richmond, Virginia

Barbara J. Byrne, DNP, RN, PPCNP-BC, Vice President of Clinical Operations, University of Wisconsin Health, American Family Children's Hospital, Madison, Wisconsin

Katherine Frontier, MS, CCC-SLP, Inpatient Speech-Language Pathologist, Children's Hospital of Wisconsin, Milwaukee, Wisconsin

Terry Griffin, MS, APN, NNP-BC, Neonatal Nurse Practitioner, St. Alexius Medical Center, Hoffman Estates, Illinois

Tondi M. Harrison, PhD, RN, CPNP, FAAN, Assistant Professor, College of Nursing, The Ohio State University, Columbus, Ohio

Mary Beth Hensel, MBA, Director, Resolve Through Sharing®, Gundersen Medical Foundation, Inc., La Crosse, Wisconsin

Stephanie Hosley, MS, RN, CPNP-PC, Clinical Instructor of Practice, Pediatric Nurse Practitioner Program, The Ohio State University, Columbus, Ohio

Karen Kavanaugh, PhD, RN, FAAN, Senior Nurse Scientist, Department of Nursing Research, Children's Hospital of Wisconsin, Milwaukee, Wisconsin

Hadley Kifner, MDiv, BCC, Pediatric Chaplain, University of North Carolina Health Care System, Department of Pastoral Care, North Carolina Children's Hospital, Chapel Hill, North Carolina

Kathie Kobler, PhD, APN, PCNS-BC, CHPPN, FPCN, APN Coordinator, Center for Fetal Care, Advocate Children's Hospital, Park Ridge, Illinois

Emilie Lamberg Jones, BSW, RN, C-EFM, CPLC, Fetal Care Coordinator, Fetal Concerns Center at Children's Hospital of Wisconsin, Milwaukee, Wisconsin

Kyle Landry, BS, School Intervention Specialist, Children's Hospital of Wisconsin, Milwaukee, Wisconsin

Steven Leuthner, MD, MA, Professor of Pediatrics and Bioethics, Department of Pediatrics, Division of Neonatology, Institute for Health and Equity, Division of Bioethics and Medical Humanities, Medical College of Wisconsin, Milwaukee, Wisconsin

Rana Limbo, PhD, RN, CPLC, FAAN, Resolve Through Sharing®, Gundersen Medical Foundation, Inc., La Crosse, Wisconsin

Mary McCarron, RN, FNP-BC, Nurse Practitioner, Milwaukee Health Department, Milwaukee, Wisconsin

Anne Chevalier McKechnie, PhD, RN, Assistant Professor, Child and Family Health Cooperative, University of Minnesota School of Nursing, Minneapolis, Minnesota

Kathleen Mussatto, PhD, RN, Nurse Scientist, Herma Heart Center, Children's Hospital of Wisconsin, Milwaukee, Wisconsin

Darryl I. Owens, MDiv, BCC, CT, CPLC, Women's Services Chaplain and Grief Counselor, University of North Carolina Health Care System, Department of Pastoral Care, University of North Carolina Hospitals, Chapel Hill, North Carolina

Jill P. Paradowski, MS, RN, Patient Care Outcomes Research, Milwaukee Health Department–Retired, Medical College of Wisconsin, Milwaukee, Wisconsin

Karen F. Pridham, PhD, RN, FAAN, Helen Denne Schulte Professor Emerita, University of Wisconsin–Madison School of Nursing, Madison, Wisconsin

Michele M. Schroeder, PhD, RN, CPNP, UnityPoint Health–Meriter Hospital, Madison, Wisconsin

Ann Scott, RN, MS, APNP, Pediatric Nurse Practitioner, Children's Hospital of Wisconsin, Herma Heart Institute, Milwaukee, Wisconsin

Traci R. Snedden, PhD, RN, CPNP, CNE, Assistant Professor, Jointly-appointed University of Wisconsin–Madison School of Nursing and School of Medicine and Public Health, Department of Orthopedics and Rehabilitation, Madison, Wisconsin

Deborah K. Steward, PhD, RN, Associate Professor and Director of the Neonatal Nurse Practitioner Program, The Ohio State University School of Nursing, Columbus, Ohio

Hallie Straka, BSN, Senior Nursing Student, The Ohio State University College of Nursing, Columbus, Ohio

Erla Kolbrun Svavarsdottir, PhD, RN, FAAN, Professor and Academic Chair of Family Nursing, Faculty of Nursing, School of Health Sciences University of Iceland, Landspitali University Hospital, Reykjavik, Iceland

Jena Tanem, MSN, RN, APNP, Family Nurse Practitioner in Pediatric Cardiology, Children's Hospital of Wisconsin, Milwaukee, Wisconsin

Audrey Tluczek, PhD, RN, FAAN, Associate Professor, Florence Blake Professor of Child and Family Nursing, University of Wisconsin–Madison School of Nursing, Madison, Wisconsin

Suzanne M. Thoyre, PhD, RN, FAAN, Francis Hill Fox Distinguished Term Professor, University of North Carolina at Chapel Hill School of Nursing, Chapel Hill, North Carolina

Lori J. Williams, DNP, RN, RNC-NIC, CCRN, NNP-BC, Clinical Nurse Specialist, Universal Care Unit and Float Team, American Family Children's Hospital and Clinical Instructor, University of Wisconsin–Madison School of Nursing, Madison, Wisconsin

Rosie Zeno, DNP, RN, CPNP-PC, Assistant Clinical Professor, Specialty Program Director, Pediatric Nurse Practitioner Program, The Ohio State University, Columbus, Ohio

Foreword

The publication of this book marks a major milestone in pediatric nursing and in our understanding of how parents become experts in the care of children with extraordinary healthcare needs. New treatments and technological advances have allowed many children with life-threatening malformations and diseases to survive. The resulting rapid rise in prevalence rates of acute, chronic, and multisystem conditions represents a growing burden to children, families, caregivers, the healthcare and education systems, and society as a whole. This epidemiological change demands attention at all levels. Parents of these vulnerable children face uncertainty about prognosis, course of disease, and even survival. For them, acute phases, life-threatening episodes, setbacks with complications, repeated hospitalizations, and extended treatment by multiple subspecialists are the norm, along with preventing acute illness, managing their child's developmental needs, and providing for a "routine" family life. In this book, the authors force us to reflect on the impact of these overwhelming challenges for parents as they acknowledge the reality and prepare to accept responsibility for the day-to-day care of their child with a severe acute, chronic, or fatal condition. This book aims to give the reader, regardless of profession and clinical specialty, the processes and tools needed to help parents become direct care experts for their child with complex needs as well as giving care to their healthy children.

Guided Participation in Pediatric Nursing Practice: Relationship-Based Teaching and Learning With Parents, Children, and Adolescents is built on decades of the authors' empirical research and clinical case examples. The authors strengthen the field "by giving voice to and a language of expression for relationship-based teaching and learning activity." Karen F. Pridham calls this uniquely and individually constructed activity "guided participation (GP)," a practice within nursing that represents a significant component of pediatric nursing. In this book, Dr. Pridham and colleagues show how concepts, principles, and assumptions underpinning GP advance the teachings of Florence Blake, Katherine Barnard, and others, who address how pediatric nursing brings together the child, the parents, and the nurse in a relationship that focuses on [and addresses therapeutically] what the child is attempting to accomplish through meaningful activities. A central activity of the nursing care process is observation and incorporation of the child's behavioral expression of strengths, limitations, and achievements as well as physical, emotional, and developmental challenges. This book describes the critical nature of clinician–parent relationships as clinicians care for children who are ill or healthy and in need of health promotional and illness prevention care; hence, the content is appropriate for all clinicians.

GP draws on, articulates with, and utilizes the theoretical perspectives of many disciplines, including cultural and educational anthropology, education science, communication science, and the science of relationships. Using descriptions rich in context and meaning, this book offers a systematic, principled, and dynamic approach that engages with the child and family in ways that support the parent's development of health- and complex-care competence. The authors advance this exceptional approach to clinician–parent interaction/work, which includes many distinctive features. They show us how shared attention and understanding between clinician and parent can enable joint problem solving and activities that lead to parent confidence and competence in health-related tasks. To make the content on GP and the associated theoretical perspectives easily comprehensible, the book uses case examples of conditions that pose care challenges, such as extreme prematurity, congenital heart disease, technological dependence, cancer, and seizure disorder. For example, Erla Kolbrun Svavarsdottir shows how GP components can be integrated with the Family Strength Oriented Therapeutic Conversations Intervention model, which focuses on family responses and adaptation to stressors in a family of a child with cancer. Jill P. Paradowski offers specific details about how public health nurses learn to use GP with parents of very-low-birth-weight infants.

Ethical debates about quantity versus quality of life for children with serious multisystem conditions abound; however, these debates are useful only in the context of relevant information. Here the book excels in describing processes that ensure incorporation of information, values, and skills. Although evidence-based practice, patient-centered care, and shared decision making (SDM) have been widely advanced by multiple groups, each has limitations in the setting of severe multisystem problems. This book illustrates how complex communication and reflection processes help parents and clinicians make shared treatment decisions that reflect both clinical realities and family values. GP juxtaposes and integrates clinician and parent information, values, and context as clinicians and parents explore together ever-changing treatment options. The concepts and process components of GP support these conversations, recognizing that parent and clinician priorities are valid only when each individual is fully informed of the perspective and information held by the other and has had the chance to integrate them both. The authors show us how, through trust, respectful dialogue/communication, and piloted observation, the clinician grows to understand the perspective of the parent and the parent grows to understand the perspective of the clinician. For example, developing joint attention and shared understanding are elegantly described—along with their pitfalls—in the case study of a fetus with prenatal diagnosis of trisomy 18, where decisions about whether and how aggressively to treat were paramount.

Kathryn Barnard, a visionary nurse scientist and pioneer in parent–infant interaction, is known for promoting special and sensitive relationships between parents and babies at risk, particularly in her research-based Nursing Child Assessment Satellite Training. Barnard helped us focus on helping the mother and infant develop turn-taking or reciprocity as they respond sensitively to each other's cues. In this book, Dr. Pridham and colleagues extend this concept by showing us vividly how the clinician and parent engage in reciprocal exchange as they learn to trust, respect, and understand each other's perspectives; respond to cues; and engage in joint problem solving. They show how the rhythm of turn-taking can be challenged or disrupted when parents have not developed a readiness but decisions about the child's treatment can't wait. Nevertheless, they also illustrate how this dynamic and fluid clinician–parent exchange facilitates engagement and creates understanding and readiness of the parent to take on the complex care of their sick child while also creating a readiness of the clinician to engage in activities that are supportive and ensure smooth transition of responsibility for care to the parent.

The organization of this text is extremely well crafted. Each chapter moves from theory to practice scenarios, building and reinforcing the GP concepts, principles, and processes central to the book. In the case examples, chapter authors provide a synopsis of the disease or condition and related-care challenges before they describe problems and approaches. Because chronic conditions differ dramatically with respect to treatments and prognoses, the background information on each condition helps the reader to visualize the circumstances as they grapple with understanding clinician–parent relationships and care challenges. The GP case examples also help the reader to analyze the specific cases. Throughout, the book is filled with rich and articulate text, clearly depicted models, informative tables and figures, references, and resources, all of which contribute to the reader's depth of understanding of GP. The editors' and chapter authors' authority in this domain is reinforced by biographies that illustrate their extensive nursing, medical, developmental, and specialized clinical backgrounds.

Few people are as qualified to edit a book on this topic as Karen Pridham and her long-standing colleagues, both of whom were her students. Dr. Pridham, a nurse scientist and clinician, is the architect of the GP process and master of its development. She is a pediatric nursing leader, internationally recognized for promoting special and sensitive relationships between clinicians and parents of infants and children who are healthy or who have severe acute, chronic, and often fatal conditions. Dr. Pridham, along with Kathryn Barnard, worked with us as we developed the visitor–mother relationship model for the New Mothers Program, now known as Nurse Family Partnership. This program also focuses on the development of sensitive relationships of parents and their children. The book builds on

Dr. Pridham's continuous commitment to the research and development of nurse–parent teaching and learning processes. The final chapter illustrates the depth of her thinking about the progress made, the important research and clinical questions that remain, and the significant potential of GP for the future.

It is with great enthusiasm that I recommend this text as the best volume to assist clinicians, theorists, and teachers as they work with parents of children who are healthy and need to maintain health or recover from acute illness or who have serious complex illness to develop an approach that is sensitive, anticipatory, diagnostic, and therapeutic. As a final note, it is essential to recognize that GP is not about evidence-based practice, patient-centered care, or decisional analysis. It is also not limited to challenges, parental coping, parent–infant interaction, and complexities of care of the seriously acutely ill or chronically ill newborn and child. It incorporates all of these conceptions, but focuses on developing a *process for teaching/learning and therapeutic interactions* carried out by specialists on behalf of parents and their children. In the book, readers are supported, as they come to understand in depth the complex interactions needed to help parents of children with multifaceted needs become competent caregivers. The tools provided help to make this an important guide for future research as well as a rich resource for advancing clinician competence.

Harriet J. Kitzman, RN, PhD, FAAN
Professor of Nursing and Pediatrics Senior Associate
Dean for Research
University of Rochester
School of Nursing
Rochester, New York

Introduction

This book is the result of a body of work on nursing care of children and their parents done by Dr. Karen Pridham, a distinguished nurse scientist and scholar, and by a number of her former students who subsequently became her colleagues and collaborators. Its focus is a model for the theory-guided practice called "guided participation (GP)," which Dr. Pridham and her team of colleagues developed with the following objective:

> *to help nurses support parents (or other caregivers) to learn what is necessary for them to know in order to protect children as much as possible from adverse consequences of illness and injury.*

Obviously, conventional teaching and learning practices may suffice for parents when their child's illnesses and injuries are commonplace. However, when the parent must become a caregiver for a child with complex and perhaps life-limiting conditions, they need much more than information . . . they need to become competent and confident as caregivers for their own child. This model addresses that specific need.

GP, to quote from Chapter 1, "has very little to do with a teacher giving information to a learner, and everything to do with the teacher working in relationship and in concert with the learner to make meaning of experience, so the learner gains confidence and competence in responsibilities and activities they face—in this case, taking care of a child with significant health issues." This simple statement belies the enormous complexity of the challenges these parents face, as you will see in the chapters that follow.

I was honored when Karen invited me to write an introduction for this book, when it was still in the planning stages. I now feel honored to contribute a very small part to what I know will become an important book, not only for nurses who care for children and their families but for professionals from many fields who share that responsibility. However, my writing was to become more challenging than I had expected. As I began to write, I found myself wanting to draw the reader's attention to so many parts of so many chapters that I soon was in danger of writing an entire chapter myself, cleverly disguised as an introduction. Instead, I will suggest two reasons why I believe this book is important, and leave you to draw your own conclusion.

First, I believe this book is important as a rich collection of clinical accounts and expert reviews on topics of significance to those who care for children with significant health issues and their parents. Each chapter reflects the fact that this field is challenging and complex, and becoming more so every day. Since children are not just small adults, professionals need both cutting-edge expertise and considerable experience to understand and treat their unique responses to serious illness and injury. And because a child's illness and injury affects not just the child, but also the parents and the entire family, the situation requires high performance collaboration across a number of disciplines. Finally, since by their very nature, children and their families grow and change, their care must be adapted to many different situations and settings, and the professionals who support them must be innovative and adaptable to meet these changing needs across time and space.

You will see ample evidence of that kind of professional expertise, perspective, innovation, and adaptability in this book. Each chapter gives the reader a unique opportunity to become immersed in the deep knowledge and wisdom, as well as the profound humanity, that I believe are so characteristic of those who care for children and families. Each chapter is written by experts with different vantage points (caring for the unborn, infants, school-age children, and adolescents across a range of health issues; different settings across the continuum from the close-in focus of hospital care to the broader perspective of community and home-based care; different professional orientations). Nevertheless, every vantage point is oriented toward a single objective: optimal adaptation of the child, parents, and the family in the context of health threats.

This collection of authors represents an impressive range of theoretical and clinical expertise, from nursing and medicine to nutrition, speech therapy, social work, and pastoral care, like the interdisciplinary teams everywhere that support children and families. Each perspective is different, but all acknowledge one central concern: Parents need to be able to protect, love, and care for their child in the face of circumstances that test the limits of their devotion, courage, and strength, and children need their parents' unconditional and unencumbered love and care, regardless of the circumstances.

There is much to learn from, and to reflect upon here.

Second, this book is important because it shows the power of GP as a theory-guided and, therefore, thoughtful and artful form of practice. While I am convinced of its power, my colleague Karen Pridham is more measured in her appraisal. In the final chapter of this book, Dr. Pridham is characteristically cautious (as a scientist should be) and humble (as she always is) about the GP model, stating that it "has promise" but is undeveloped from theoretical, research, and health systems perspectives. She argues that "much research must yet be done" to understand how GP functions, how it contributes to healthcare outcomes, and under what conditions it is effective. Those indeed are appropriate questions to ask and answer.

However, as a nurse scientist with some understanding of the challenges parents face in becoming parents, as well as the ways in which professionals are and are not helpful in that process, I have a slightly different opinion. From my perspective as a perinatal nurse researcher and grounded theorist, I agree that there is more research to be done to demonstrate the utility of GP. However, I regard GP as a theoretically robust and pragmatically applicable middle-range theory *now*.

GP is *theoretically robust* because it is built upon not only what is generally known from research on the transition to parenthood but also on extensive clinical observations about the specific experiences of parents with seriously ill children. Parents in this situation must adapt relatively quickly to the reality that their child has a significant health condition that will change all of their lives, and that will test them in every way imaginable, far beyond the "normative" challenges inherent in the transition to parenthood. And because the parent must almost certainly become the primary caregiver for their child (and the primary decision maker if the child's life is short), this theory logically places the parent as the primary focus and requires the professional to step away from his or her usual position of "sage at center stage" into the position of "guide at the side," to use contemporary educational jargon. In this theoretical context, the professional provides guidance and support that is informed as much by his or her relationship with, and connectedness to, the parent as it is by his or her clinical expertise. Formal professional power and status and predetermined clinical protocols still may figure into the equation, but the theory's gravitational pull is still back to the relationship between the parent and the professional, with the parent at the center.

GP is also *pragmatically applicable* as a middle-range theory. This means that a middle-range theory can profitably be used by one actor (i.e., the professional) to guide his or her actions and interactions, and the actor can do so with some confidence that the actions will have meaning for (i.e., be understood by) another actor (i.e., parent) in the specific situation, and that the risk (i.e., of saying or doing something seriously "wrong") is very low, as long as the theory is sufficiently specific to and grounded in a limited social sphere. I believe GP as a middle-range theory is well specified and deeply grounded in experience with parents of children with significant health issues. The specificity of the theory is evident in that it identifies and describes:

- Core issues that explain the behavior of parents and professionals alike (nurturing and protecting, relating and guiding, maintaining life quality)
- Competencies that parents must learn for themselves and for their child over the illness trajectory (being with their child, knowing and relating, communicating and engaging, doing tasks, problem solving, and regulating emotions)

■ Processes that professionals can use to guide and support parents to attain those competencies over the illness trajectory (getting and staying connected, joining and maintaining attention, bridging, structuring the task/learning, and transferring responsibility)

■ Ancillary materials to support GP practice and research are accessible through Springer Publishing Company at www.springerpub.com/pridham. Throughout the chapters the link appears with this icon ▶. Supplemental material includes additional case studies, GP competence checklists for nurses and for parents, nutrition education for infants, and a Mom and Baby video. An online continuing education course will also be available (https://CE.ICEP.WISC.EDU/GUIDED-PARTICIPATION).

My conclusion is based on the fact that this book contains many examples of how professionals have used it to guide their practice in ways that appear to make a positive difference for parents and, by extension, for their children. And I am equally reassured by instances in which authors decided that they made some mistakes in applying the model in their practice. In these instances, the consequences were manageable; *as the model predicted*, the professional had already attended carefully to the critical process of building and maintaining their relationship with the parent, *as the model directed*. As Dr. Limbo writes earlier in this front matter, "human connectedness helps solve problems," but in the context of GP this is not connectedness in the everyday, greeting-card sense, but rather connectedness in an intensely thoughtful, purposeful, and disciplined sense.

In the end, I am convinced that GP as theory-guided artful practice *works* because it is built upon the careful observations and keen insights of Dr. Karen Pridham and her team of colleagues and collaborators over 30 years of work. As a result of those years of observation, analysis, and practice, I believe this body of work leads inevitably to a single conclusion: Because it is in the nature of parents and infants to strive for wholeness and balance in spite of the shocks and losses they must endure, it is therefore the responsibility of those working with parents, children, and families to support that striving by guiding, teaching, and trusting, rather than leading, lecturing, and intruding. To paraphrase Dr. Sue Thorye, Dr. Pridham's former student and now distinguished colleague (Chapter 5): "As guides, we keep in mind the parent/child/family system is designed to function well; with thoughtful care using principles of guided participation, it will."

Katharyn A. May, PhD, RN, FAAN
Professor and Dean Emerita
School of Nursing, University of Wisconsin–Madison
Madison, Wisconsin

Acknowledgments

We are deeply grateful to the authors who contributed to this book, all with commitment, inspiration, and collaborative spirit. They expanded our thinking about guided participation (GP) as they developed their chapters and linked them to the work of other authors in the book. Writing for and editing the book was a GP activity for both the editors and authors. We learned more than we had anticipated when we started the book project. We learned about GP from the perspectives of multiple disciplines that we may not have tapped into without the opportunities this book gave us.

The book project began several years ago when Elizabeth Nieginski, Springer Nursing Publisher, and Karen Pridham met serendipitously at the Springer booth at the American Academy of Nursing meeting which was near Karen's poster. With the understanding of what we were trying to accomplish in regard to GP, Elizabeth, assisted by Rachel Landes, also of Springer Publishing, nurtured and guided the book project with the three of us editors, myself, Rana Limbo, and Michele Schroeder, to a satisfying completion. We are thankful to Elizabeth for the very thoughtful editorial leadership and pursuit of mutual goals that kept the book on course and true to its aims. We also extend special thanks to Rachel Landes, who worked closely with us to produce the book, and to all of the Springer staff involved in its production.

The many families the three of us editors have had the privilege of working with brought GP to life in clinically focused research. The families, many of them with the project for a year or more, made GP a tangible practice we could grasp. Teaching–learning of the participatory type that we were reading about in the literature and studying for clinical implications became operational, dynamic, credible, challenging, and exciting as we experienced GP with parents and extended family members through many health-related life events and situations with their child. Some children were highly vulnerable to poor health due to extreme prematurity or complex congenital heart disease, while some children were healthy and born full term. Regardless of the infant's condition, parents—mothers, in particular, but increasingly fathers—opened their lives to us. Parents shared the details of caring for their infants and young children with us patiently and earnestly, as if they knew how much it mattered to us to learn about the vicissitudes and issues of their caregiving, particularly in feeding their infants. Feeding, it turned out, was the epicenter of parenting thought and emotion, and revealed parents' internal working models in forms that could be discerned in their accounts of parenting experience and studied over time. The families provided the substance of this book and reason for writing it. Through their participation in extensive and ongoing interviews and observations, they were, in a real sense, collaborators in the production of the book.

We heartily thank the institutions for whom we worked and with whom we were affiliated during the writing of the book and for the organizations that gave us funds and resources to do the work that directly supported this book. The University of Wisconsin–Madison School of Nursing supplied funding support through the Florence Blake Research Fund and gave technical assistance and resources for manuscript preparation. Brian Coulter, Bob Silva, and Renee Schmitt need special mention. Resolve Through Sharing®, Gundersen Medical Foundation, Inc., supported us in numerous ways: with materials, graphic design, and staff time, including that of materials expert Melissa Koch. We are grateful to Resolve Through Sharing director Mary Beth Hensel for her enthusiastic support of requests we made involving the book—and for her willingness to also serve as an author. The unwavering, flexible support from Sherry Casali (Michele's UnityPoint Hospital–Meriter supervisor) of time and mental space needed to bring the book to completion is gratefully acknowledged. The encouragement of our colleagues was invaluable and sustaining. Lisa Miller volunteered her time to prepare online supplemental materials, specifically the Guided Participation Modules, the beginnings of an online course.

Our families deserve special thanks. Life goes on while editing and writing a book. At times it was challenging to juggle attention to family members and the timeline of the book. It was hard to write about issues concerning caregiving while family members patiently put up with the scarcity of our presence. Yet they remained genuinely enthusiastic about the book and their interest kept us energized and moving along on the process. Their commitment to us is embodied in this book.

To you, the reader, we acknowledge with thanks your attention to the chapters of this book. The extent to which you share or disagree with us in our understanding of GP is an important source of motivation to the development of knowledge.

Section I

GUIDED PARTICIPATION THEORY IN NURSING

1

Guided Participation Theory for Teaching and Learning in Clinical Practice

Karen F. Pridham, Ann Scott, and Rana Limbo

Learning about guided participation for clinical practice with parents and children may connect us with the learning we did as children. Beginning in infancy and early childhood, all of us experienced guided participation with parents or other adult caregivers and with siblings or peers (Rogoff, 1990). Guided participation is the application of principles and methods of teaching and learning, which qualifies it as a practice. Parents use guided participation to help babies learn to stay put while diapers are changed and to play reciprocating games. Guided participation gains complexity as infants become toddlers who are expected to learn self-care skills like toileting or dressing.

Take learning to tie shoes. Parents initially work with the child to help develop capacity to tighten the laces, fold the laces into a bow, cross the bow, thread one lace through the created bow, and finally, tighten the laces to form a bow that is tight enough to hold the shoes on. Finally, after numerous attempts over many days and weeks, the parents' abilities to teach and the child's abilities to learn result in becoming competent in "doing the task." At some point, parents recognize that preparing for a school day no longer requires their help in getting the child's shoes on. Responsibility for teaching and learning has been passed to the child (guided participation process of "transferring responsibility"), who is now the central figure in accomplishing a task that increases the child's competence and confidence. Both parent and child have positive emotions that reflect how a guided participation approach to teaching and learning results in success in skills building. This example, though simple, is familiar to the universe of parents and children, whether about tying shoes or performing some other aspect of self-dressing. Because of its simplicity and universality, a child's learning self-dressing skills can provide an answer to the question, "What is guided participation?" A child's learning self-dressing skills can also serve as an exemplar for broader application of guided participation (e.g., learning to communicate more effectively with one's manager) and the longer span of caregiving (e.g., nurturing and protecting an elderly relative), including in a clinical context.

In this chapter and throughout much of the book, nursing is the primary discipline through which guided participation is threaded, becoming a practice within the larger, more encompassing practice of nursing. As a "practice within a practice," guided participation is central to pediatric nursing in which "relationship" is the central focus of all interactions between and among the child, the child's parent or parents, and the nurse (Blake, 1954). As the nurse engages in the conceptual and practical challenges of teaching and learning practice (Lave, 1993) in the context of the family, he or she is practicing what we refer to as *guided participation*, which must be viewed, we caution, within the principles, methods, and goals of nursing practice itself.

A view of guided participation as a practice tailored to the principles and methods of the larger discipline makes clinical disciplines in general host disciplines for guided participation practice by clinicians. Clinicians are all professional persons who work directly with people for healthcare. This book includes chapters that describe guided participation from the perspective of clinicians other than nurses, including a physician, nutritionist, speech and language pathologist, and hospital chaplains. We know clinicians in disciplines other than nursing, including child life, counseling psychology, and social work, who are practicing guided participation, but whose work was not included in this book. Each discipline tailors the goals, issues, and methods to the types of outcomes that are the focus of the discipline.

Doing guided participation is helping another person become competent enough to engage in a socially important activity by providing expertise and working alongside the learner (Pridham, Limbo, Schroeder, Thoyre, & Van Riper, 1998). A process that occurs often in everyday life with more or less sophistication and complexity, guided participation for clinical practice can be made more accessible with exploration of its theory and principles of practice. Central to guided participation is the dynamic process of teaching and learning that occurs in the context of a relationship, generally in the setting of the activity (Rogoff, 2003; Rogoff & Lave, 1984). Recall your memories of guided participation with a child in your home or perhaps a hospital or clinic room where you were caring for a child and working with parents. Keep in mind that guided participation may be spontaneous or scheduled, momentary or ongoing, over many encounters. The constant feature of guided participation, and its necessary element, is an understanding of what learners must gain competence in for fully carrying out responsibilities in their own environments.

The attention and understanding concerning matters of mutual interest or concern stem from a relationship. In the context of pediatric nursing and nursing care of children, guided participation refers to learning through participation and guidance within a culture that supports health. The relationships of child, parent, and nurse are at the heart of this culture (Blake, 1954). The purpose of this chapter is to provide theory and principles for a clear understanding of guided participation and enlarged capacity for developing its practice.

As disability in childhood and adolescence grows in prevalence in the United States and other countries (Halfon, Houtrow, Larson, & Newacheck, 2012), more parents and their offspring have caregiving and self-care responsibility relevant to health. This responsibility is a function of and qualified by developmental transition, environmental adversity, resource availability or deficit, and healthcare practice and caregiving expectations in the community. Continuing learning is necessary to maintain or promote health and to prevent or limit disability and secondary illnesses. The substance, processes, and outcomes of this learning have been highlighted as participatory and guided for engagement in promotion and protection of health, including mediation of the effects of adverse environments and toxic stress (Shonkoff, Richter, van der Gaag, & Butta, 2012; Shonkoff, 2014).

Protection of children from adverse environmental and experiential effects on health and development requires caregivers who are skilled in problem solving, planning, monitoring, and emotion regulating, including control of impulses (Shonkoff et al., 2012; Shonkoff, 2014). Guided participation is designed to develop these executive and self-regulating competencies, among other categories of competencies—physical, cognitive, social, behavioral, and moral. These competencies are integral to promoting health, preventing acute and chronic illness, alleviating or reducing illnesses secondary to an acute or chronic illness, and adjusting and adapting old patterns of living and behaviors (Coker et al., 2016; Moore, Bethell, Murphey, Martin, & Beltz, 2017). Learning that occurs through guided participation is documented in descriptive case studies and quantitative research and in several clinical trials (Limbo & Lathrop, 2014; Limbo & Pridham, 2007; Pridham et al., 2005; Pridham, Limbo, & Schroeder, 1998; Schroeder & Pridham, 2006; Thoyre, Hubbard, Park, Pridham, & McKechnie, 2016).

This book concerns a form of guided participation we developed for the clinical practice of nursing of children, including infants, toddlers and preschool children, school-age children, and adolescents, all referred to as "children." On occasion, we have used the acronym, GP, instead of spelling out the full name. In general, guided participation, in this book, refers to the caregiving that parents, surrogate parents (e.g., extended family members, older siblings, day-care staff), or clinicians do on behalf of children. Guided participation is, for the most part, an informal type of learning that occurs outside of school settings, and is often described as instruction in an everyday practice offered by someone who has experience or expertise in a socially important activity or task to a less- or nonexperienced person, sometimes referred to as a novice. We have used "teacher" or "guide" in place of "expert" and "learner" in place of "novice" to suggest that the teacher and learner may need to draw on each other's expertise, and that both may be learners, often in relationship to each other. Guided participation refers to interactions that are deliberately structured or intended to assist development of competencies relevant to health.

Ann Scott, RN, MSN, CPNP, APNP (pediatric nurse practitioner, pediatric cardiology, the Herma Heart Center, Children's Hospital of Wisconsin), wrote the following case to both document the extensive teaching parents of an infant, Ben, born with a complex congenital heart defect require to manage care at home and to be a source of ideas about initiating guided participation with parents as they engage in learning to feed their infant prior to going home. Keep Ben in mind as you read this chapter. We will come back to him before we leave it.

FEEDING AND THE LEARNING IT REQUIRED FOR PARENTS AND BABY BEN

Complex congenital heart disease (CCHD) has severe and continuing implications for parents. In addition to the stress all parents' experience in caring for a healthy infant, parents of infants with CCHD face additional stressors. Periods of transition such as the birth of the infant (especially in the context of a prenatal diagnosis of CCHD), surgical intervention, and preparing for discharge home often increase stress. The parents of an infant with CCHD are often forced to adjust their expectations of what they were hoping for their infant (Lee & Rempel, 2011; Pridham, Harrison, Krolikowski, Bathum, Ayres, & Winters, 2010; Pridham, Harrison, McKechnie & Brown, 2017; Rempel, Ravindran, Rogers, & Magill-Evans, 2013). The nurse plays an integral role at these periods of transition. This case study will focus on the period of preparing for hospital discharge.

Babies with congenital heart disease are required to achieve many milestones prior to hospital discharge including hemodynamic stability, successful feeding, and stable weight gain. Feeding often proves to be challenging for the infant with CCHD, as well as the parents. The healthcare team is responsible for developing a feeding plan that safely provides optimal nutrition and results in adequate weight gain. This feeding plan may conflict with how the parents had been hoping to feed their infant. In addition to providing nutrition, feeding an infant is also an important time for parents to engage with their infant through physical contact, eye contact, and other social interactions.

Case Example 1.1

Baby Ben was prenatally diagnosed with CCHD consistent with single-ventricle physiology. Immediately after birth, he was stabilized and transferred to the neonatal intensive care unit. He continued to be stable from a cardiorespiratory standpoint. Speech therapy was consulted and Ben was allowed to breast and bottle-feed in addition to receiving total parenteral nutrition (TPN). At 3 days of life, he was transferred to the cardiac intensive care unit prior to undergoing the first stage of the palliative surgery at 6 days of life. Following cardiac surgery, Ben was fed only with TPN. Once stabilized postoperatively, trophic nasogastric (NG) feeds were started and he was slowly advanced to bolus feeds. He tolerated full volume bolus NG feeds, and oral feeds were reinitiated. The speech therapy team continued to work on oral feeding skills with Ben and his parents, Marya and Len. Due to inadequate oral intake, the decision was made for gastrostomy tube (GT) placement. After GT placement, feeds were slowly advanced to goal feeds and caloric density was increased to promote weight gain. Baby Ben continued to do well from a cardiorespiratory standpoint, and, with optimization of his cardiac medication regimen, was discharged home about 2 weeks after GT placement.

GT placement is often difficult for parents as it does not always align with how they were hoping to feed their infant and with their thoughts and feelings about their goal of protecting their child's body. The nurse practitioner (NP) played an integral role in preparing Ben's parents for these challenges and providing them with support and resources. The NP, with the speech team's recommendations, encouraged the parents to keep working with Ben on his oral feeding skills. The NP also encouraged physical and eye contact while Ben was receiving GT feedings.

Throughout hospitalization, the team of NPs prepared Ben's parents for discharge and participation in the home monitoring program (HMP). Babies with single-ventricle physiology are at high risk for mortality between the first two palliative surgical procedures (the interstage period). Our center utilizes a HMP to detect subtle physiologic changes that may indicate declining clinical status. The HMP requires extensive parental training and education prior to discharge, which is provided by the NP team. Daily information is monitored and recorded by the infant's parents, including oxygen saturations, weight, and 24-hour enteral intake. Ben's parents were instructed to contact the HMP team if there was a breach in any of the preestablished criteria: oxygen saturation (SpO_2) less than 75% or more than 90%, weight loss of 30 g or failure to gain 20 g over 3 days, and enteral intake of less than 100 mL/kg/day. In addition, the parents received weekly phone calls from the HMP team, and Ben had a minimum of biweekly clinic visits.

Ben's case raises questions about guided participation practice and how it fits into the preparation and education of parents, for example: (a) When, where, and how does guided participation begin? (b) What are the issues, and what issues get priority for discussion?, (c) What does guided participation sound and look like? (d) How is it different from giving parents the information they need to take good, safe care of their child?

(e) What are the goals of guided participation, and how are they supported or accomplished? (f) What is the process of guided participation? and (g) What are the outcomes it is intended to deliver?

What questions did Ben's case raise for you? As you read about the theory and practice of guided participation in this chapter, including its structure, processes, and outcomes, keep Ben's case in mind along with ideas about how guided participation can be described as a prominent, intentional, and goal-directed component of care.

A CLINICAL CONCEPT OF GUIDED PARTICIPATION

Guided participation draws on five conceptual origins: (a) theory of education (teaching–learning); (b) the development and maintenance of human relationships; (c) social–cultural activity; (d) internal working model of the mind, a metaphor for the expectations, intentions, goals, and emotions that are operative when engaged in the task and relationship issues of an activity, all of which have implications for development of caregiving competencies; and (e) the systems of behavior we label parenting, caregiving, child feeding, healthcare using, or some other form of behavior, its function revealed in social activity expressed in a historical context. Discussion of teaching–learning, relationship, internal working model, and caregiving components of guided participation will be followed by practice features consistent with theory.

Guided participation is a type of participatory education or teaching–learning practice (Bransford, Brown, & Cocking, 2000) distinguished by its setting in everyday social–cultural activity (Rogoff, 2003; Rogoff, Mejia-Arauz, Correa-Chavez, 2015). Guided participation draws on five theoretical traditions. These are:

1. The central function of experience in learning (Dewey, 1938)
2. The mediating function of social interaction in constructing greater understanding of what is known from what has already been learned, that is, the concept of the zone of proximal development (Vygotsky, 1978)
3. An anthropological and social–cultural concept of learning in informal or formal settings in everyday life, outside of school settings, structured to develop competencies for an activity or practice important to social life (Rogoff, 2003; Rogoff & Lave, 1984), for example, parental management of care of an infant with CCHD
4. Boyd's (1968) specification of teaching–learning as orientation (issues), processes, and outcome (competencies)
5. Bowlby's (1982) concept of internal working model to describe and explain the motivated activity through which learning occurs

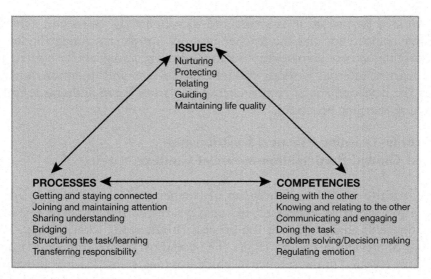

FIGURE 1.1 Guided participation issues, processes, and competencies.

Figure 1.1 shows guided participation as a relationship among issues, processes, and competencies. These three dimensions are used for assessing and structuring teaching–learning activity.

The internal working model is a concept of cognitive, emotional, and volitional activity of the mind engaged in goal-directed activity. This concept is a central component of Bowlby's (1982) attachment theory, generated from scholarly and clinical work to describe and explain a child's development of a relationship with the primary caregiver, generally the mother. Motivation for closeness and security in the child evolves to motivation for caregiving as the child grows older and becomes an adult. The expectations, intentions, and goals that characterize the operation of a motivation such as caregiving are cognitive and emotional functions (Bowlby, 1982; Bretherton & Munholland, 2016). The internal working model of a behavioral system operating in the context of a social–cultural activity such as caregiving can be described in terms of relationships involving self and others and tasks central to the activity that is oriented and directed by a socially driven motivation.

An internal working model makes a socially cultural activity such as caregiving tangible, specific, and personal in the expectations and intentions that are expressed in a social–cultural context (Rogoff, 2003). The assessment of internal working models in the context of expressed or discerned motivation is a prime source of knowledge of issues that matter or mean something to a person or that are directing a person's activity or work, again in a specific social–cultural context and particularly in a setting of socially important functions and responsibilities (Lave & Wenger, 1991; Wertsch, 1988), describe the structure of social–cultural activity and, following Vygotsky, its importance for mental functioning and learning.

Guided participation is structured to support the learner in achieving greater competence and the teacher in more knowingly aiding the learner. Because the activity involves motivation, meaning, and goals for both teacher and learner, internal working model expectations and intentions intersect with the development of competencies, the issues being addressed, and the teaching–learning processes.

Teaching–Learning Practice: Relationship-Based Guided Participation in Social Context

Salient features of the relationship of teacher and learner for guided participation are trust expressed in sensitive responsiveness and respectful confidence in engagement in the process (Bretherton, 1985; Hinde, 1995; Hinde & Stevenson-Hinde, 1988). The collaborative relationship (Rogoff, 1998) is revealed in the teacher or guide listening to the learner about what learning means and what is relevant to becoming more skilled. Guided participation may involve problem solving an issue faced in real life and making a decision about it. Collaboration of teacher and learner is at the core of cocreating ideas about what is going on, processes that can be used to understand the situation and to take action to solve the problem, and reflections on what it means.

When the teaching–learning explicitly or implicitly concerns the relationship of parent and child, guided participation may operate on parallel processes. One process has to do with the parent and guide. A second process, parallel to the first, has to do with what parents are learning about their relationship with their child. A process used in guided participation to specifically and intentionally support the relationship has been referred to by attachment relationship theorists as "holding in mind" (Pawl, 1995; Winnicott, 1960).

Caregiving: Social–Cultural Activity Central to the Nursing Care of Children

Caregiving of children, applying Bowlby's (1988) and Solomon and George's (1996) theory, elaborated with the studies of Ainsworth, Blehar, Waters, and Wall (1978), anticipates and reciprocates a child's bids for closeness and security with sensitive and responsive behavior (Bretherton, 1994; Bretherton & Munholland, 2016; George & Solomon, 1999). Viewed from a social–cultural vantage point, caregiving requires the commitment of both teachers and learners to the learner's development of competencies. When the health of a child is at issue, the expectations and goals of the healthcare culture articulate with those of the family and community. When guided participation for development of competencies in caregiving of children is the objective, both learner and teacher—the less and more expert—are called to be with each other in ways that enhance sensitive responsiveness to the behavior of the other and to the behavior of the child (Bretherton & Munholland, 2016).

The relational competencies of being with and knowing the other (Hinde, 1995), specifically the parent or parent surrogate, are integral to guided participation for caregiving of children.

GUIDED PARTICIPATION PRACTICE

Clinicians may assume they are doing guided participation when initiating and maintaining open-ended discussion about what is going on for parents, what is on their minds, and what they are doing about it. Guided participation, however, is a practice (Lave, 1993). In addition to expectation of active engagement of parents and children in learning, guided participation is oriented to the learner's life circumstances or issues and, in that context, is directed to increasing competencies for addressing these circumstances with improved, maintained, or promoted health.

The processes used in guided participation are consistent with these practice expectations and goals. Shown in Figure 1.1, guided participation processes for development of child caregiving competencies are designed and organized for intersubjectivity of learner and teacher. The concept of intersubjectivity concerns shared attention to and mutual or shared understanding of an issue (Bruner, 1985; Vygotsky, 1978; Wertsch, 1984). Intersubjectivity is needed for the operation of guided participation processes. The guided participation processes identified by Rogoff (1990, 1995) and found in our own clinical practices include teacher and learner getting and staying connected through interpersonal communication, joining and maintaining attention to what is salient to the issues at hand (Bruner), bridging or connecting what is known to what is new or anticipated, and transferring responsibility for what is learned with the goal of full participation in caregiving activity specific to the issues (Rogoff, 1990). Connecting refers to cognitive (e.g., as in "connecting the dots" or concepts or ideas), emotional, and social actions. All of these processes may require deliberate structuring for learning, referring to organizing, and applying resources to support bridging. Structuring includes use of self to scaffold learning, that is, to advance the learner toward a more advanced, complex, or realistic understanding of how things are, need to be, or could be (Vygotsky, 1978; Wood, Bruner, & Ross, 1976). Guided participation can be recognized by these processes occurring in relation to each other. Although not necessarily applied in a linear manner, the processes when taken together distinguish guided participation practice from merely personalizing teaching or engaging learners in a participatory teaching–learning activity.

The process of bridging sharply differentiates guided participation from giving information as the approach to teaching and learning. The intention of bridging is to support a learner in making connections between what is known or unknown or misconstrued and in need of revision or reconstruction (Rogoff, 1990). Bridging is a function of experience, recalled, simulated, or relived, as through video playback of interaction with a child, or imagined. Bridging supports learners in reflecting on how things were, are now, or could be with new ways of thinking and behaving. Wondering with the learner is a strategy teachers may use to facilitate reflection and make connections; for example, wondering with a parent what her child was saying when he behaved, the way he was observed behaving, or what she might have been feeling when her child behaved that way (Slade, 2005).

Strategies and techniques used in the process of bridging may be drawn from many sources with the goal of advancing the learner's understanding and behavioral competencies. Through the use of bridging strategies and techniques, the guided participation supports learning in what Vygotsky (1978) coined the zone of proximal development. This concept represents the competence a learner may achieve with guidance. The teacher observes and assesses what the learner already knows and keeps it in mind along with an image or knowledge of the desired competence (Hedegaard, 1990).

Features of guided participation that distinguish it as a teaching–learning practice are shown in Table 1.1. You might use this list of features, along

TABLE 1.1 Guided Participation Practice

Distinguishing Features	Definitions and Explanations
A process intended and designed to address health-relevant issues	The goal is developing caregiving competencies.
Focused on activity	The activity may be a task that has limited longevity, a responsibility that has indefinite duration, or an anticipated response to an event with uncertain probability of occurrence. The activity may be as complex as a practice, e.g., feeding an infant very prematurely born or with CCHD.
Guided participation may focus on relational, cognitive, behavioral, or emotion regulating competencies	Being with and knowing and relating to the other, i.e., the one cared for, are two categories of relational competencies. Doing the task, e.g., giving good care, communicating and engaging, and problem solving, which encompasses goal setting and decision making, is a behavioral competency. Regulating emotion includes competencies in the emotional domain.
Guided participation may be highly regulated or not specified, prescribed, or thought out in advance	Helping parents learn to feed a preterm or medically vulnerable infant who is learning to nipple feed is an example of guided participation in highly regulated conditions to maintain the infant's safety. The goal shared by parents and clinicians is for parents to be able to take an infant who knows how to feed home as quickly as possible. The processes of achieving the goal, however, may be challenging, and negotiation among parents and clinicians may be needed.

(continued)

TABLE 1.1 Guided Participation Practice (*continued*)

Distinguishing Features	Definitions and Explanations
Supports learning for dealing with highly impactful events or conditions likely to affect physical and mental health	Among the conditions or events that may call for guided participation are the diagnosis of a severe chronic illness, the death of a child, recognition of disability, or exposure to disabling communicable disease.
May need to be engaged rapidly in emergent, highly stressful situations	Goals in an emergent situation may be to maintain already existing competencies, aid rapid and focused development of new or not well-developed competencies, or attend to the relationship by communicating empathy and building trust.
May be initiated by a learner or by a teacher	If the learner is viewed as needing to engage in guided participation, gaining joint attention and developing shared understanding may need attention to assure being "on the same page" in respect to identifying issues of mutual concern.
May make use of a variety of strategies or techniques drawn from multiple sources to help a learner develop competencies	Motivational techniques are an example of what might be used in guided participation when a learner has competing goals (Miller & Rollnick, 2013). Goal clarifying may aid choosing a goal to adhere or commit to.
A parent or another caregiver may use guided participation with the other parent or another caregiver to aid development of caregiving competencies	Teacher and learner functions may flip between parents. Guided participation quality may be a function of how supportive parents are of each other in caregiving for their child.

CCHD, complex congenital heart disease.

with the definitions and explanations of the items on the list, to estimate how your own practice of teaching and learning compares.

Guided Participation for Caregiving: A Case Example of Teaching and Learning Through Communication

A relationship is integral to the process of guided participation, and development of competencies for carrying out caregiving responsibilities and activities is the reason for doing it. Guided participation for caregiving dynamically makes use of the opportunities at hand, on the fly, or in the moment. It is not protocol driven, with objectives laid out in advance. Instead, it is motivated to develop competencies for taking care of a child. Focus on Ryan, an infant, and his parents, Mat and Delores, and his toddler brother, Simon.

Ryan is 8 weeks old and 7½ weeks postoperative palliative surgery for a complex congenital heart defect. He has been home 3 weeks. He is offered a nipple feeding before every day-time feeding. The bulk of his feeding is provided through a GT. Mat and Delores are happy to have another son, although they had hoped for a girl. Ryan will be a companion for almost 2-year-old Simon. Ryan's parents wonder if their infant's breathing is like it should be—it seems fast, particularly when he is trying to nipple feed. Ryan receives a low level of supplemental oxygen via nasal cannula around the clock. Both parents are concerned that Ryan gets the nutrients he needs.

Mat views Ryan as being very fragile and does not participate in his son's feedings. Delores also views Ryan as fragile and in need of protective care, but is committed to giving him the best care possible. Both Delores and Mat agree that it would be good if he would participate in feeding Ryan. Delores is getting too little sleep, and Mat is aware of her need for help with child care. Mat says that he does not think he can manage care of a young infant, and Delores does a better job of feeding than he can do. At the moment, Mat helps Delores by taking Simon off her hands when he comes home from work on the day shift.

Reflecting, a Guided Participation Activity for Bridging and Connecting

The questions that follow are intended to aid readers in bridging (i.e., making connections) with what they already know with new or extended ways of thinking about guided participation. Try the questions out for yourself, and make a note of additional questions that come to mind.

- What would guided participation offer this family? What makes it suited as an approach to teaching and learning for these parents?
- What are potential challenges in implementing guided participation with these parents? Where might some hurdles be encountered or the zone of proximal development get too distant to easily navigate?
- When in Ryan's case would you initiate guided participation with his family, and how?
- Do you see a place in which "wondering" would be an appropriate bridging strategy? How would you frame your statement about wondering for parents' response?
- How would you name the caregiving issues, including those the parents have named and those that you may think could be present? Remember that issues are not necessarily problems, but may also be goals or desires.

Refer to the guided participation framework in Figure 1.1 that identifies issues, processes, and competencies we have found to be applicable across populations of parents and children, health-related situations, and events and conditions with implications for health. A dictionary of categories and examples of processes and competencies may be accessed through the Springer Publishing website at **www.springerpub.com/pridham**, Chapter 1.

Here is a summary of a discussion Ryan's parents had with each other and with the nurse when Ryan was next seen at the clinic. Mat acknowledged

Delores's charge that he lacked experience in feeding his infant son, either orally or by gastrostomy. He was still not sure gastrostomy feeding was the right thing to do. The gastrostomy feeding bewildered him, although he had learned the technique before Ryan's discharge from the hospital. When asked by the nurse what was on his mind about Ryan's feedings, Mat said he was trying to figure out what Ryan experienced during the feeding, what gave him pleasure in feeding, and how his pleasure and interest in feeding could be increased.

Mat continued that he did not think he could make a difference for his son's feedings. He wanted him to have some joy in feeding, but he thought the gastrostomy feedings made no difference to Ryan. Oral (nipple) feedings were a struggle for both him and his son, Mat reported. Mat agreed to the nurse's offer to spend time with him and Delores to learn more about what Ryan was communicating through his behavior and how his behavior could best be responded to support a positive feeding experience for all three of them.

From this vignette, name the issues for teaching–learning that you hear expressed and that you think need to be addressed. Then identify what you, as the nurse, would focus attention on with Ryan's parents and how you would suport Mat and Delores in making connections. What connections would you want to support Ryan's parents in making, both for the feeding and for their relationship? An example of a connection concerns Ryan's eye contact with his parent feeder and what that might mean, both for Ryan and for his parents. Bridging might tap into varied aspects of the situation, for example, criteria of successful feeding, differences between parents in criteria, and recognition of new criteria based on progression in oral intake and relationship that the parents could adopt.

IMPLICATIONS OF GUIDED PARTICIPATION FOR CLINICAL PRACTICE

Guided participation, when planned and assessed comprehensively in respect to relationship, technical care, communication, and emotion regulation, can be entered at many different points in clinical care and in respect to many different issues, either foremost in the minds of the parents or child, if old enough to be engaged in care, or in the minds of the clinicians working with them. Guided participation, when implemented throughout a clinical service, could be a vehicle of person- and family-centered care (Harrison, 2010). A list of parenting competencies, accessed through **www.springerpublishing.com/ pridham**, Chapter 1, was developed to support assessment of issues for guided participation.

Return to the case of Ben and his parents, Marya and Len (this chapter). The transition to care at home begins well before discharge. In Baby Ben's case, the preparation concerned clinical goals of safety in respect to adequacy of growth, fluid and nutrition, and cardiorespiratory function. The clinical goals required reliably performed competencies in technical care and in communicating with clinicians. The NP team was also working with Ben's parents in supporting development of competencies in relating to their infant, maintaining health, and in regulating their emotions. What guided participation processes would you bring into play if Marya said, "I will be afraid to sleep at night when we take Ben home," or if Len said, "I will be worrying that Marya has enough patience to feed Ben the way he needs to be fed while I am at work and her maternity leave was used up." What issues would you want to be sure to introduce if you were a member of the NP team working with the family? How would you assess joint attention and develop shared understanding for the issues that merit guided participation?

The chapters that follow document guided participation for a broad spectrum of families who have children requiring pediatric nursing care. Applicable to the gamut of clinical settings and types of health problems and goals experienced by children and their families, guided participation is practiced in a variety of ways. The structures and processes, depending on the issues, processes, goals, populations, resources, and time lines involved, will differ. Guided participation practice, however, will be recognizable through principles common to its broad-based applications. These principles are focused on developing competencies through participation in socially meaningful activities and practices with a guide (teacher) who reciprocates in teaching and learning while advancing the learner's making connections and extending understanding in the zone of proximal development (Rogoff, 1990, 2003; Rogoff, Turkanis, & Bartlett, 2001). Broadly envisioned, guided participation, from the perspective of the family or clinician, is a journey continuing through the years of infancy, childhood, and adolescence along a path that requires continutiy of support for relationships and focuses on development of competence in caregiving and self-care. A checklist of nurse competencies, accessible through **www.springerpublishing.** **com/pridham**, Chapter 1, was developed through our work with families and nurses in the context of guided participation practice.

Guided participation practiced with reflection and cognizance of developing beyond what is known at this point but that could be known with support—the zone of proximal development—facilitates learning for both teacher and learner. The late architect, Zaha Hadid (*New York Times*, December 24, 2016, C6), expressed this idea in claiming that one learns from what one teaches and shows learners what they can achieve beyond what was thought possible.

For many families, guided participation in a primary or tertiary clinical setting is of necessity a team practice. On the whole, intra- and interdisciplinary members of the clinical team need to be brought into guided participation as a clinic-based practice for the purpose of picking up the issues and processes and advancing or supporting the competencies for any child and family unit. Guided participation requires that medical and healthcare as well as social service issues are being attended to in conjunction with teaching–learning for development of caregiving and self-care competencies.

Our concern with guided participation as a teaching–learning practice that needs attention to stability of the environment, the social well-being (Tomlin, Weatherston, & Pavkov, 2014) and mental health of participants, and ongoing access to reflective supervision will be apparent in the chapters of this book. Our goal is to bring guided participation into evidence-based practice (Taylor, Preifer, & Alt-White, 2016).

Cases for Guided Participation Practice

Additional case studies involving infants and young children are available online through the Springer Publishing website at **www.springerpub.com/pridham**, Chapter 1. These documents are titled Case Study Carl, Case Study Emma, and Cases Concerning Feeding Issues. A guide for getting started on guided participation with a family new to one's teaching–learning practice is also shown in the online supplemental materials.

REFERENCES

Ainsworth, M. S., Blehar, M. C., Waters, E., & Wall, S. (1978). *Patterns of attachment*. Hillsdale, NJ: Lawrence Erlbaum.

Blake, F. G. (1954). *The child, his parents and the nurse*. Philadelphia, PA: J. B. Lippincott.

Bowlby, J. (1982). *Attachment and loss. Vol. 1. Attachment* (2nd ed.). New York, NY: Basic Books.

Bowlby, J. (1988). *A secure base*. New York, NY: Basic Books.

Boyd, R. D. (1968). General principles of teaching at the university level. In L. E. Bone (Ed.), *Library education: An international survey* (pp. 223–245). Champaign, IL: University of Illinois.

Bransford, J. D., Brown, A. L., & Cocking, R. R. (2000). *How people learn: Brain, mind, experience, and school*. Washington, DC: National Academies Press.

Bretherton, I. (1985). Attachment theory: Retrospect and prospect. In I. Bretheron & E. Waters (Eds.), *Growing points of attachment theory and research* (pp. 3–35). Monographs of the Society for Research in Child Development, 50(1–2, Serial No. 209).

Bretherton, I. (1994). The origins of attachment theory: John Bowlby and Mary Ainsworth. In P. Ornstein, R. Parke, J. Reiser, & C. Zahn-Waxler (Eds.), *A century of developmental psychology* (pp. 431–471). Washington, DC: American Psychological Association.

Bretherton, I., & Munholland, K. A. (2016). The internal working model construct in light of contemporary neuroimaging research. In J. Cassidy & P. R. Shaver (Eds.), *Handbook of attachment: Theory, research, and clinical applications* (3rd ed., pp. 63–88). New York, NY: Guilford Press.

Bruner, J. S. (1985). A historical and conceptual perspective. In J. V. Wertsch (Ed.), *Culture, communication and cognition: Vygotskian perspectives* (pp. 21–34). Cambridge, UK: Cambridge University Press.

Coker, T. R., Chacon, S., Elliott, M. N., Bruno, Y., Chavis, T., Biely, C., . . . Chung, P. J. (2016). A parent coach model for well-child care among low-income children: A randomized controlled trial. *Pediatrics, 137*, e20153013. doi:10.1542/peds.2015-3013

Dewey, J. (1938). *Experience and education*. New York, NY: Collier Books.

George, C., & Solomon, J. (1999). The development of caregiving: A comparison of attachment and psychoanalytic approaches to mothering. *Psychoanalytic Inquiry, 19*, 618–646.

Halfon, N., Houtrow, A., Larson, K., & Newacheck, P. W. (2012). The changing landscape of disability in childhood. *The Future of Children, 22*, 13–42.

Harrison, T. M. (2010). Family-centered pediatric nursing care: State of the science. *Journal of Pediatric Nursing, 25*, 335–343.

Hedegaard, M. (1990). The zone of proximal development for instruction. In L. C. Moll (Ed.), *Vygotsky and education: Instructional implications and applications of sociohistorical psychology* (pp. 349–371). Cambridge, UK: Cambridge University Press.

Hinde, R. A. (1995). A suggested structure for a science of relationships. *Personal Relationships, 2*, 1–15.

Hinde, R. A., & Stevenson-Hinde, J. (1988). *Relationships within families: Mutual influences*. Oxford, UK: Clarendon Press.

Lave, J. (1993). The practice of learning. In S. Chaiklin & J. Lave (Eds.), *Understanding practice: Perspectives on activity and context* (pp. 3–32). Cambridge, UK: Cambridge University Press.

Lave, J., & Wenger, E. (1991). *Situated learning: Legitimate peripheral participation*. Cambridge, UK: Cambridge University Press.

Lee, A., & Rempel, G. R. (2011). Parenting children with hypoplastic left heart syndrome: Finding a balance. *Journal of Specialists in Pediatric Nursing, 16*, 179–189. doi:10.1111/j.1744-6155.2011.00289.x

Limbo, R., & Lathrop, A. (2014). Caregiving in mothers' narratives of perinatal hospice. *Illness, Crisis, & Loss, 22*, 43–65.

Limbo, R., & Pridham, K. F. (2007). Mothers' understanding of their infants in the context of an internal working model of caregiving. *ANS: Advances in Nursing Science, 30*, 139–150.

Miller, W. R., & Rollnick, S. (2013). *Motivational interviewing: Helping people change* (3rd ed.). New York, NY: Guilford Press.

Moore, K. A., Bethell, C. D., Murphey, D., Martin, M. C., & Beltz, M. (2017). Flourishing from the start: What is it and how can it be measured? *Child Trends Research Brief, 2017–16*, 1–14.

Pawl, J. H. (1995). The therapeutic relationship as human connectedness: Being held in another's mind. *Zero to Three, 15*(4), 2–5.

Pridham, K. F., Brown, R., Clark, R., Limbo, R. K., Schroeder, M., Henriques, J., & Bohne, E. (2005). Effect of guided participation on feeding competencies of mothers and their premature infants. *Research in Nursing & Health, 28*, 252–267.

Pridham, K. F., Harrison, T., Krolikowski, M., Bathum, M. E., Ayres, L., & Winters, J. (2010). Internal working models of parenting: Motivations of parents of infants with a congenital heart defect. *Advances in Nursing Science, 33*(4), E1–E16. doi:10.1097/ANS.0b013e3181fc016e

Pridham, K. F., Harrison, T. M., McKechnie, A. C., & Brown, R. (2017). Motivations and features of co-parenting an infant with complex congenital heart disease. *Western Journal of Nursing Research*, 193945917712693, e-publication ahead of print. doi:10.1177/0193945917712693

Pridham, K. F., Limbo, R., & Schroeder, M. (1998). Support of family caregiving for children with special needs. In J. C. Westman (Ed.), *Parenthood in America: Proceedings of the conference held in Madison, Wisconsin, April 19–21, 1998*. Madison: University of Wisconsin–Madison General Library System.

Pridham, K. F., Limbo, R., Schroeder, M., Thoyre, S., & Van Riper, M. (1998). Guided participation and development of care-giving competencies for families of low birth-weight infants. *Journal of Advanced Nursing, 28*(5), 948–958.

Pridham, K. F., Schroeder, M., & Brown, R. (1999). The adaptiveness of mothers' working models of caregiving through the first year: Infant and mother contributions. *Research in Nursing & Health, 22*, 471–485.

Rempel, G. R., Ravindran, V., Rogers, L. G., & Magill-Evans, J. (2013). Parenting under pressure: A grounded theory of parenting young children with life-threatening congenital heart disease. *Journal of Advanced Nursing, 69*, 619–630. doi:10.1111/j.1365-2648.2012.06044.x

Rogoff, B. (1990). *Apprenticeship in thinking: Cognitive development in social context*. New York, NY: Oxford University Press.

Rogoff, B. (1995). Observing sociocultural activity on three planes: Participatory appropriation, guided participation, and apprenticeship. In J. V. Wertsch, P. Del Rio, & A. Alvarez (Eds.), *Sociocultural studies of mind* (pp. 139–184). Cambridge, UK: The University of Cambridge.

Rogoff, B. (1998). Cognition as a collaborative process. In W. Damon (Series Ed.), D. Kuhn, & R. S. Siegler (Vol. Eds.), *Handbook of child psychology, Vol. 2: Cognition, perception, and language* (5th ed., pp. 679–744). New York, NY: John Wiley & Sons.

Rogoff, B. (2003). Learning through guided participation in cultural endeavors. *The cultural nature of human development* (Chap. 8, pp. 282–326). Oxford, UK: Oxford University Press.

Rogoff, B., & Lave, J. (1984). *Everyday cognition: Its development in social context*. Cambridge, MA: Harvard University Press.

Rogoff, B., Mejia-Arauz, R., Correa-Chavez, M. (2015). A cultural paradigm—Learning by observing and pitching in. *Advances in Child Development and Psychology, 49*, 1–22.

Schroeder, M., & Pridham, K. F. (2006). Development of relationship competencies through guided participation of mothers of preterm infants. *Journal of Obstetric, Gynecologic, and Neonatal Nursing, 35*, 358–368. doi:10.1111/j.1552-6909.2006.00049.x

Shonkoff, J. P. (2014). A healthy start before and after birth: Applying the biology of adversity to build the capabilities of caregivers. In K. McCartney, H. Yoshikawa, & L. B. Forcier (Eds.), *Improving the odds for America's children: Future directions in policy and practice* (pp. 28–39). Cambridge, MA: Harvard Education Press.

Shonkoff, J. P., Richter, L., van der Gaag, J., & Butta, Z. A. (2012). An integrated science framework for childhood survival and early childhood development. *Pediatrics, 129,* e460–e472. doi:10.1542/peds.2011-0366

Slade, A. (2005). Parental reflective functioning: An introduction. *Attachment & Human Development 7,* 269–281.

Solomon, J., & George, C. (1996). Defining the caregiving system. Toward a theory of caregiving. *Infant Mental Health Journal, 17,* 198–216.

Taylor, M. V., Priefer, B. A., & Alt-White, A. C. (2016). Evidence-based practice: Embracing integration. *Nursing Outlook, 64,* 575–582. doi:10.1016/j.outlook.2016.04.004

Thoyre, S. M., Hubbard, C., Park, J., Pridham, K. F., & McKechnie, A. (2016). Implementing co-regulated feeding with mothers of preterm infants. *MCN: The American Journal of Maternal Child Nursing, 4,* 204–211. doi:10.1097/nmc.0000000000000245

Tomlin, A. W., Weatherston, D. J., & Pavkov, T. (2014). Critical components of reflective supervision: Responses from expert supervisors. *Infant Mental Health Journal, 35,* 70–80. doi:10.1002/imhj.21420

Vygotsky, L. S. (1978). *Mind in society: The development of higher psychological processes.* Cambridge, MA: Harvard University Press.

Wertsch, J. V. (Ed.). (1984). *Culture, communication and cognition: Vygotskian perspectives.* New York, NY: Cambridge University Press.

Wertsch, J. V. (1988). *Vygotsky and the social formation of mind.* Cambridge, MA: Harvard University Press.

Winnicott, D. W. (1960). The theory of the parent-infant relationship. *International Journal of Psychoanalysis, 41,* 585–595.

2

Relationship-Based Approach to Caring for Children With Serious Illness

Kathie Kobler

As the trajectory of care unfolds for infants and children with serious illness, healthcare professionals and palliative care teams strive to optimize quality of living while minimizing suffering for the entire family. The American Academy of Pediatrics (AAP) calls for teams to establish relationship with such families in a manner that fosters joint decision making for the child's well-being (AAP, 2013). Guided participation (GP) offers healthcare professionals useful strategies to facilitate the identification of child/parental goals, foster effective communication, and guide critical decision making. GP processes and strategies can be especially useful when guiding parents and healthcare teams during the in-between/liminal times of prognostic uncertainty (Carter, 2017). This chapter explores how healthcare professionals can integrate GP competencies, processes, and strategies into care of infants and children within the framework of initiating, maintaining, and transitioning relationship.

Of note, when using GP in clinical settings, it is assumed that the healthcare professionals (guides or teachers) are seeking to understand the internal working model of the family (learners) and act as guides to address the issue at hand (Pridham, Limbo, Schroeder, Thoyre, & Van Riper, 1998). Yet within the context of navigating a child's serious illness, parents and/ or the child are experts in their family's values, goals, and expectations.

Successful integration of GP requires clinicians to humbly balance their understanding of a child's status and future disease progression while holding in mind that it may be the child who serves as expert and guide for the parents and team.

INITIATING RELATIONSHIP

For healthcare professionals, there is always a first introduction or first interaction with a child and the family that occurs through relationship, learning what is meaningful and significant to another (Pridham et al., 1998). As such, healthcare professionals should be mindful of their own expectations, beliefs, hopes, fears, and motives prior to meeting the child/family for the first time (Limbo, Kavanaugh, & Kobler, 2017). Taking a self-inventory provides insight to one's own internal working model and what might be carried into the new relationship. The PRAM model (Limbo & Kobler, 2013) offers a framework for self-inventory as one pauses, reflects on what is at the forefront of one's thoughts, acknowledges feelings, and is mindful beginning a new patient interaction. In such moments of reflection, the healthcare professional may consider questions such as:

- What is happening in my personal life right now that may impact my interactions with this child and family?
- What do I know about this child's situation?
- What personal thoughts, feelings, values, or biases come to mind when I anticipate meeting the child and family?
- What expectations do I have for this child's care?
- What information from other team members should I hold in mind, or lay aside, when I first connect with the family?
- How does this child's situation remind me of past experiences with other children? What did I learn from those experiences that I might carry with me or lay aside at this time?

Taking time for self-awareness helps team members to ground themselves by using the GP strategy of holding in mind personal concerns or limitations that may arise during the child's care (Duncan & Kobler, 2016).

First Interactions With the Parents

GP begins as a healthcare professional works to establish joint attention, with the goal of aligning personal motives and understandings with the family (Pridham et al., 1998). Parents of children with serious illness hold strong beliefs about their core responsibilities to be a good parent for their child, which may include ensuring the child feels loved, staying at the child's side, unselfishly making decisions in the child's best interest, and advocating for the child's needs with the healthcare team (Hinds et al., 2009;

Feudtner et al., 2015). When establishing relationship with parents, it may be helpful to ask questions and make statements such as:

- "Help me to know what it means to you to be a good parent for your child."
- "In what ways may I support you as you parent your child?"
- "Please tell me about your child, and what is important to you for his or her care."

Some parents may respond with concrete information, such as valuing honest and timely communication. Other parents view caring for the child is their sole responsibility and may not wish for intensive support (October, Fisher, Feudtner, & Hinds, 2014), which is important to discern before engaging in discussions about the child's care.

Learning how the parents prefer to take in medical information is key to getting connected in relationship (Duncan & Kobler, 2016). Using a GP approach, the healthcare team may also inquire how parents have worked through complex situations before as a family, how they relate to each other in daily interactions, and what gives them strength as a parent and as a family, thus providing further insight to their internal working model. Failure to assess a parent's communication preferences may lead to an inability to join and maintain attention. For example, one young couple refused all attempts by the neonatal team to discuss their baby's critical condition. It was only after the palliative nurse stated "I wish to care for you in a way that is important to you as a couple. Please help me to know how you'd prefer to receive updates from the neonatal team" that the parents related they were waiting for their elder uncle, the family patriarch, to arrive from their homeland. Only in his presence would the couple connect with the team to discuss their child's medical needs.

Initial attempts to establish relationship with a family may also involve deciding to slow the pace of communication, offering a protective respite to parents who may be feeling overwhelmed. This approach embodies the GP competency of being present for the parents, and may include statements such as:

- "I'm glad for the opportunity to meet you, and I respect that you've already talked with many team members today. I'm here to introduce myself, and I'm wondering if you would prefer to wait until another time for a longer visit."
- "While the team has information to share, please know that we are also ready to pause our discussion when you feel that you've heard enough for today."
- Or if meeting the family when other team members are sharing extensive information, the healthcare professional may take a GP approach by stating, "We just covered a lot about your child. I'm wondering, what do you need to happen next?"

One parent responded to a similar request saying, "You can talk all you want about what's wrong with my child, but I'm going to tell you right now I won't hear a word. I'm just too sad today." Her response allowed the palliative team to acknowledge the mother's feelings, rather than the team's initial goal of sharing updated medical information. Taking the responsibility of pacing initial interactions, while protecting parental limits of knowledge intake, increases the likelihood of establishing a trusting relationship with the family.

Connecting With the Child

GP can also help the healthcare professional to connect with a child in a way that beings relationship founded on trust. With each new patient encounter, the healthcare team should first address any distress the child is experiencing before venturing further in conversation or interactions. If the child is old enough, asking him or her directly about what measures will address their comfort, or fostering parents' ability to nurture their child by asking for their assistance in optimizing comfort, will set a respectful stage for all subsequent interactions.

In addition to optimizing the child's physical comfort, the healthcare team can work to create safe boundaries, letting the child regain a sense of control in how interactions should unfold. For one little girl, protecting personal space during her first clinical exam meant letting her decide where to first place the stethoscope bell so her palliative team could assess breath sounds. This invitation to assist the team and control stethoscope placement continued with all her future examinations. In a similar fashion, the GP process of bridging was used as an older teen chose safe phrases to use when she was having, as she described, one of "those days." Per her request, the safe phrases became a signal to her palliative team that she preferred to talk later in a more private setting.

Initiating relationship and getting connected with children requires an investment of the clinician's time and patience to learn the child's individual personality and preferences. GP questions such as "What is most important to you right now?" or "What are you hoping happens today?" can provide insight into the child's internal working model and begin a caring relationship. When asked such a question, one young boy responded, "I'm hoping you all start wearing masks so I don't have to smell your coffee breath and catch your germs. You know I have cancer, right?" His honest declaration led the way to cocreating how and when the healthcare team could respectfully enter his hospital room. Once the boy saw that the team honored his requests (and freshened their breath!), he was willing to trust and stay connected when complicated issues arose in his care.

Lastly, acute moments often arise in clinical settings, requiring an accelerated need to establish connection and gain trust of both parent and child. In such situations, team members may convey their goal of providing care that meets the family's needs by delivering difficult news in a kind fashion, building in pausing points during communication, acknowledging heightened emotions, and asking what is most important for the team to address first. These GP strategies of holding the family's well-being in mind foster relationship even amid emotionally charged, emergent situations.

MAINTAINING RELATIONSHIP

Implementing GP in clinical settings provides the opportunity for the guide (healthcare team) to bring a learner (family) into full participation in care over time, with the goal of anticipating and preventing both difficulties that may arise (Pridham et al., 1998). As one mother shared with her child's nurse, "Thank you for knowing in advance what I would need to think about for my child; you gave me your courage when I had none." Shifts in the child's condition give rise to a myriad of opportunities for the healthcare team to provide ongoing guidance, expertise, and support while incorporating a GP approach to care.

Ongoing Assessment

Fostering secure attachments with the family is essential to providing quality care (Papadatou, 2009), especially when a child's health status is tenuous or uncertain. Ongoing assessment of parental well-being is one way of staying connected, as a child's long medical journey puts parents at risk for masking emotions when they are really experiencing a high level of emotional discontent with the situation at hand (Hexem, Miller, Carroll, Faerber, & Feudtner, 2013). A GP approach to understand the parents' internal working model might include these assessment questions:

- What is your understanding of your child's condition?
- Based on your understanding, what do you expect to happen next?
- What are your hopes? Your worries?
- What sustains you or gives you strength?
- What would help you know what to do? (Limbo et al., 2017; Pridham et al., 1998; Waldman & Wolfe, 2013)

One mother, who had conveyed an ongoing cheerful attitude at her son's intensive care bedside, responded to such an inquiry by confiding to the palliative nurse, "I may look like I've got it together, but I'm not sleeping at all and feel like a hot mess on the inside." Parent and child responses to such questions will provide insight into that which is tangible, understood, and valued (Pridham et al., 1998), guiding the healthcare team in determining priorities for next steps in supporting parent and child.

Healthcare professionals using a GP approach to staying connected should be prepared to creatively meet the family's expressed needs or preferences for care, even if such requests require the team to think outside of their comfort zone. For example, when asked what is most important, parents who recently emigrated from another country shared that their baby boy's neurodegenerative disorder progression might be halted if they could perform a healing tradition of applying bat's blood to the forehead. Knowing that bat's blood was not a safe option, the palliative and neonatal intensive care teams collaborated to provide a space where parents could substitute chicken blood in a manner that would minimize the risk of infection while honoring the family's tradition for healing.

Facilitating Decision Making

Parents report valuing accurate information that is shared in an honest, compassionate, and timely manner; they also value time to reflect and process news of their child's changing condition (Xafis, Wilkinson, & Sullivan, 2015). Healthcare teams can use GP processes of structuring information gathering and monitoring progress to aid parents in understanding significant shifts in their child's medical condition. As parents often struggle with knowing what to ask healthcare teams (Xafis et al., 2015), a GP-focused assessment may facilitate a shared understanding and entrance into tender conversations, and foster a shared understanding. The healthcare professional might ask a question like "What is weighing on your heart right now?" Or acknowledging when parents let out a loud sigh, by saying "That sounded important. I'm wondering what you're thinking about right now?"

One parent responded by softly whispering, "I'm afraid that the moment I've dreaded since he was born with this terrible disease will come true, like the time we have left together is very short." Her admission of concern served as a bridge for the team and parent to honestly share perceptions about the child's current condition, and eventually paved the way to shifting from adding additional medical interventions to focusing solely on the child's comfort.

The ability for the healthcare team and family to jointly set new goals for the child's care is often impacted by parents' emotions and hopeful patterns of thinking (Hill et al., 2014). The GP strategy of facilitating opportunities for reflection can help parents and the team identify practical goals to honor what is most important (Pridham et al., 1998). For example, after time had passed following news of a child's cancer progression, her family was asked, "If we could find a way to keep one thing the same right now for your family, what would that be?" The child and her parents answered in unison, "We miss sitting down to dinner as a family; please help us to do that before things change again!" Following the expression of this new goal, the palliative and oncology teams creatively used the GP process of transferring responsibility, helping the family brainstorm ideas that eventually led to a family picnic on the hospital grounds.

In the face of a child's deteriorating medical condition, healthcare professionals may struggle how to respond when parents state they are hoping for a miracle. Parents are not always asked about their hopes, and they can hold simultaneously incongruent beliefs of hoping for a cure while also believing such a cure may not be possible (Kamihara, Nyborn, Olcese, Nickerson, & Mack, 2015). Parental hope is a dynamic process, requiring ongoing assessment by the team to guide care and maintain relationship (Limbo et al., 2017). GP approaches can ascertain and acknowledge the family's overall hope while also drawing out additional, and perhaps more attainable, hopes that parents may be holding in their hearts (Arzuaga, 2015; Limbo et al., 2017). Healthcare professionals can ask parents "What do you believe is ahead for your child?" (Mack & Joffe, 2014), and once their main hope is expressed can follow with additional probes, asking gently, "And what else do you hope for? And what else?" (Feudtner, 2009).

Answers can provide insight to the parents' internal working model and feasible interventions that will honor hope and sustain the parent–child relationship. For example, one mother resisted the intensive care team's attempts to communicate her son's multisystem organ failure and dependence on ventilator support. The primary nurse eventually asked, "How do you expect your son will be 6 months from now?" The mother immediately smiled, sharing her belief that she will be sitting under the Christmas tree, helping her son to open presents. The nurse wisely acknowledged the mother's hopes, adding respectfully, "And what else do you hope for?" This guided approach, within the context of an established, trusting relationship, led to the mother acknowledging aloud for the first time that her son may die before December. The nurse then helped the mother to consider other choices, eventually transferring responsibility as the family made special memories by celebrating a summertime Christmas in the child's intensive care room.

Listening to the Child's Voice

End-of-life decision making is a process dependent upon relationship between the child, family, and team (Papadatou, 2009). Healthcare professionals and parents alike are challenged to understand a child's perspective, and parents especially may hold conflicting feelings of wanting to help draw out their child's voice, while also wishing to protect the child from harm (Kars, Grypdonck, de Bock, & van Delden, 2015), which requires watching carefully for moments when the child and parents are open to an honest discussion (Duncan & Kobler, 2016). One mother learned of her young daughter's fears about dying when overhearing a conversation between the child and her twin. The mother gently joined in her children's discussion, afterward sharing with the palliative team relief that "we could finally face together what was being kept inside." When sharing how much she valued the opportunity to bring comfort and reassurance to her twins, this mother also gratefully reminded the palliative team of how they helped her to prepare having such a conversation.

Waiting for such moments to arise is a true reflection of the GP process of transferring responsibility for all who care for and about the child. For one young man, transferring responsibility unfolded when his primary cardiologist provided a private email address after the teen admitted he felt more comfortable writing about his feelings. This led to a fruitful discussion in written word with a trusted physician, eventually resulting in a clear end-of-life care plan identified and directed by the young man.

When working with children transitioning to end of life, the healthcare team may choose to support the child by focusing on the GP competency of regulating emotions, especially when the parents state that they prefer not to talk about end-of-life care because of cultural or religious values. Focusing on regulating emotions may also help with the tender work of assisting a child confront the terminal nature of their medical condition. For example, upon hearing a young teen with terminal cancer announce, "Do not cry in front of me!" the palliative team worked to draw out the meaning of his statement, asking, "Help us to know more so we can make sure the team honors your request." This invitation led to the teen confiding with a trusted team member how he felt responsible for his family's grief, and was especially worried about his mother's well-being after his death. The team member then incorporated the GP competency of knowing and relating to self/others by helping the child identify ways to share and process his feelings of guilt, grief, and loss.

In another case, focusing on the GP competency of regulating emotions meant meeting a sibling's request to "walk and not talk" following his sister's death. The nurse walked with the child to another part of the hospital, letting the child choose the direction and transferring responsibility for their journey, anticipating that he might need to find a private space. Eventually, the child chose a safe spot in a dimly lit room overlooking the city lights, and finally uttered aloud feelings of disbelief at his sister's unexpected death.

Staying Connected When Expectations Differ

GP processes are helpful in situations where differing expectations about the child's care occur between the parents, between parents and their child, or between the family and team members jeopardize relationship (Feudtner, 2007). Such experiences of conflicting views may arise when all involved hold tight to their personal goal of wanting what they believe is best for the child. Healthcare clinicians may use invitational phrases such as "Help me to understand" or "I am curious about," as well as avoiding using the word "but" during conversation to shed light on the conflicting viewpoints at hand (Feudtner, 2007). The GP process of joining and maintaining attention can redirect communication toward identification of common core values or goals upon which to continue collaborative decision making.

Staying connected in relationship may also be challenged when parents ask the team to "do everything" for their child while the team members perceive the child to be suffering and would prefer limiting further medical interventions. The GP process of bridging can aid in drawing out the parents' perspective by saying "You said some very important words. What does 'do everything' means to you?" For many parents, "doing everything" is closely linked to their feelings of responsibility to provide and care for the child, and less about specific medical interventions that the team might provide. Using a GP approach, the healthcare team can both affirm parents' love for their child and confirm the team's commitment to collaborative care (Gillis, 2008).

GP can also play a critical role when rifts in relationship arise between the parents and team members. For example, parents shared with the chaplain that they no longer wished to interact with the child's attending physician. Holding in mind the GP competency of knowing and relating to self/ others, the chaplain stated, "Our team strives to care for families in ways that are most meaningful to them, and we are very open to learning when we have fallen short of expectations. When you are ready, can we talk further about your request?" This acknowledgement and invitation paved the way for the parents to honestly present their concerns, and allowed the physician an opportunity to respectfully share his desire to repair the relationship and maintain connection with the child and family.

TRANSITIONING RELATIONSHIP

As the child's serious illness progresses, the healthcare team and family will experience moments of change from existing, familiar situations to new levels of interaction. When significant shifts in care unfold, relationship with the team is impacted, as healthcare professionals often report missing their daily engagement with a child and parents (Jankowski, 2013).

Anticipating Shifts in Care

Transitions in relationship may occur when a child returns to a relative period of stability, requiring less frequent encounters with the healthcare team. Discharge from the hospital to home, completion of intensive therapies, or a change to adult providers when the child reaches young adulthood all result in different levels of relationship between the team and family. Healthcare professionals may use a GP approach to help families anticipate and navigate change. Teams may work with families to determine alternative methods of staying in touch when daily interactions cease, thus facilitating a way to reconnect when future crucial shifts in a child's status occur (Duncan & Kobler, 2016).

Preparing for End-of-Life Care

The most permanent change in relationship occurs when a child transitions to dying, and all who care for the child collaborate to identify priorities as death approaches. The only way a healthcare professional may understand a child or family's internal working model in such complex situations is to ask with respect and kindness, "I'm wondering how I can best support you at this time," or "What is important for you to accomplish right now?" One child responded by asking the nurse for some small-sized sticky notes so she could "mark who gets to use my stuff when I'm gone." While this task was difficult for the parents to watch, they supported their daughter's wish to choose how and when her most precious possessions would be shared with others after death. Please refer to subsequent chapters in this book for more in-depth discussion about integrating GP into the care of infants, children, and families at end of life.

Honoring Relationship With Ritual

Throughout all of history, humans have turned to ritual to acknowledge significant moments and significant life events (Limbo & Kobler, 2013). Whether formatted upon sacred tradition or rising up informally during special moments of connection, ritual offers all participants the opportunity to connect, make meaning, and experience transformation in mind and heart. As noted by Limbo and Kobler (2013), "Ritual flows from relationship. Relationship forms a bridge from suffering to hope. Hope transforms."

All aspects of the GP approach are relevant to cocreating ritual with children and families, as when healthcare professionals inquire "Holding in mind all that is happening right now, how would you like to acknowledge this moment?" or "As you anticipate what is next for your child, what would be important to accomplish?" One mother, whose daughter was experiencing a prolonged hospitalization, responded by asking the primary nurse to help her child listen in by phone when the parents read a bedtime story to her siblings at home. Through creative use of technology, the nurse facilitated a nightly opportunity for the child to connect with her family while listening to her mother or father read well-loved storybooks. Another family decorated colorful fabric squares to mark everyday moments and special occasions with their child. When the child died, the squares were sewn together into a quilt that was used to cover his casket at the funeral.

Ritual can also play an important role for healthcare teams in acknowledging and processing their experiences of caring for a child with serious illness, especially after a child's death (Kobler, 2014; Limbo & Kobler, 2013). Those working to bring ritual to grieving teams may incorporate GP processes and strategies to cocreate an experience that will allow the healthcare professional to recall past meaningful moments with the child, while also acknowledging their feelings of loss and grief. For example, the palliative nurse and chaplain spent time listening to healthcare team members share how they felt connected in relationship to a beloved patient who died. Team members told stories of sharing popsicles with the child when she was lonely, or offering brightly colored stickers to her when she completed her daily therapies. With their permission, popsicles, stickers, and other linking items were used during a team ritual to acknowledge the child's death and honor the ways she impacted her team members' lives.

CONCLUSION

GP offers healthcare professionals an effective framework to initiate, maintain, and transition relationship with the children and families in their care. Readers are encouraged to explore the wisdom in the chapters that follow, each one highlighting creative and powerful ways to incorporate GP competencies, processes, and strategies to help families live well and treasure special moments within the context of significant health challenges.

REFERENCES

American Academy of Pediatrics Section on Hospice and Palliative Medicine and Committee on Hospital Care. (2013). Pediatric palliative care and hospice care commitments, guidelines, and recommendations. *Pediatrics, 132*(5), 966–971.

Arzuaga, B. H. (2015). Clinical challenges in parental expression of hopes and miracles. *Pediatrics, 135*(6), e1374–e1375.

Carter, B. S. (2017). Liminality in pediatric palliative care. *American Journal of Hospice and Palliative Medicine, 34*(4), 297–300.

Duncan, J., & Kobler, K. (2016). Communication in pediatrics. In C. Dahlin, P. J. Coyne, & B. R. Ferrell (Eds.), *Textbook in advanced practice nursing* (pp. 597–608). New York, NY: Oxford University Press.

Feudtner, C. (2007). Collaborative communication in pediatric palliative care: A foundation for problem-solving and decision-making. *Pediatric Clinics of North America, 54*(5), 583–607.

Feudtner, C. (2009). The breadth of hopes. *New England Journal of Medicine, 361*(24), 2306–2307.

Feudtner, C., Walter, J. K., Faerber, J. A., Hill, D. L., Carroll, K. W., Moellen, C. L., . . . Hinds, P. S. (2015). Good-parent beliefs of parents of seriously ill children. *JAMA Pediatrics, 169*(1), 39–47.

Gillis, J. (2008). We want everything done. *Archives of Disease in Childhood, 93*(3), 192–193.

Hexem, K. R., Miller, V. A., Carroll, K. W., Faerber, J. A., & Feudtner, C. (2013). Putting on a happy face: Emotional expression in parents of children with serious illness. *Journal of Pain and Symptom Management, 45*(3), 542–551.

Hill, D. L., Miller, V., Walter, J. K., Carroll, K. W., Morrison, W. E., Munson, D. A., . . . Feudtner, C. (2014). Regoaling: A conceptual model of how parents of children with serious illness change medical goals. *BMC Palliative Care, 13*(9), 1–8.

Hinds, P. S., Oakes, L. L., Hicks, J., Powell, B., Srivastava, D. K., Spunt, S. L., . . . Furman, W. L. (2009). "Trying to be a good parent" as defined by interviews with parents who made Phase I, terminal care, and resuscitation decisions for their children. *Journal of Clinical Oncology, 27*(35), 5979–5985.

Jankowski, J. B. (2013). Professional boundary issues in pediatric palliative care. *Pediatrics, 31*(2), 161–165.

Kamihara, J., Nyborn, J. A., Olcese, M. E., Nickerson, T., & Mack, J. W. (2015). Parental hope for children with advanced cancer. *Pediatrics, 135*(5), 868–874.

Kars, M. C., Grypdonck, M. H. F., de Bock, L. C., & van Delden, J. M. (2015). The parents' ability to attend to the "voice of their child" with incurable cancer during the palliative phase. *Health Psychology, 34*(4), 446–452.

Kobler, K. (2014). Leaning in and holding on: Team support with unexpected death. *MCN: The American Journal of Maternal-Child Nursing, 39*(3), 148–154.

Limbo, R., Kavanaugh, K., & Kobler, K. (2017). Honoring relationship and hope. In K. Kobler & R. Limbo (Eds.). *Conversations in perinatal, neonatal, and pediatric palliative care.* Pittsburgh, PA: Hospice & Palliative Nurses Association.

Limbo, R., & Kobler, K. (2013). *Meaningful moments: Ritual and reflection when a child dies.* La Crosse, WI: Gundersen Lutheran Medical Foundation.

Mack, J. W., & Joffe, S. (2014). Communicating about prognosis: Ethical responsibilities of pediatricians and parents. *Pediatrics, 133*(S1), S24–S30.

October, T. W., Fisher, K. R., Feudtner, C., & Hinds, P. S. (2014). The parent perspective: "Being a good parent" when making critical decisions in the PICU. *Pediatric Critical Care Medicine, 15,* 291–298.

Papadatou, D. (2009). *In the face of death: Professionals who care for the dying and the bereaved.* New York, NY: Springer Publishing.

Pridham, K. F., Limbo, R., Schroeder, M., Thoyre, S., & Van Riper, M. (1998). Guided participation and development of care-giving competencies for families of low birth-weight infants. *Journal of Advanced Nursing, 28*(5), 948–958.

Waldman, E., & Wolfe, J. (2013). Palliative care for children with cancer. *Nature Reviews Clinical Oncology, 10,* 100–107.

Xafis, V., Wilkinson, D., & Sullivan, J. (2015). What information do parents need when facing end-of-life decisions for their child? A meta-synthesis of parental feedback. *BMC Palliative Care, 14*(19), 2–11.

Section II

GUIDED PARTICIPATION FROM THE PERINATAL PERIOD THROUGH INFANCY

3

Preparing for the Birth of an Infant With a Congenital or Genetic Condition

Anne Chevalier McKechnie and Emilie Lamberg Jones

PARENTS' EXPERIENCES FOLLOWING FETAL DIAGNOSIS OF A CONGENITAL OR GENETIC CONDITION

An upward trend in detection through early ultrasounds and genetic screenings is resulting in an increasing population of parents affected by the fetal diagnosis of a congenital or genetic condition (Gould, Figueroa, Robinson, & Reichard, 2011). These parents are dealing with unexpected pregnancy outcomes, preparing to care for medically vulnerable infants, and struggling to meet needs that go beyond clinical explanations of diagnosis and treatment. A diagnosis also forces parents into making major decisions that were either never anticipated or required much earlier than expected. It is clear that under these circumstances, parents encounter heightened and changing needs for support, and have varied abilities to comprehend and make use of diagnosis-related information (Jones, Statham, & Solomou, 2005; Leuthner, Bolger, Frommelt, & Nelson, 2003; McKechnie, 2013; McKechnie & Pridham, 2012; McKechnie, Pridham, & Tluczek, 2015, 2016; McKechnie, Tluczek, Pridham, Lamberg Jones, & Thoyre, 2014; Rempel, Cender, Lynam, Sandor, & Farquharson, 2004). While parents want to manage distress and be able to understand and make the best decisions regarding diagnosis and treatment, challenges remain. During this early and uncertain time, the focus tends to be on the fetal or anticipated infant condition. Parents often conceal or gloss over their own needs, thinking of them as low priority, or guarding against others' potential judgments of their psychological fitness and caregiving competencies (McKechnie, 2013; McKechnie, Johnson, Baker, Docherty, & Thoyre, 2015). Parents also want to put their efforts into developing caregiving skills and competencies to best support the growth and development of the child. Yet caregiving readiness can be compromised by parental distress, lack of understanding, and inadequate support.

Recent research (McKechnie, 2013; McKechnie, Johnson, et al., 2015; McKechnie & Pridham, 2012; McKechnie, Pridham, et al., 2015; McKechnie et al., 2016; McKechnie et al., 2014) reporting on parents' experiences following fetal anomaly diagnoses can be informative for nurses' assessments and use of guided participation (GP). Consequent to and sometimes interrelated with the shock and grief of the diagnostics news, parents have described navigating the transition to parenting a new infant that diverges from the norm. Parents can develop a range of strategies in response to perceived severity of and changes in fetal health, their own experiences of loss, and interactions with others (McKechnie, 2013; McKechnie, Pridham, et al., 2015; McKechnie et al., 2014). The quality of support can also influence parents' experiences and the strategies developed to deal with adverse events (McKechnie, Johnson, et al., 2015). Parents who described ample support in terms of partner involvement, emotional and instrumental help from family and friends, and information from healthcare providers appeared to develop strengths in managing child health. Those parents who recounted processing emotions, gaining diagnosis-related knowledge, and engaging in healthcare also emphasized their abilities to address diagnosis-related challenges over time, mobilize people and resources, and collaborate with their healthcare providers to address their own and their child's needs (McKechnie, Johnson, et al., 2015). Yet for some parents, the paths to meeting the challenges are very steep. It has been suggested that dealing with expectations of healthcare provider that are unmet, struggling to reconcile illness and nonillness care, and perceiving little agency as parents can parallel concerning symptoms of anxiety, depression, and trauma (McKechnie et al., 2016). Since parents' responses to a fetal diagnosis and their subsequent needs and efforts to manage healthcare vary, it is necessary to assess this variation so that nurses and physicians can provide family-centered, tailored care. Such care is needed to effectively support these parents in reducing their distress, navigating a transition to parenthood after a fetal diagnosis, and managing healthcare during an early, formative time as they are developing their internal working models for parenting an infant with a complex condition.

PREPARATION AND TRANSITION TO CAREGIVER AND CO-PARENT

Parents are developing as caregivers and can begin working together as a couple during the early transition to parenthood before birth. Caregiving can be recognized for an individual parent as the complement to child attachment, and should not be underestimated in importance for family and child health. A mother's development as a parental caregiver after a fetal diagnosis involves prenatal preparation with added concerns and amplified motivations directed toward maintaining infant health compared to those of a mother preparing for a healthy infant (McKechnie, 2013). Infant health can become a centerpiece of family attention, with positive and negative consequences for the parent–infant dyad, the couple, and the family.

Although much less is known about caregiving development for fathers or same-sex partners, their roles as co-parents have garnered attention (Farr, Simon, & Bruun, 2017). Co-parenting, defined as two parents working together to care for a child, is related to individual parental caregiving development (McHale & Lindahl, 2011). Co-parenting was recently described as taking shape during the prenatal time frame after a fetal diagnosis and influencing longer term co-parenting strengths (McKechnie, Rogstad, Martin, & Pridham, 2017). A couple's work toward having a shared meaning of the fetus' and future child's health condition and co-parenting-related communication that fosters emotional support, information sharing, and agreement could endure through the early years and apply to changing caregiving issues. Thus, in addition to the tumult after a fetal diagnosis, the prenatal time is still a time to prepare, begin the transition to parenting the infant, and initiate co-parenting. Although a fetal anomaly diagnosis can be emotionally draining for parents, the prenatal time can prompt the need to develop key competencies. Nurses and other healthcare professionals can find the opportunities for sensitive assessments and GP to support optimal outcomes.

NURSES AS GUIDES

Nurses have incorporated GP into perinatal bereavement care provided to families for decades (Limbo & Kobler, 2010; Pridham, Limbo, Schroeder, Thoyre, & Van Riper, 1998). This approach to care can be extended to the population of parents who experience loss even though the infant is expected to live. One of the first, and most important, assessments to be made is to determine the extent of the clinical relationship a parent wants with the nurse. This assessment must be a recurrent one throughout the prenatal time as rapport is established and as the parents' needs change. The GP process with parents can then be tailored appropriately. This process is, by necessity, shared between the nurse and parents. GP can be slow or quick to evolve based on timing of the fetal diagnosis, emergent conditions, and subsequent need for immediate decisions. Although it is understood that nurses have limited time, without such attention the healthcare team could be left unaware of a parent's needs and at risk for providing less effective care.

Three-Part Nursing Assessment Before Birth

Throughout the nursing care encounters with parents dealing with a fetal anomaly diagnosis, the nursing assessment is interconnected with the use of GP processes. The three-part assessment is focused on (a) *issues*—the nurse attends to the most salient issues by clarifying the situation and what is new, (b) *competencies*—the nurse determines the couple's competencies regarding knowledge, skills, and/or perspective-taking that are needed in respect to the goals that the issue reveals, and (c) *processes*—the nurse identifies the most effective place to join parents in the GP process to attend to the issue and develop or incorporate each parent's competencies to accomplish a set goal.

To use the three-part assessment sensitively and with accuracy, the first and all subsequent discussions require the nurse's careful listening. To do this, the nurse focuses on simply listening, and reserves questions or education that substantially redirects the conversation for later when a foundation for a nurse–parent relationship has been formed. Careful listening happens with (a) attentiveness to the content of what is being said, and (b) sensitive observation of expression of emotion and physical or behavioral nuances that could be tied to the description of issues the parents are working on. The nurse could observe extreme emotions expressed (e.g., crying, yelling), or in contrast, emotional shutdown with little to no emotions expressed. Thus, listening to the words used, listening for emotion behind the words, as well as listening for what is needed the most at that time, is essential. This kind of comprehensive listening takes practice.

Be aware of and check out the potential for misunderstandings and assumptions based on the appearance, age, and socioeconomic status of a parent or couple. Use words and phrases that support parents' continued talking, such as "I see," "uh-huh," or "really." Avoid using words or phrases that convey evaluation, judgment, or correction, such as "great," "excellent," "yes," or "you are doing a good job." Asking open-ended questions can elicit a range of issues, reveal key competencies needed, and determine the most appropriate process to engage parents in. While taking notes is always helpful for the nurse to keep track of potential issues to follow up on in the short and long term, doing so could be interpreted by parents in different ways. Seeing the nurse take notes during a conversation could raise a barrier if the parent or couple considers it as creating a social distance, nerve-wracking, or even offensive. Alternatively, note-taking could demonstrate to the couple that the nurse is paying close attention and values what is being shared by them. Validating the nurse's intention can be a useful technique to help minimize misunderstanding. Details of interactions warrant careful consideration when highly sensitive nursing care incorporates GP in the context of a nurse–patient relationship.

GP Processes Before Birth

The nurse's recurrent three-part assessment for GP expands on and sensitizes nursing practice. The GP processes that are central before birth include (a) getting and staying connected, (b) joining and maintaining attention, and (c) bridging (see book's frontispiece). The two cases in this chapter offer specific examples of how nurses can approach assessment and use the GP processes to facilitate prenatal preparation, the development of parental caregiving, and the beginnings of co-parenting for parents after a fetal anomaly diagnosis.

Case Example 3.1

Jess and Albert are partnered and both 19 years old. They live in a rural community where Jess works part time at a bank and Albert works as a mechanic and a farmer and takes on extra side jobs. Albert has been attending all the clinic appointments with Jess even though the travel time is long, his work hours can extend into the middle of the night, and he does not get enough sleep. Due in about a month, their first child will be a boy with gastroschisis, a malformation of the abdominal wall allowing the intestines and other organs to protrude outside the body.

It has been several weeks since the diagnosis was made. Albert is primarily focused on driving Jess to and from appointments in a safe and on-time manner so he can find out if the pregnancy and fetus are "still okay." Both Jess and Albert have asked questions to the healthcare providers in hopes of "short, simple answers" that they can understand. Since instead they received long, complicated answers, they saw their efforts to engage in these discussions as not useful to them. So, now they have decided not to ask many questions because, as Albert said, they just need to know "the basics."

During the clinic appointment, Jess and Albert sit together with solemn expressions. They really expected to have a healthy pregnancy and infant. Early in the conversation with the nurse, Jess says she has been feeling angry, "I don't deserve this. It's not like I was doing drugs. I am a pretty healthy person." She explains how she has been struggling with her negative emotions. She is very worried that her emotional stress will impede fetal brain development and bring about "bad energy" that could put her infant into the category of the "5% who die." Albert interjects, admitting that the diagnosis is a strain. He cannot believe this problem is happening to them and explained that every day he needs to limit the time spent thinking about the diagnosis and related issues. He says he will wait to see what he really needs to worry about.

Jess is thinking that their son will need to be hospitalized for up to 6 months while Albert is expecting him to be hospitalized for 40 days. Jess is worried that their baby will suffer in pain, and because of this, she sees her own personal problem of being sad as nothing to concern herself with. Albert does not quite see himself in the role of being a parent yet, pointing out that since he is "technically not a parent until after birth," he is waiting to see what will happen. Both believe that eventually after treatment their son can have a normal life. Albert remembers being told that he could even be "an Olympic athlete." Albert anticipates that when they see their son undergo the treatments, they will never take him for granted.

Jess and Albert acknowledge that although they are young and inexperienced with parenting, they see themselves as responsible and capable enough to handle the situation. The current personal challenge they are dealing with has to do with the ability and willingness of their family members to provide them with support. The couple is not emotionally close to their family, and most family members are also geographically distant. The two family members currently living in their small community include Albert's sister, who has decided to move away, and Jess's mother, who has been unsupportive and insensitive. Albert sees himself acting as a buffer to minimize the impact of her hurtful remarks on Jess.

As a couple, they agree that the previous experiences of healthcare providers not tuning in to what they need and not answering their questions in a way that is meaningful to them have often resulted in them leaving an appointment with the idea that they are "just a number" in the system.

Three-Part Assessment and Using GP

After encouraging both Jess and Albert to share what was on their minds, and carefully listening, key issues arose that would need to be addressed with this couple. To understand and clarify the issues, the nurse included reflective statements such as "It sounds like you have been feeling worried" and "There is a lot involved in understanding a surprising and complex diagnosis—maybe you have not felt fully included in what all is going on." To pursue the assessment, the nurse also posed questions such as "What are you most worried about lately? What is still not clear to you?" and "What are your goals for today?"

Issues

Together, the nurse and the couple identified several issues. Based on the assessment and clinical knowledge, however, the nurse prioritized three issues in the following order. First, there is a need to engage in relationship building between the nurse as part of the healthcare team and this couple. The goal is to establish a trustworthy bidirectional relationship for purposes of individualizing care. For this couple, such care should include plain language to convey information, invite dialogue, and ensure that the couple's needs are considered in the interaction, especially regarding education about the fetal and future child's condition. Second, there is a need to explore how emotions are being regulated by this mother and father, and how they are managing emotions as a couple. The goal would be to tap into emotion regulation through the different experiences of each parent, in terms of worry, guilt, and preparing to become a parent, in order to bring each parent into an awareness of their own and their partner's state of being, whether feelings, thoughts, or actions (McKechnie & Pridham, 2012). The third issue to examine is the support needed by these parents to adapt. The nurse should consider the emotional support parents will need to manage the strain and fear of having a child with a life-threatening condition, and also the instrumental support parents will need to meet day-to-day needs such as who will go to the grocery store, make meals, mow the lawn or shovel the snow, or do the laundry. This couple's time away from home is spent attending up to three appointments per week during pregnancy and later will involve extended time with the hospitalized infant. The goal would be to identify the support needs of the parents, the support available to these parents, and to ensure that the necessary support is in place to meet the challenges of caring for an infant with a life-threatening condition in both short and long terms.

To give a sense of what can be accomplished during the time allowed in one clinic appointment, the highest priority issue of relationship building will be the focus. Related to this issue, the nurse will need to assess the individual parent and couple competencies present and those needed to reach the goal of a trustworthy bidirectional relationship. Once the competencies are examined, the nurse can bring the couple into the GP process.

Competencies

Through the nurse's assessment, the competencies of each parent and the couple can be acknowledged and brought forward to manage the circumstances. The strengths of this couple include their willingness to share with the nurse what they know and think about the diagnosis as well as their personal circumstances that are posing additional challenges for them. If the nurse needs further clarification or emphasis on the strengths for the couple, a request could be "Tell me what you and your partner are handling well together?" To focus on the competencies needed requires recognizing insufficiencies that are amenable to change in order to reach the goal. In this case, the couple could work on competencies related to expressing agency as parents. Expressing agency as parents has been described in terms of their efforts to gain an understanding of the diagnosis, confidence in decisions made, and a readiness for infant caregiving in the parent role (McKechnie et al., 2016).

Process—Getting and Staying Connected

The focus for getting connected with this couple is on trust, respect, and working toward a bidirectional relationship. What must be considered first is that this couple has and will continue to experience strain from hours of traveling due to the health complications. Therefore it is particularly important for the nurse to begin with addressing their basic physical needs, which could simply mean a bathroom break, some water, and a comfortable, quiet room.

Once the basic physical needs are addressed, the nurse can move on to support a readiness to build trust. Very intentionally using plain language, the nurse should acknowledge that the couple has been through a great deal in the past few weeks, and the nurse can point out that other members of the healthcare team might have missed the opportunity to connect with them. Now sitting with the couple, the nurse highlights the privilege she has in working with them. It is crucial to deliver the message clearly and with emphasis, which demonstrates that the nurse and other members of the healthcare team would like to do their best to meet their needs. The nurse–mother relationship is often the first and easiest path to follow. The nurse should be mindful and even cautious of this default relationship-building focus. Since GP in this case is to be used with the couple, eliciting responses from both Jess and Albert is essential.

Fostering agency, meaning for these parents to engage in and take on the responsibilities for maternal–fetal healthcare, could prove foundational for their development of parental agency after birth. How members of the healthcare team respond to a parent's presence and participation in care has also

Getting and Staying Connected. This process is often the starting point, and requires a nurse's intentional efforts to create and maintain the space and the time for parents to share what is on their minds. Structuring the environment for parents begins with attending to the physical needs (e.g., offering water or a snack, minimizing the need to wait, or relocate from room to room), and then the social and ethical needs (e.g., addressing the parent by preferred name, guarding against the rushed rhythm of a busy clinic/hospital, ensuring privacy and confidentiality). In such an environment, the nurse can initiate discussion and listen for what is on the minds of the parents or collectively concerns the couple. Thinking and feeling are intertwined but separate. How a parent or couple is doing with regulating emotions can also be assessed through body language and behaviors that are either observed or recounted. This assessment will inform the nurse about readiness to engage in the GP process. If ready, the nurse can discern what is known and understood by the parents and where the gaps need to be filled—likely a very familiar role for the nurse. Beyond filling knowledge gaps, the nurse will begin to identify the parents' expectations and intentions related to the goals they are working toward reaching. Sharing an explicit understanding of the work that has been done and needs to be done to reach the mutually set goals of the nurse and parent(s) is the key to determining the competencies needed.

been related to how parents engage in expressing agency (McKechnie et al., 2016). To provide a useful experience, the nurse can ask the parents to talk about the tests and procedures that are on their minds. These parents should be encouraged to ask questions of the nurse with the expectation that the question will be answered in a manner that is useful to them. Work could then shift to extending beyond the relationship between the couple and nurse to others on the healthcare team. The nurse can explore how they see themselves and healthcare providers working together, as well as what problems they foresee. With some relationship building accomplished, the nurse will continue to act as a guide and partner to stay connected with this couple. The next steps involve supporting and acknowledging each parent's readiness to work on and practice behavior related to developing the competency of expressing agency.

Process—Joining and Maintaining Attention

With a mutual goal of establishing a trustworthy bidirectional relationship, joining attention is used to identify strategies that Jess and Albert could develop to better understand the health problems now and those anticipated in the future, and to gain some control over and satisfaction with the decisions made. Strategies that help the couple feel ready to take on parenting after birth should also be developed.

Two approaches could be used to facilitate success for these parents and allow them to see themselves as experts and advocates for their yet-to-be-born infant. Since this couple is young and inexperienced with the healthcare system, the nurse can offer to sit in on one or more of the frequent consultations these parents have with specialists. During these consultations, the nurse can ask the questions that might be on their minds. In this way, the nurse models how to ask questions without the effects of intimidation. The nurse can also ask for clarifications and, being persistent, if necessary, for rephrasing to enable understanding. The parents can be brought into the discussion and invited to ask more questions. The other approach is to suggest that Jess and Albert bring a family member or friend who is more removed from the circumstances and can be an "extra set of ears" and potentially take notes. Involving a family member or friend can be valuable for the couple since they will have the same information from the healthcare team, ideally then be "on the same page," and can provide long-term support when the couple is at home.

Joining and Maintaining Attention. This process involves seeking understanding and attention to issues and related goals. The purpose is not to gain an immediate mastery of the current situation, but rather to establish starting or reentry points for communication. The mother, father, and the nurse together examine culturally sensitive, interpersonal meaning of the diagnosis for the couple and their communication styles to support caregiving development and co-parenting. This process relies on identifying strengths and areas of concern that are collaboratively determined by the parents, with their expertise of being in the family and experience of the transition of becoming a parent to this infant, and the nurse, who brings clinical expertise.

Continuing GP

In addition to the issue of building a bidirectional relationship, the issues of emotional regulation and support will need discussion. There is a need to grieve over the loss of a "normal" pregnancy. This is a loss, and parents might feel angry—potentially, a necessary emotion to experience before a parent can gain other competencies. It is important to note that these parents are ready to support each other, and believe that they can address grief, guilt, and anger. The nurse will need to continue to observe and work with these parents as they deal with uncertainty and reach or try to reach acceptance in their own ways. During future interactions with the parents, the nurse can discern each parent's state of being. It has been posited that a parent's state of being is related to caregiving development and readiness to parent the infant (McKechnie & Pridham, 2012). While the stage of caregiving development could be a function of the physical and psychological experience of pregnancy, the processing of grief is a necessary consideration in this context. Addressing emotion regulation could offer insights into the current stage of caregiving development and how to facilitate movement and readiness for parenting and co-parenting. There could be challenges ahead if Albert maintains his compartmentalized views related to logistics and the insensitivity of family members. Bringing Albert into the GP process is essential for the health of this family. It could be particularly important for the nurse to look for opportunities to facilitate joy that is normative. For example, placing an emphasis on what is healthy and "normal" about the fetus rather than the pathology on imaging for serial monitoring. If parents are ready, they can make a conscious decision to find the joy through this, and other ways, as they are becoming parents.

Emotional support from within the family and from the healthcare team has been limited for this couple. In the short term, looking for the who and how of putting in place people for the parents to talk to and lean on will be essential. The instrumental support needed will include accepting help from friends and the community temporarily during the infant's hospitalization and transition home. In this case, instrumental support can also mean care coordination that will cluster appointments to minimize travel time and missed work. Long-term considerations might include support groups and early family and child development services. Meeting instrumental support needs over time might involve lifestyle changes, even moving closer to an urban center.

Case Example 3.2

Tracy is 39 years old and learned of a fetal diagnosis of hypoplastic left heart about 6 weeks prior to this appointment. Her partner John has not attended any appointments with Tracy. They live in a mid-sized town where Tracy is a graduate student commuting to a nearby university, and John works at a small business. Tracy sits confidently as she speaks with the nurse very articulately about her recent experiences and how she and her "life partner are not on the same page." John wanted very much to terminate the pregnancy after the diagnosis was made. John's mother echoed his opinion since she had experienced the death of John's older brother shortly after he was born with a heart defect. Tracy slumped back in the chair as she acknowledged having dealt with her own deep conflict about what the right path was supposed to be for her. She is quick to recover, emphasizing that time has passed quickly with the pregnancy progressing and birth pending.

Tracy's confidence returns as she describes how her perspective has shifted so that now she sees herself as developing a relationship with her "daughter" although not yet born. John is having trouble, however, with this shift and what will need to happen next. Tracy explains that John is not talking about the diagnosis with anyone. She believes that he is not yet "giving his voice" to the problems they have encountered with the pregnancy because "he is suffering a lot more" than she is now. Surprisingly though, Tracy brings up that John would like to create the nursery room with a pirate theme. Tracy seems hopeful that John will engage more with her and the baby after birth.

Tracy opens up about her experiences in a stepwise manner. She sees her coping skills as well developed, and recognizes going through four turning points which have resulted in how she currently views her daughter. Initially, there was the diagnosis that came as a complete surprise and moved her in directions that she would never have considered before. The aftermath of the diagnosis involved feelings of ambivalence, accompanied by emotional struggles after the decision to terminate. Tracy searched for a feasible way to have the procedure. As the possible pathways for termination dwindled, she returned to gathering information about the diagnosis and prognosis, and the possibility that she might have to continue pregnancy.

To imagine the possibility of continuing pregnancy and having this baby, she sought out infant heart disease–specific parenting groups online and in person. Filling the need for emotional support, she became closer with a few good friends. With these close friends wanting to be helpful, a question was posed to Tracy about the name she had chosen for her expected baby. They wanted to pray for her expected baby by name. Tracy experienced a second turning point as she named her daughter, Violet. Reflecting on this name, she regretted choosing such a delicate and feminine name. She expressed confidence, saying that her daughter will "be a strong girl and she'll figure it out" when it comes to the adversity and daily life with her heart disease.

Tracy realized the third turning point when she was attending a parenting group where she learned that a couple went to great lengths to adopt a toddler with the same kind of heart disease that her daughter would have. Based on the couple's story, she developed a deeply meaningful, new perspective that a child with such severe heart disease could be wanted so much, and loved as much as a healthy child.

The fourth turning point came when Tracy believed that she had exhausted her search for a termination procedure. She found no healthcare facility in her state providing the procedure during the gestational age. She then determined the time and money needed to travel out of state and concluded it was not feasible to afford the healthcare costs without insurance coverage for the procedure. The option of perinatal hospice had also been presented to Tracy so that she and her infant would be supported with palliative care and her Violet's short life celebrated. But Tracy felt that once Violet was born, she would want to pursue curative therapies despite her concerns about Violet's long-term prognosis. Thus, Tracy decided to continue pregnancy with plans to deliver Violet where she would have immediate access to pediatric cardiology care and start her path toward surgical treatment of the heart defects. Consequently, John and some family members see her as selfish for bringing a child into the world despite the pain and suffering the condition could inflict. Their comments raised questions for her about what her motives were and how she will manage the dread of seeing her daughter go through the surgeries and pain. In spite of these circumstances, she emphasizes her conscious decision to change strategies and immerse herself in becoming a mother, after earlier not wanting to "bond" as she sought termination.

Tracy explains that she is reading all the disease-related materials she can access, and that she is planning and hoping for the best outcome. She sees herself as a capable advocate for her daughter not yet born, emphasizing, "I'm already a parent of a kid with special needs." She recounted how sensing pity from others triggered intense reactions. Although she believes technological advances will lead to a good quality of life for her daughter, her worries mount up much higher than for a "normal mother." Even before birth, Tracy is thinking about what her daughter's life will be like when she is an adult in her 20s. She imagines in detail what the future might hold, and the goals and strategies that could be applicable. Sitting with the nurse, Tracy leans in to explain that she is not a particularly religious person, but thinks of herself as "chosen" to provide special care for this child—that she is the one to provide more than would be needed if she were a healthy child. She believes that as an educated and motivated mother, this child will have every advantage.

Three-Part Assessment and Using GP

Through several previous interactions in person and over the phone, the nurse and Tracy developed a trustworthy bidirectional relationship. The nurse knew that Tracy considered all the possibilities and initially chose to pursue termination. Yet as time passed, the experience appeared to fit with a "choice lost" (Sandelowski & Jones, 1996) due to insufficient access to services and health insurance limitations regarding second-trimester pregnancy termination. Tracy is now working to navigate her emotions and prepare to be a competent mother. To understand and clarify the issues in this context, the nurse included reflective statements such as "It sounds like you have been dealing with so many emotions" and "There is a lot to consider as you are preparing to be a mother to Violet—maybe you have not yet had a chance to talk about it." To pursue the assessment, the nurse also posed questions such as "How you are handling the ups and downs lately? What kind of support do you need now?" and "Considering the goal of feeling at peace, what do you think would help you?"

Issues

The focus here again will be on the same three types of issues as identified in the first case. In this case, however, the issues are characterized differently and prioritized based on how the nurse assesses Tracy's needs early the discussion. First, the nurse will attend to emotion regulation concerning Tracy's lingering questions about continuing pregnancy and bringing her daughter into a world to endure suffering so that she could be a mother. The goal is for Tracy to feel at peace knowing that she will be a mother who is caring and competent and will, therefore, be able to protect and nurture her daughter. Second, Tracy needs emotional and instrumental support. The tension with, or perhaps the absence of, John as a partner and co-parent will need attention. Lack of support from family members could come to the fore, especially after Violet's birth. The goal is to buffer against depression and trauma that Tracy is at high risk for encountering by ensuring that she does not feel alone. The third issue is related to trusting in and relying on the bidirectional relationship that Tracy has with the healthcare team. The nurse and other members of the healthcare team have recognized Tracy's ability to think about and plan for the future. The concern, as well as the goal, has to do with how she will sustain her emotional endurance.

Between the appointments scheduled on this day at the clinic, the nurse and Tracy have a little more time than usual for discussion. This factor contributes to the nurse's assessment to explore the issue of emotion-regulation as prioritized. Although Tracy has many developed competencies, she will likely need some guidance to find peace with her past decisions and to move ahead without the weight of guilt she has alluded to.

Competencies

Tracy has many competencies to draw on, especially given her social–emotional strengths. She has already faced deeply critical messages from those close to her and sought out support groups to get through an adverse time. There are competencies needing development, although needing a more nuanced approach. The nurse can direct attention to develop competencies having to do with shifting perspectives. Working together, the nurse can help Tracy see how her emotions fit within a range of what is normal and expected, and to see how the care for Violet will be a process rather than one outcome of an infant suffering.

The process of getting and staying connected with Tracy has been used many times before, and at this time, only requires checking in to ensure that her physical, social, and ethical needs are met. In a private setting, the nurse will engage Tracy in joining and maintaining attention and will move into bridging to reach a mutually set goal of finding peace in herself as a mother who can protect and nurture Violet.

Process—Joining and Maintaining Attention

Attention to the issue of finding peace relies on the rapport that the nurse has with Tracy. The nurse can highlight the ways in which Tracy has bonded with Violet even before birth, and in such a short time. The nurse can deliver a clear message that loving parents might consider pregnancy termination, and share clinical experiences from working with mothers like Tracy. It is important to specify that regardless of the degree of action toward termination, many mothers have explained that such a consideration was not about wanting or not wanting to have a child, but rather about the ethical grappling with wanting to avoid long-term pain and suffering. By offering examples, the nurse can facilitate the normalizing of complex emotions and could allow the feelings of guilt to rise to the surface for further discussion. Mothers' experiences of guilt can be expected in this context (McKechnie, 2013).

Gaining a view of oneself as a competent mother can be useful because this view is not very compatible with harboring guilt. The nurse will help Tracy see additional areas to develop her competencies as a good mother and valued member of the healthcare team. There might be an unrealized ability for Tracy to engage in reviewing options now and as needed in the future for the healthcare management. Healthcare management during the prenatal time can be preparatory and strategies can be formed and used both before and after birth.

Joining and Maintaining Attention. The issues most needing attention are those that are perplexing, need resolving, or must be accomplished. While it is possible for either the nurse or the parents to initiate discussion and explore the issues, the nurse remains the guide. The nurse brings the mother and/or her partner into a conversation about what they are feeling now, might feel in the near future, and also what they need to be thinking about now and in the near future. The discussion may turn to the diagnosis, urgent decision making that might need to be made, the parents' psychosocial status, and communication styles, and why competence in specific areas is needed and important. Encouraging joint attention to an issue in this way is essential for achieving intersubjectivity, or a shared understanding of the meaning or subjective experience of the situation.

Process—Bridging

The next process is to intentionally work toward bridging what Tracy knows, and has clear competencies in doing, with new ways of reflecting on her decisions and new information for Tracy—allowing for new strategies to take shape. To provide the care that could be needed for emotion regulation, the possibility of mental health services is explored. The clinic where Tracy is receiving her maternal–fetal care is part of a large quaternary care center that employs numerous specialists including counselors, psychologists, and psychiatrists. Mental health services are included in the clinic's care and so would not present a financial burden. Tracy can appreciate the need for such services but did not think she would need them. Her infant is the one to worry about, not her. The nurse explains that the complexities and duration of her emotions can take a toll. She also points out that resources are akin to tools in a tool box, and used as needed for small adjustments or big problems. Tracy agrees that it is possible she might not be aware of how much her experiences have impacted her and will meet with the staff psychologist who specializes in women's health.

There could also be a need to invite Tracy to engage with additional specialists to allow her to see how she can be a nurturing and protective mother. The nurse can be very explicit in explaining that palliative care is not only for patients in hospice. It should have been communicated with

***Bridging.** This process requires a nurse to encourage parents to make connections between what they have felt, thought, and known to new information that could be used to strengthen a competency. The nurse considers the zone of proximal development (Vygotsky, 1978, 1987), or the parent's current psychosocial and cognitive resources, to guide parents in progressing beyond what they could do independently to a higher level. To make progress, the nurse identifies how and what the mother and/or her partner learned and what to expect in regard to their infant, as well as how and what they are learning about themselves and each other and what this situation means for each of them. Making these connections with new information facilitates dealing with issues and resolving present or future problems. The nurse needs to be careful to foster connections rather than disconnections from parents' familiar culture and practices. The nurse and parent or couple can then work together to develop competencies for dealing with issues related to communication, decision making, co-parenting, and social circumstances. In this way, parents become more competent in understanding and making meaning of the diagnosis, identifying, reflecting on, and regulating their own and their partners' emotions, and communicating in preparation as caregivers for the child. Parents should be encouraged to contribute individual or shared experiences so that the nurse can use a relevant experience to give context to feedback and direction during the GP process.*

Tracy earlier that involving the palliative care specialists within the team directing treatment and the overall care plan could be a beneficial option. The nurse gave a clear message that this infant's pain management and quality of life are going to be very important to the healthcare team. Tracy will be able to work with the healthcare team to manage her daughter's pain. The nurse assured Tracy that Violet will be cared for so that she will not suffer in pain. Upon hearing this, the tears welling up in Tracy's eyes cleared with a smile, signaling that there was still work to be done to reconcile her choice to continue pregnancy and the scenario of pain management for little Violet. There was also the opportunity to bring up the lactation specialists. Since Tracy had intended to breastfeed and pump her breast milk, lactation specialists could support her in contributing to Violet's health and development in this special way. Tracy could gain preparatory information now and the tangible skills after the birth to be a confident mother feeding her infant. The nurse and Tracy agreed that an appointment should be made with the healthcare team and additional specialists to discuss pain management and feeding. Tracy appeared to relax and suggested that she could also talk with other parents who had these concerns and made it through their infants' staged surgeries and months of hospitalization.

Continuing GP

In addition to the issue of emotion regulation and the goal for Tracy to see herself as having a strong foothold as a competent, good mother, the emotional and instrumental support will shore up her efforts and contribute to the best outcome. The nurse or other member of the healthcare team could ask Tracy "Who are the people around you?" and "How can I have this discussion with them as well?" These questions could provide a mechanism for Tracy to invite family members and close friends to join her for an appointment, or to agree to a phone call. Healthcare providers could change the narrative they have created and rally support for Tracy. Her ongoing involvement in the parent support groups could also reduce fear by seeing how families manage a child's heart condition and live life to the fullest.

The issue of the bidirectional relationship that Tracy has established with the healthcare team will need to be sustained. Instead of the typical mother who might imagine where her child will go to college, this mother has mentally extrapolated illness-related concerns and quality of life worries into her daughter's early adult life. Tracy is in the midst of an acutely difficult transition, and managing care and handling circumstances practically following Violet's birth will likely call for her steadfast presence and action. While acknowledging her work to see possible futures, directing her thinking to a shorter term might help to conserve her emotional energies for a crucial time. Her trust in the healthcare team will make it more likely that she considers such guidance.

CONCLUSION

GP can be a particularly valuable approach used by nurses to assist parents and couples as they are becoming parents after a fetal anomaly diagnosis. With the nurse as guide, a three-part assessment leads to identifying and prioritizing the issues that are either on parents' minds or that need work. Parents' competencies are engaged and developed as the nurse employs the appropriate GP processes to reach a set goal. Supporting parental efforts to achieve an adaptive transition to parenthood while managing healthcare is necessary for optimal infant and family outcomes.

REFERENCES

Farr, R. H., Simon, K. A., & Bruun, S. T. (2017). LGBTQ relationships: Families of origin, same-sex couples, and parenting. In N. R. Silton (Ed.), *Family dynamics and romantic relationships in a changing society* (pp. 110–136). Hershey, PA: IGI Global.

Gould, S. W., Figueroa, T. E., Robinson, B. W., & Reichard, K. W. (2011). Recent advances in the prenatal diagnosis and subsequent management of congenital anomalies. *The Journal of Lancaster General Hospital*, 6(1), 5–9.

Jones, S., Statham, H., & Solomou, W. (2005). When expectant mothers know their baby has a fetal abnormality: Exploring a crisis of motherhood through qualitative data-mining. *Journal of Social Work Research and Evaluation*, 6(2), 195–206.

Leuthner, S. R., Bolger, M., Frommelt, M., & Nelson, R. (2003). The impact of abnormal fetal echocardiography on expectant parents' experience of pregnancy: A pilot study. *Journal of Psychosomatic Obstetrics and Gynaecology*, 24(2), 121–129.

Limbo, R., & Kobler, K. (2010). The tie that binds: Relationships in perinatal bereavement. *MCN: The American Journal of Maternal/Child Nursing*, 35(6), 316–321.

McHale, J. P., & Lindahl, K. M. (2011). *Coparenting: A conceptual and clinical examination of family systems*. Washington, DC: American Psychological Association.

McKechnie, A. C. (2013). *Becoming a parent after a prenatal diagnosis: A model of preparing heart and mind within the caregiving system* (PhD dissertation). University of Wisconsin—Madison. Retrieved from ProQuest Dissertations & Theses Global database.

McKechnie, A. C., Johnson, K. A., Baker, M., Docherty, S., & Thoyre, S. (2015). *Adaptive leadership of parents caring for their children born with a life-threatening condition*. Paper presented at the 39th Midwest Nursing Research Society Annual Conference, Indianapolis, IN.

McKechnie, A. C., & Pridham, K. F. (2012). Preparing heart and mind following prenatal diagnosis of complex congenital heart defect. *Qualitative Health Research*, 22(12), 1694–1706. doi:10.1177/1049732312458371

McKechnie, A. C., Pridham, K. F., & Tluczek, A. (2015). Preparing heart and mind for becoming a parent following a diagnosis of fetal anomaly. *Qualitative Health Research*, 25(9), 1182–1198. doi:10.1177/1049732314553852

McKechnie, A. C., Pridham, K. F., & Tluczek, A. (2016). Walking the "emotional tightrope" from pregnancy to parenthood: Understanding parental motivation to manage health care and distress after a fetal diagnosis of complex congenital heart disease. *Journal of Family Nursing*, 22(1), 74–107. doi:10.1177/1074840715616603

McKechnie, A. C., Rogstad, J., Martin, K. M., & Pridham, K. F. (2017). An exploration of co-parenting in the context of caring for a child prenatally diagnosed and born with a complex health condition. *Journal of Advanced Nursing*, 74(2), 350–363.

McKechnie, A. C., Tluczek, A., Pridham, K. F., Lamberg Jones, E., & Thoyre, S. (2014). *Embraced, avoided or de-emphasized: How expectant parents managed technological information about their fetal diagnoses*. Paper presented at the 38th Midwest Nursing Research Society Annual Conference, St. Louis, MO.

Pridham, K. F., Limbo, R., Schroeder, M., Thoyre, S., & Van Riper, M. (1998). Guided participation and development of care-giving competencies for families of low birth-weight infants. *Journal of Advanced Nursing, 28*(5), 948–958.

Rempel, G. R., Cender, L. M., Lynam, M. J., Sandor, G. G., & Farquharson, D. (2004). Parents' perspectives on decision making after antenatal diagnosis of congenital heart disease. *Journal of Obstetric, Gynecologic, and Neonatal Nursing, 33*(1), 64–70.

Sandelowski, M., & Jones, L. C. (1996). "Healing fictions": Stories of choosing in the aftermath of the detection of fetal anomalies. *Social Science & Medicine, 42*(3), 353–361.

Vygotsky, L. S. (1978). *Mind in society: The development of higher psychological processes.* Cambridge, MA: Harvard University Press.

Vygotsky, L. S. (1987). Thinking and speech. In R. W. Rieber & A. S. Carton (Eds.), *The collected works of L. S. Vygotsky* (N. Minick, Trans.) (pp. 37–285). New York, NY: Plenum.

4

Guided Participation for Mothers Learning to Feed Their Prematurely Born Infant: Goals and a Community of Learners

Lisa F. Brown

This chapter focuses on guided participation (GP) beginning in a NICU for learning of feeding skills of mother and infant, both learners, and of a feeding practice for mothers of very prematurely born infants getting started at nipple feeding. In this chapter, as a nurse researcher and expert NICU nurse, I write about mothers' learning in relation to a sociocultural activity, infant feeding, with high clinical importance for the well-being of mothers and infants and for the growth and development of the infant. Using GP as my framework, I analyze the dialogue I had with three mothers who had a very prematurely born infant either in the NICU or early in the mother's care of the infant at home. My analysis includes issues, processes, and competencies examined in the context of the goals that mothers and clinicians concurrently held. I pay particular attention to the mother's goals for feeding her infant and assesses their impact on the learning of feeding skills and the development of a feeding practice. As part of my analysis, I reflect on my response to mothers, and wonder how the GP session might have gone if I had responded in a different manner. I chose to include the audio-recorded and transcribed verbal content of my GP discussions with mothers, revealing the potential for change in teaching–learning practice that could occur.

THE FUNCTION OF GOALS IN GP

Learning, a practice important to the well-being of members of a community, is a sociocultural activity (Rogoff, 2003). "Humans develop through their changing participation in the sociocultural activities of their communities, which also change" (Rogoff, 2003, p. 11). Learning, practiced through GP, brings learners and guides in the activity together to accomplish the development of the learner's skill in the activity. The aim of learning is for the learner to become skilled enough to be in charge of performing the activity. The learner's change in participation from being peripheral, perhaps in the role of observer, to being a central performer of the activity occurs through the guide's more or less gradual transfer of responsibility for the activity (Lave & Wenger, 1989; Rogoff, 1990). As learners become the central participants in a socially important activity and contribute their voices to the development of skills in an activity, the activity itself, including the teaching and practice processes and strategies of the guides, is likely to develop and even change in character. The learning goals of the learner and how the guide (teacher or facilitator) works with the learner in relation to learner and practice goals may contribute to both the learner's development of skills for the activity and in the socially important activity itself.

Goals Expressed in the Process of Learning Skills for Infant Feeding

The goals and functions of a mother's practice of infant feeding are generally determined by experts in infant nutrition and feeding and codified in NICU policy. From a clinical standpoint, the functions and goals of a mother's feeding activity are an infant who feeds efficiently, safely, and effectively in respect to the amount of nutrients consumed and the growth achieved and in respect to a mother who is sensitively perceptive of the infant's cues of need and effectively responds to them (Lau, 2016; Thoyre, Shaker, & Pridham, 2005). Mothers, however, may have commitments to personal goals toward which they are striving and on which satisfaction with the feeding experience depends (Hill & Feudtner, 2016).

Goals are a component of a mother's internal working model (IWM) of caregiving focused on feeding. Goals shape expectations and orient and direct intentions. A mother's personal goals may correspond or conflict with the goals set in place by NICU policies and procedures, or mothers may struggle with the infant's seeming lack of interest in feeding or slow progress on the clinician-specified goals.

The goals of mothers of very young, vulnerable infants who are learning to feed their infant, initially in an NICU and later by themselves at home in the company of the memories they have of NICU learning, are central to this chapter. Four ideas about GP as a teaching–learning activity for beginning feeding in the sociocultural environment of the NICU are useful to keep in mind when reading this chapter as ideas applicable for learning a new practice in any new environment. The first idea is that learning occurs in a learning community, even one not publicly recognized for its learning projects. The second idea is that focusing on the goals of persons who are working at learning is critical to understanding the support, guidance, and participation needed to learn parent-desired and clinician-expected functions of infant caregiving, for example, an infant's feeding. The third idea is that the learner's goals are likely to change as the learner develops competence, including new understanding of the infant's behavior and awakened appreciation and pleasure in the infant as a person. The fourth idea focuses on the guide who is likely to be viewed by learners as an expert with unquestionable competencies and definitive, authoritative answers to questions. In the process of a learner's development of competence and potential change of goals, the guide's goals or concept of the function of GP for this parent may also change or evolve.

GP and Mothers' Goals for Feeding a Prematurely Born Infant

GP can assist mothers in identifying, thinking about, and working toward their goals with their infants. A NICU is a community of learners (Rogoff, Matusov, & White, 1996), both mothers and nurses working together to nurture the infant, primarily through the activity of feeding, but also through actions of relating and being with the baby (Schroeder & Pridham, 2006). Nurses support mothers' learning and development of competencies through their knowledge of how prematurely born infants develop feeding skills and their attention to what mothers and infants are ready to learn. A baby, however, is a person who is new to both members of the learning community, mother and nurse. Mothers, through being with the baby during gavage and nipple feedings, optimally repeatedly and for sustained periods of time, are making observations, experiencing feelings that shape the relationship, and figuring out how the baby responds to them as a person (Thoyre, Park, Pados, & Hubbard, 2013). Through a nurse guide's structuring and supporting a mother's sharing of her experience, the nurse has a larger opportunity to learn who the baby is and who the mother and infant are as a dyad, and is, therefore, in a better position to guide the mother's learning. The mother, as a consequence, becomes a collaborator in the learning activity. Through this collaboration, the mother learns to participate in becoming competent and in taking on responsibility as primary caregiver for feeding and relating to her infant. Her goal may be interpreted as what she chooses to learn or focuses on learning.

GP for the development of feeding skills is by its nature a collaborative process in the NICU. Goals that are shared are at the heart of collaboration. Goals are important to discern, identify, and state because they determine the lens both mother and nurse guide use to process conversations with each other for learning and shape how both think about and structure the infant's care in the NICU. The joint effort both mother and guide put into the infant's feeding depends on goals they both share. Some mothers may have difficulty stating goals because of lack of opportunity to share their ideas about what they would like to do or think they should do (Belenky, Clinchy, Goldberger, & Tarule, 1986). In a collaborative teaching–learning model, goals that are clear to mother and nurse and subscribed by both to some extent are conditions required for GP to proceed effectively (Rogoff et al., 1996).

Understanding Mothers' Goals for Feeding a Prematurely Born Infant

If GP is collaboration toward understanding and working to accomplish the shared goals of parent and nurse, processes of clarifying, negotiating, and revising goals may be needed. These facets of GP process contribute to commitment to the teaching and learning nurse and mother are engaging in and to alignment with each other in taking the same direction and orientation. The goals, made specific to a mother and maximally beneficial through refinement and elaboration with a nurse guide, support the overarching goal of development of caregiving competencies, including competencies for feeding a prematurely born infant. In this chapter, I present accounts of taking on caregiving responsibilities beginning in the NICU of three mothers (Amy, Beth, and Erin). Each of these mothers expressed goals for caregiving, specifically feeding a prematurely born infant who was learning to nipple feed in the NICU. The mothers' accounts include clinician perspectives and activities. My acquaintance with the mothers began when they became participants in the research I was conducting. The conversations I had with them about their experiences in learning to successfully feed their infant are documented in Tables 4.1 to 4.9. In these conversations, I identified GP issues, processes, and competencies.

Case Example 4.1

Amy (Dan's mother) identified bottle feeding and taking Dan home as her top two goals. At times these two goals were incompatible because Dan and Amy needed to learn to feed safely before he could go home. Conflicting goals may become a prominent first-order issue to deal with so that the nurse can be helpful to the mother in accomplishing her goal or goals.

Dan was born at 23 weeks gestational age and developed chronic lung disease and reflux. He was on 1/8 L of oxygen via nasal cannula, and had problems with nipple feeding in the past. After several infections, several episodes of feeding intolerance, and several recent episodes of choking, Dan was placed on continuous nasogastric (NG) tube feedings. My goal in working with Amy was to help her see feeding safety as a goal that would support a second goal, that is, to strengthen her relationship with her baby through the sense of confidence and competence that safe feeding would support.

Amy and I developed and maintained joint attention around her goal of helping Dan learn to feed. I listened for the issues that Amy brought up and dwelled on when I asked her what she was noticing about Dan and how she was feeling about how he was doing. Feeding was the most prominent issue in Amy's report concerning both her baby and herself. Dan was in the hospital a little over 28 weeks. The doctors wanted to put in a gastrostomy tube (G-tube) but Amy refused. Toward developing shared understanding, I tried to wonder and reflect with Amy about her strong aversion to Dan having a G-tube, but she was not ready. In Table 4.1, I have documented our conversation concerning caregiving issues with the GP processes we were engaged in and the competencies that were the objective of the processes. The processes are shown in Figure 1.1 (see Chapter 1). Parental competencies for infant caregiving are accessible through this link **www.springerpub.com/pridham,** Chapter 1.

Amy was getting very upset and boisterous. I was afraid that Dan's nurse would come in to check on us and discontinue our time together. I didn't think I would get anywhere with Amy concerning her feelings about Dan having a G-tube at this point. I decided to put this topic on hold and come back to it at a later date. I attempted, successfully, to bring Amy's level of emotion down (competency: regulate emotion) so she could continue to engage in GP with me about Dan's feeding skill and supporting its development. In Table 4.2, I refocused the conversation on a topic concerning supporting Dan in developing skill in feeding that I knew was of interest to the mother. This skill concerned persisting at feeding without difficulty in sucking, swallowing, and breathing.

Amy and I had been working on reading Dan's stress cues during feeding. These cues included spilling formula from the corner of his mouth, gulping when swallowing, and breathing rapidly throughout, making Dan often stop feeding to catch up in breathing. We worked on strategies Amy could use to help Dan feed. These strategies included giving Dan a breathing break every three to five sucks or placing him in an elevated side-lying position to feed. Amy recognized Dan's cues of stress, but her two goals were, at this stage of Dan's learning to feed, not mutually supportive. She wanted Dan to finish his bottles and wanted him to be able to go home. These two goals resulted in her continuing to feed Dan beyond the point of knowing she should stop and give Dan a rest from feeding. Amy's continuation of the feeding resulted in her baby showing physiological and behavioral signs of

TABLE 4.1 Guided Participation Conversation: Issues, Processes, and Maternal Competencies—Part 1. Mother Amy and Baby Dan in the NICU

Conversation Concerning Caregiving (Issues)	Guided Participation Processes	Maternal Competencies
Amy: Dan choked again yesterday and the doctors want to put in a G-tube.		Communicating (takes initiative in raising issues)
Nurse: How do you feel about that?	Gaining joint attention	
Amy: I told them NO! I don't want him to have a G-tube!		(Expresses rejection of medical plan for a G-tube and conflict with medical team)
Nurse: Why? What does having a G-tube mean to you or to Dan?	Bridging/making connections: Sharing understanding	
Amy: I don't know. I just know HE DOESN'T NEED ONE! [Mother is getting agitated and raises her voice.]		Caregiving (unable to express why baby does not need a G-tube) Communicating (having difficulty regulating emotion)
Nurse: This is upsetting you. I wonder where that feeling is coming from.	Bridging/making connections	
Amy: Yeah, they are not cutting on my baby! The next thing you know he will have another infection, be back on a vent, and not feeding. He don't need no damn G-tube and he doesn't want one! He just got a little tired yesterday.		Knowing and relating to baby Communicating (informs more specifically of her concern)
Nurse: So, you are afraid he will get sick again with a G-tube? Is that the worst thing that could happen if he got a G-tube?	Bridging/making connection: Sharing understanding	
Amy: There is no need to talk about a G-tube BECAUSE HE'S NOT GETTING ONE!		Communicating (discontinues conversation about G-tube)

G-tube, gastrostomy tube.

TABLE 4.2 Guided Participation Conversation: Issues, Processes, and Maternal Competencies—Part 2. Mother Amy and Baby Dan in the NICU

Conversation Concerning Caregiving (Issues)	Processes	Maternal Competencies
Nurse: Okay. You mentioned earlier that he got tired.	Joining and maintaining attention	
Amy: Yeah, he was almost finished. Only 7 mL left! [Mom took a breath and seemed to calm herself.] She began to tell me about Dan's last feeding: "Dan had started spitting it out [the formula], squirming, and turning his head away from the bottle, so I stopped feeding for a little while. Dan fell asleep for a minute. When he woke up and opened his eyes I tried to feed him. He choked! I rubbed his back but the nurses had to come in and turn up his oxygen. I went over the 30 minutes I was told to limit the feeding to. Dan was just tired. He chokes when he gets overly tired."	Bridging/making connections	Emotion regulating (brought her level of tension and anger down by refocusing on how baby was feeding) Problem solving/ decision making/ learning (made connections concerning her own actions and the baby's response) Knowing and relating to baby
Nurse: How do you think he felt when he choked?	Bridging/making connections	
Amy: [long pause] Scared.		Knowing and relating to baby
Nurse: How did you feel when he choked?		
Amy: I was a little scared. I kept rubbing and patting him. His heart rate came back up but his pulse ox wouldn't come up. I forgot to turn up the oxygen. When the nurse came in she reminded me that when something like that happens to give him more oxygen.		Communicating (expressed what frightened her) Problem solving/ decision making/ learning (what should be done when baby shows stress cues, including cardiovascular and respiratory signs of difficulty)

(continued)

TABLE 4.2 Guided Participation Conversation: Issues, Processes, and Maternal Competencies—Part 2. Mother Amy and Baby Dan in the NICU (*continued*)

Conversation Concerning Caregiving (Issues)	Processes	Maternal Competencies
Nurse: So why was it important that he finish his bottle yesterday?	Bridging/making connections (yesterday's feeding experience and why Amy wanted baby to finish his bottle of formula)	
Amy: He had been finishing his bottles and the doctor said if he kept it up he could go home.		Communicating (expressed goals: Baby take the prescribed amount of formula so mother could take him home)

distress and the feeding having to be discontinued. The conversation I had with Amy concerning stress cues, strategies to support effective feeding, and goals for feeding is shown in Table 4.3.

At this point in our GP conversation, Amy made the connection, in the context of my asking the question about her goals for feeding Dan, that her goal of taking Dan home was interfering with her goal of Dan's gaining competence in feeding, making it safe for her to take him home. Amy needed to commit to the goal of feeding competence as her top priority. She indicated in our conversation her recognition of the connection between the two goals.

After a swallow test to determine if Dan had an anatomical problem that explained his feeding difficulty, the speech therapist developed guidelines for feeding Dan. Amy learned to feed Dan through his NG tube in case Dan tired during nipple feeding. Almost 6 weeks later, Dan was ready for discharge. Dan was 1½ months postterm age when he went home. However, almost 2 weeks later he was back in the hospital for suspected aspiration.

Amy and I had developed a relationship in which mutual trust was evident. The events that follow show evidence of reciprocity in our communication. Amy was comfortable enough being with me to assert her position and communicate how she felt things needed to go for Dan. The conversation that follows, in Table 4.4, occurred in hospital after Dan's readmission.

TABLE 4.3 Guided Participation Conversation: Issues, Processes, and Maternal Competencies—Part 3. Mother Amy and Baby Dan in the NICU

Conversation Concerning Caregiving (Issues)	Processes	Maternal Competencies
Nurse: You've stated two goals—feeding and taking Dan home. How would you prioritize your goals?	Bridging/making connections: Structuring the conversation for examination of goals	
Amy: I need to concentrate on feeding first because if we get that down, he will be able to go home. I just got a little carried away with the thought of taking him home soon.	Bridging/making connections: Identifying the priority goal	Problem solving/decision making/learning (identified links, including antecedents and consequences, and her own role in how well her baby feeds)

TABLE 4.4 Guided Participation Conversation: Issues, Processes, and Maternal Competencies—Mother Amy and Baby Dan in the Hospital After Readmission

Conversation Concerning Caregiving (Issues)	Processes	Maternal Competencies
Amy: They think he aspirated a little. They also said he's not growing as fast as they want so (starts to tear up; hands me two fact sheets, one on gastrostomy and one on fundoplication) but I still don't want it.		Communicating (provided information about what had happened and what her desire is)
Nurse: Okay. I know this is a sensitive subject for you, but you once told me the worst thing that can happen if he has the surgery was he could end up with an infection and back on the ventilator. What's the worst thing that can happen if he doesn't have surgery?	Bridging/making connections: Bringing expectations to light; contrasting worst case with and without the surgery; structuring a way to think things through	
Amy: If he doesn't have surgery, he could still wind up here and on a vent.		Problem solving (identified plausible outcome)

TABLE 4.4 Guided Participation Conversation: Issues, Processes, and Maternal Competencies—Mother Amy and Baby Dan in the Hospital After Readmission (*continued*)

Conversation Concerning Caregiving (Issues)	Processes	Maternal Competencies
Nurse: You said you were scared when his monitors went off. What do you think he was experiencing when all of that was going on?	Bridging/making connections between the baby's physical experience of aspiration and the emotional experience	
Amy: I'm sure he was scared too.		Knowing and relating to baby (identified baby's emotional experience)
Nurse: What else? Do you think he might have been uncomfortable or in pain?	Bridging/making connections: Reflecting (wondering about the baby's experience)	
Amy: Yeah, it is uncomfortable to throw-up and sometimes it can be painful.		Knowing and relating to baby (identified what the baby could have experienced, physically; related her own experience to what baby could have experienced)
Nurse: How often does he throw-up?	Bridging/making connections: Extending the information about the baby's experience of feeding; enlarging the scope or significance of the feeding difficulty	
Amy: At least a couple of times every day and some days after every meal.		Problem solving (has observed and can recall and give details of the baby's feedings)

(*continued*)

TABLE 4.4 Guided Participation Conversation: Issues, Processes, and Maternal Competencies—Mother Amy and Baby Dan in the Hospital After Readmission (*continued*)

Conversation Concerning Caregiving (Issues)	Processes	Maternal Competencies
Nurse: Do you think he will eventually connect pain and eating?	Bridging/making connections: Identifying possibilities, anticipating outcomes	
Amy: Probably.		
Nurse: How do you think he will start to feel about eating?	Bridging/making connections: Extending the possible consequences of feeding and throwing up	
Amy: The doctor said if this keeps up he probably won't want to eat		Communicating (recalled and applied what doctor had told her)
Nurse: I know you have very strong feelings about the doctors cutting on Dan but after the procedure he should only be in the hospital a few days. You will be able to take him home and take care of him. You will be the one making sure he doesn't get an infection and end up back here on a vent. I wonder what Dan would want?	Bridging/making connections: Developing expectations and goals	
Amy: [hunches her shoulders as if to express "I don't know."]		
Nurse: If Dan could talk what do you think he would choose? Having the surgery and not being uncomfortable or in pain every day and risking the possibility of getting an infection. Remember it is only a possibility. It is not a certainty that he will get sick. Or do you think he would choose to not have the surgery and be in pain or uncomfortable and scared every time he eats?		

(*continued*)

TABLE 4.4 Guided Participation Conversation: Issues, Processes, and Maternal Competencies—Mother Amy and Baby Dan in the Hospital After Readmission (*continued*)

Conversation Concerning Caregiving (Issues)	Processes	Maternal Competencies
Amy: He would probably want the surgery [she starts to cry].		Knowing and relating to baby (expressed a sense of the baby as a person with desires of his own)

CPAP, continuous positive airway pressure.

As I wondered with Amy about the source of her feelings, I learned her grandmother died during surgery a few years ago. Amy was able to make the connection between her fear of surgery and her grandmother's death. Amy also realized that letting Dan have the surgery was the best thing for him.

One of my goals in GP with mothers of premature infants was to help them to learn their babies' cues or signals of need and to respond sensitively and effectively to the identified need. A challenge for GP practice in relation to this kind of goal is the fleeting nature of infant and maternal behavior that could be shared for bridging and making connections. Stopping a feeding to question a mother about what is happening disrupts the natural course of the feeding and may be distressing to infant and mother. Neither guide nor mother is likely to be able to recall significant seconds of the feeding for later teaching–learning processes. One solution to the problem of both guide and mother having an opportunity to attend to the same facet of the feeding without disrupting it was a method of video recording with playback developed for GP practice. Guidelines for use of video recording as a teaching–learning tool may be accessed in the document, "Interview About Feeding the Baby" through this link: **www.springerpub .com/pridham,** Chapter 4.

In the following GP case study of Beth and her infant daughter, Abbie, I used video playback with focus on selected facets of a feeding to support bridging and making connections. The GP was based on identification and naming of a troublesome, challenging, or rewarding facet of the feeding. My aim for the GP was, in this case, to support learning concerning breastfeeding a prematurely born infant. The learning would be focused on how breastfeeding could be best supported in respect to the microbehaviors of infant and mother in interaction (see Thoyre, Park, Pados, & Hubbard, 2007, for a description of cue-based assessment of the feeding of a young infant).

Abbie was born at 34 weeks gestation and did not require supplemental oxygen through her NICU stay. She was a healthy premature infant. Abbie spent 2 weeks in the hospital learning how to breastfeed prior to discharge home. Her mother did not view her as good at breastfeeding when she took Abbie home. My first GP session with Abbie and Beth was scheduled for a home visit when Abbie was 1-month corrected age. Beth stated her goal as wanting Abbie to be a better breastfeeder.

During the feeding I observed, Abbie was on and off the nipple frequently. She did not latch on to the nipple as if she wanted to feed. She wiggled and fussed throughout the feeding. Beth tried repositioning Abbie from cradling her to using a more controlled football hold. Beth tried feeding Abbie on the opposite breast, and then tried burping her. None of Beth's strategies resulted in Abbie latching on or staying latched on for more than a few minutes. After 15 minutes of the feeding interaction, Beth told me the feeding was over. By stopping the feeding, Beth demonstrated competency in knowing and responding to her baby's preferences. She was also interacting with the baby in a way that indicated she was connecting with the baby and what the baby was experiencing.

I made this assessment of Beth's maternal competencies in feeding as I replayed the video recording I had made during the feeding and talked with Beth about it immediately after the feeding. My assessment raised the question, however, of what explained Abbie's not latching onto the breast nipple well at a time Beth had thought she was hungry. As we watched the video recording, I wondered with the mom what was going on with Abbie. Beth stated this had not been a normal feeding. The conversation, analyzed in GP terms, follows in Table 4.5.

Abbie latched on and breastfed without problems. Beth was able to see how sensitive Abbie was to her emotions during feeding. Beth also reflected on her feelings, expressed them, and calmed down, bringing her tension to a manageable level. In the process of GP, Beth had clarified her goal for the experience that involved her feeding her baby. She realized that she had made positive presentation of herself, her infant, the feeding, and the home environment as the goal, and relaxed when it became clear that this goal thwarted the goal of helping Abbie to breastfeed successfully.

Erin's goal was to learn Jordan's early cues of respiratory difficulty so she could nipple feed him safely. Jordan was born at 27 weeks gestation. He was diagnosed with a grade III intraventricular hemorrhage (IVH) on the left and a grade IV IVH on the right. He also had periventricular leukomalacia, apnea of prematurity, respiratory distress syndrome, and gastroesophageal reflux disease. At 35 weeks postmenstrual age, he began nipple feeding. Jordan drooled a lot during feeding and he had difficulty in coordinating sucking, swallowing, and breathing. He became lethargic during feedings and could never finish his feeding in the recommended 30 minutes or less. He became pale, apneic, and bradycardic during feedings.

TABLE 4.5 Guided Participation Conversation: Issues, Processes, and Maternal Competencies—Mother Beth and Baby Abbie at Home at 1 Month Following a Breastfeeding

Conversation Concerning Caregiving (Issues)	Processes	Maternal Competencies
Nurse: You stated that was not a normal feeding. I wonder what's going on with Abbie today.	Joining and maintaining attention	
Beth: I'm not sure what's going on. She's never acted like this before. It took forever to get her to latch on and then she would only take a couple of sucks and come right off. I know she's still hungry because of the way she's sucking on her pacifier. She never takes her pacifier after a feeding.		Knowing and relating to baby; problem solving (making comparisons in terms of specific infant behaviors)
Nurse: Do you think the feeding was different because I was here or because I was videotaping?	Making connections: Differences in this feeding from other feedings made by nurse's presence	
Beth: No, I don't think you bothered her at all. You sat quietly on the floor and she didn't even look your way or pay any attention to the video camera. I'm not sure what's going on with her.		Problem solving (identifying evidence for the nurse's presence not being the reason for the difference in the infant's behavior)
Nurse: Did you have trouble like this feeding in the NICU?	Making connections: Comparing this feeding with earlier feedings	

(continued)

TABLE 4.5 Guided Participation Conversation: Issues, Processes, and Maternal Competencies—Mother Beth and Baby Abbie at Home at 1 Month Following a Breastfeeding (*continued*)

Conversation Concerning Caregiving (Issues)	Processes	Maternal Competencies
Beth: I had trouble getting her to latch on, but once on she was on. This was different.		Beth is continuing to contrast feedings (now and in the past) with the aim of identifying what made this feeding different. Beth was managing the ambiguity or uncertainty about what was going on/what explained the baby's behavior
Nurse: I've videotaped you and Abbie in the hospital feeding, so how was this different?	Making connections: Assisting in the search for information	
Beth: I'm not sure.		
Nurse: I was wondering if you were nervous having me in your home videotaping?	Making connections	
Beth: Well [long pause], I guess I was a little nervous having you here. I made sure I cleaned the house last night because I knew I wouldn't have time this morning. I still ended up feeling rushed this morning because I wanted to make sure the baby was dressed nice. I had to fix my face and comb my hair. I wanted to make sure everything in the video looked nice and presentable.		Communicating (expressing openness to the ideas that others offer; using information from others)
Nurse: Babies can be very sensitive and tuned into their mother's feelings. Do you think Abbie sensed your nervousness?	Making connections	

(*continued*)

TABLE 4.5 Guided Participation Conversation: Issues, Processes, and Maternal Competencies—Mother Beth and Baby Abbie at Home at 1 Month Following a Breastfeeding (*continued*)

Conversation Concerning Caregiving (Issues)	Processes	Maternal Competencies
Beth: She probably did.		Problem solving (accepting the possibility of the connection concerning her own actions and the baby's responses)
Nurse: [replaying the video recording] For instance, what was going on right here?	Bridging/making connections: Sharing the focus of attention (mom is repositioning)	
Beth: I thought if I repositioned her into the football hold she would feed better but she just looked at me and started crying.		Problem solving (recalling her intentions, her action, and its outcome)
Nurse: How were you feeling when you were trying to reposition her?	Making connections: Asking Beth to recall and share her emotional response when she repositioned her baby	
Beth: I was getting more and more nervous and upset.		
Nurse: How do you think Abbie was feeling?	Making connections: Asking mother to identify Abbie's emotional response to being repositioned	
Beth: She was looking at me and she was getting more and more upset.		Knowing and relating to baby (attributing feelings about the repositioning; relating to Abbie as a person)
Nurse: Do you think she sensed your feelings and started mirroring them back to you?	Making connections: Structuring questions for Beth to make the connection between her feelings and Abbie's response	

(continued)

TABLE 4.5 Guided Participation Conversation: Issues, Processes, and Maternal Competencies—Mother Beth and Baby Abbie at Home at 1 Month Following a Breastfeeding (*continued*)

Conversation Concerning Caregiving (Issues)	Processes	Maternal Competencies
Beth: Probably because I was ready to cry and she started crying. [Baby starts to fuss.] Okay, Abbie, do you want to try this again?		Problem-solving (identifying a relationship between her feelings and her baby's emotion) Communicating (talking with baby about her feeding readiness) Regulating emotion (Beth had moved from the tension of earlier feeding to readiness to start feeding again in a calm manner)
Nurse: How are you feeling now? Are you still nervous?		
Beth: No, I'm more relaxed now. Talking about it helped. Actually, talking about it makes me feel kind of silly for being nervous. Isn't that right, Abbie? Mama was just being silly. Come on, let's go! Let's eat!		Being with baby (displays comfort with experience and positive feelings about starting the feeding again) Caregiving with skill (managing challenges in feeding—Beth picked up on baby's cues of readiness to feed and continued the feeding)

Jordan received a G-tube when he was about 40 weeks postnatal age. He was discharged from the hospital when he was 2½ months old, age corrected for prematurity. While in the hospital, most of Jordan's feedings were given by pump over 1 hour. When Erin took her baby home, she was very experienced in feeding via G-tube and less experienced in bottle-feeding. When I arrived at Erin's home for the 3-month assessment of feeding, she was outside smoking a cigarette. Table 4.6 details Erin's spontaneous conversation with me about how she had adjusted her life to meet Jordan's needs.

During the feeding, Jordan drooled, gulped, had audible swallows, and showed signs of working hard to breathe, including nasal flaring. As the feeding continued, he lost tone in his upper extremities and his drooling increased. Erin stopped the feeding after 10 minutes in response to Jordan's signs of fatigue. Table 4.7 details Erin's problem solving during the video playback of the feeding.

Following this conversation, Erin told me about how she had fed Madea, her great grandmother when she was sick. She connected Madea's loud swallow and the water rolling out of the side of her mouth when the cup was turned up too far with Jordan's drooling and audible swallows.

TABLE 4.6 Guided Participation Conversation: Issues, Processes, and Maternal Competencies—Part 1. The Nurse Questions Erin

Conversation About Caregiving (Issues)	Processes	Maternal Competencies
Erin: You caught me?	Getting and staying connected	
Nurse: I caught you?		
Erin: Yeah, I'm trying to quit. I've cut down a lot because I don't smoke in the house. Plus, I'm usually too tired to drag myself out here or it is too cold to stand out here and smoke.		Knowing and relating to the baby as a person (providing environmental supports; making changes in her habits to protect baby's health)
Nurse: It sounds like coming outside to smoke has become a good deterrent to your smoking.	Joining and maintaining attention: Supporting plans the caregiver identifies	
Erin: Yep! And I'm sure Jordan's happy not to have to breathe in my smoke. I know it is healthier for him this way [baby begins to cry]. Well it sounds like someone's ready for you. Come on in and I will wash my hands and get his bottle ready. [Erin uses a hand sanitizer and leans over the crib and starts to talk to Jordan]. Where's your binkie? Shh, don't cry. Here use your hand while mommy warms your bottle.		Giving care to the child (comforting, nurturing, and protecting)

TABLE 4.7 Guided Participation Conversation: Issues, Processes, and Maternal Competencies—Part 2. Erin's Problem Solving

Conversation about Caregiving (Issues)	Processes	Maternal Competencies
Erin: He's tired. I will give the rest [of the feeding] through his G-tube.		Knowing and relating to baby (supports the baby's physiologic stability; responds appropriately to events that disrupt feeding, including infant fatigue)
Nurse: Okay. I will get the video ready [for playback] while you settle him. Can I talk while you settle him?	Structuring the task for learning	
Erin: Sure.		
Nurse: Did you hear the noise he was making while swallowing? I was wondering what you thought about it?	Joining and maintaining attention: Focusing on a specific aspect of the feeding	
Erin: He's always done that. He's just greedy.		Knowing and relating to your baby (mother has made an observation of baby's feeding behavior, but has made a flawed attribution of its source)
Nurse: Greedy?	Bridging/making connections: Raising a question to encourage Erin's reflection on and exploration of Jordan's behavior	
Erin: Yeah, it's like he can't get it fast enough when he first starts feeding.		Problem solving (has an idea /formulates a hypothesis about what is going on)
Nurse: Is that why you took the bottle out of his mouth?		

(continued)

TABLE 4.7 Guided Participation Conversation: Issues, Processes, and Maternal Competencies—Part 2. Erin's Problem Solving (*continued*)

Conversation about Caregiving (Issues)	Processes	Maternal Competencies
Erin: Yeah, I wanted to slow him down before he choked.		Problem solving (gives a reason for behavior—protecting Jordan, showing she is thinking about how she can prevent choking)
Nurse: How about we take a look at that spot on the video?	Joining and maintaining attention: Focusing on the specific aspect of the feeding in question, replaying the video recording	
Erin: Can I see that again?		
Nurse: Of course, why don't you take the remote control so you can look at it as much as you want? [Erin replayed the video recording several times.]		
Erin: Huh.		
Nurse: What are you thinking?	Bridging: Supporting Erin in making connections between what she is noticing about Jordan's feedings	
Erin: I don't think he was being greedy.		Problem solving (identifying an alternative explanation for Jordan's behavior)
Nurse: What do you see?	Bridging/making connections: Supporting Erin in stating her idea of an explanation for Jordan's behavior	

(continued)

TABLE 4.7 Guided Participation Conversation: Issues, Processes, and Maternal Competencies—Part 2. Erin's Problem Solving (*continued*)

Conversation about Caregiving (Issues)	Processes	Maternal Competencies
Erin: I'm not sure but he … he looks like … um … [long pause]. He looks like he is spitting the formula out of his mouth with each swallow.		Communicating expressing her idea or hypothesis about what was going on
Nurse: What do you make of that? Do you think he could be getting too much formula in his mouth so he's getting rid of the extra?	Making connections: Suggesting an idea for Erin to consider	
Erin: Yeah, because it [the formula] is kind of flowing out [of his mouth].		Communicating (affirming the hypothesis the nurse offered, and providing an observation that affirmed her agreement)

G-tube, gastrostomy tube.

TABLE 4.8 Guided Participation Conversation: Issues, Processes, and Maternal Competencies—Part 3. The Nurse Questions Erin

Conversation about Caregiving (Issues)	Processes	Maternal Competencies
Nurse: Did the doctor change Jordan's formula last week?	Sharing the focus of attention	
Erin: No, he was colicky so I changed it a couple of days ago. The [brand of formula] says it is designed to help avoid spit-up, fussiness, and gas and it seems to be working.		Problem solving/decision making (making a decision about the formula to feed based on only one aspect of Jordan's needs)

TABLE 4.9 Guided Participation Conversation: Issues, Processes, and Maternal Competencies—Part 4. The Nurse Continues to Question Erin

Conversation about Caregiving (Issues)	Processes	Maternal Competencies
Nurse: Have you talked to the doctor or the dietician to let them know you've switched formulas?	Bridging/making connections: Identifying clinicians as a source of help with Jordan's feeding issues	
Erin: No.		
Nurse: You are going to call the doctor to tell him you've changed the formula … right?	Transferring responsibility: Helping Erin to know that clinicians needed to be involved in the decision about Jordan's formula	
Erin: Do you think I should?		
Nurse: Yes! [formula brand] is designed for premature babies. Plus, you've decreased his calorie intake by going from a 22-calorie formula to a 20-calorie formula. You want to make sure he's getting the nutrients he needs since he was born preterm and you also want to make sure his calorie intake is sufficient for adequate growth. If he's colicky the doctor could decide to change his formula or give you instructions on other things you can do to help him. For example, hold him upright when feeding to prevent him from swallowing air, burp him often, or feed smaller amounts more frequently.	Making connections: Erin needed information about Jordan's nutritional needs and how to support his feeding to reduce spitting up and fussiness	
Erin: Okay. I will call him.		Communicating: (expressing agreement to take the recommended step)
Nurse: So, you will call the doctor today … right?	Transferring responsibility (making the expectations clear)	
Erin: Yes, I promise I will call him today.		Communicating (Erin agreed, with commitment to act on the nurse's direction)

During the visit, Erin completed a 24-hour dietary recall. Jordan was on (formula brand), a 22-calorie formula, in the hospital but now she was feeding him (a different formula), a 20-calorie formula. In Table 4.8, the nurse questioned Erin about the change in Jordan's formula.

Jordan's primary physician had prescribed a higher calorie formula because his rate of growth was slow and his weight percentile was falling on the growth chart. The dietary intake Erin had recorded was low for an infant Jordan's corrected age. Erin, making an attempt at problem solving, had identified Jordan's problem with spitting up and fussiness as colic and quickly had decided the solution was a change in formula. She had not adequately assessed the problem, nor had she examined potential outcomes of her solution to it. In addition, her problem solving was done without the consultation of clinicians who could bring more knowledge of infant nutrition and growth to bear on what Erin saw as Jordan's problem. In Table 4.9, the nurse continued to question Erin about the change in Jordan's formula.

When I called Erin later that evening, she told me the doctor had put Jordan back on (formula brand) 22. She also stated that the doctor wanted to see Jordan the next day. In the meantime, he advised her to burp Jordan more often during feedings.

This was a clear example of identifying an issue that was not anticipated. I knew feeding Jordan safely was an issue, but I did not predict Erin's problem solving and decision making skills to present this particular problem. This was an issue that I wanted to target directly because I thought Jordan's well-being was being jeopardized. However, reflecting on our conversation, I should have modified the GP to extend Erin's thinking. It may have been more helpful to her if I had wondered with her how changing from a 22-calorie formula to a 20-calorie formula might affect Jordan's growth.

GOALS AND COLLABORATIVE TEACHING AND LEARNING IN AN NICU: REFLECTION ON GP

The three case studies are reported the way they happened. In hindsight, I would have liked it if I had stated some things differently. When I felt I had pushed a little too much (e.g., with Amy in relation to the G-tube) or when I should have been a little more tactful in my response (e.g., to Erin concerning her changing Jordan's formula), I made a mental note of it and learned from the experience. The mother's response was an impetus to reconstruct my response. I was learning through reflection. Thankfully, I had developed a relationship with all three mothers so there was little likelihood of having disturbed or destroyed the relationship with the mother. The *important thing is to reflect or be mindful of the GP process and keep* going with the goal in mind.

CONCLUSION

This chapter concludes with Dr. Pridham's assessment of how Dr. Brown emphasized the critical role of goals in using GP with three mothers and their babies around teaching and learning related to feeding.

Lisa Brown's case studies have raised important ideas about goals in GP practice. The ideas that follow are ones that were significant to me to reflect on:

- Making goals explicit within a GP session is critical. GP is a collaborative process of working together to achieve a mutually desired outcome.
- GP may be advanced by support in revealing goals, a component of the process of joining and maintaining attention, for example, with a statement like, "Help me understand what you are attempting to do here—or wanting to happen."
- GP process can be used to make operative goals clear and to get them expressed so they can be worked on as the issue of the process.
- Effective GP depends on knowing one's own goals and the goals of the other person in the teaching–learning experience.
- When multiple goals are operating, they may need some exploration of how they relate to each other, the priority of goals, and how they need to be sequenced in the activity of interest.
- Processes of bridging and making connections can be used to determine the priority and compatibility of goals. Reflecting or wondering can be used to work through the consequences of putting a goal in operation. The following question can be asked: "What would happen if ...?"

REFERENCES

Belenky, M. F., Clinchy, B. M., Goldberger, N. R., & Tarule, J. M. (1986). *Women's ways of knowing: The development of self, voice, and mind.* New York, NY: Basic Books.

Hill, D. L., & Feudtner, C. (2016). Hope, hopefulness, and pediatric palliative care. In B. P. Black, P. M. Wright, & R. Limbo (Eds.), *Perinatal and pediatric bereavement in nursing and other health professions* (pp. 223–247). New York, NY: Springer Publishing.

Lau, C. (2016). Development of infant oral feeding skills: What do we know? *American Journal of Clinical Nutrition, 103*(2), 616S–621S. doi:10.3945/ajcn.115.109603

Lave, J., & Wenger, E. (1990). *Situated learning: Legitimate peripheral participation.* Cambridge, UK: Cambridge University Press.

Rogoff, B. (1990). *Apprenticeship in thinking.* New York, NY: Oxford University Press.

Rogoff, B. (2003). *The cultural nature of human development.* Oxford, UK: Oxford University Press.

Rogoff, B. A., Matusov, E., & White, C. (1996). Models of teaching and learning: Participation in a community of learners. In D. R. Olson & N. Torrance (Eds.), *The handbook of education and human development: New models of learning, teaching and schooling* (pp. 388–414). Cambridge, MA: Blackwell.

Schroeder, M., & Pridham, K. F. (2006). Development of relationship competencies through guided participation for mothers of preterm infants. *Journal of Obstetric, Gynecologic, and Neonatal Nursing, 35,* 358–368.

Thoyre, S., Park, J., Pados, B., & Hubbard, C. (2013). Developing a co-regulated, cue-based feeding practice: The critical role of assessment and reflection. *Journal of Neonatal Nursing, 19*(4), 139–148. doi:10.1016/j.jnn.2013.01.002

Thoyre, S. M., Shaker, C. S., & Pridham, K. F. (2005). The early feeding skills assessment for preterm infants. *Neonatal Network, 24*(3), 7–16.

5

Guided Participation Approach to Supporting Mothers and Very Preterm Infants During Early Development of the Dyad's Feeding Skills

Suzanne M. Thoyre

This chapter describes a guided participation (GP) approach to supporting mothers and very preterm infants in gaining competence in the challenging activity of early breast and/or bottle-feeding. While transitioning to full oral feeding, and in the months thereafter, very preterm infants are in a unique developmental period of skill development, which requires understanding and support of emergent systems that are dynamically coalescing to accomplish feeding. Within a GP approach to care, mothers learn to observe and give meaning to subtle changes in sucking, swallowing, breathing, and communicative behavior during feeding so their feeding care matches the needs of their child and builds their sense of self as a supportive and sensitive mother (Pridham, 1998; Schroeder & Pridham, 2006).

Guiding mothers to understand novel indicators of their child's capacities requires a relationship of trust with the mother whereby the guide joins with the mother in learning about her child and herself as a mother. During guided feedings, the mother directly experiences providing the type of support her child needs to experience stability and practice functional feeding skills. Reflecting on the feeding as it unfolds, and once it is complete, extends the mother's understanding of her child. The mother's sense of self as loving and supportive and able to join with her child is affirmed throughout. Jointly planning how feedings can be improved in the future helps the mother develop an adaptive approach to feeding. Guiding mothers in the context of a hospital setting where several providers will be the guide is an aspect of GP that requires further effort. The infant's group of nurses and feeding specialists will need to orchestrate joining together as a team to share what they are learning about the infant and the mother so the mother and infant experience a seamless and consistent process of learning.

COMMON ISSUES FOR VERY PRETERM INFANTS AND THEIR MOTHERS

Research over the past 20-plus years has increased our understanding of the physiologic dynamics of feeding for the infant who begins oral feeding prior to term age. During this time, systems that contribute to feeding skill, such as the respiratory system and the state system, are immature and moving toward maturity at different rates of development. Contributing to the dynamics of feeding are the competencies the feeder brings to support the infant during feeding and their ability to adapt as the infant's skills change across any single feeding and over the days, weeks, and months to follow. A case can illustrate the issues that are common for feeding for both the very preterm infant and their mothers during the hospital period.

Case Example 5.1

Annie was born to a 37-year-old mother, Sarah, who has a college degree, a full-time job, and lives with her husband, Tim. This was their first child. Annie was born early at nearly 31 weeks gestation due to complications of her mother's hypertension. She was severely growth restricted at birth, with a birthweight of 680 g. Her mother pumped breast milk for her and Annie began to feed orally when she was 34 weeks postmenstrual age (PMA). As was the practice in the nursery caring for Annie, breastfeedings were offered when Sarah was able to visit, and bottles were introduced by the nurses on week 2 of oral feeding. At 36 weeks PMA, Sarah returned to work and gradually stopped pumping breast milk and offering her child the breast, stating she preferred to bottle-feed Annie once she was home. At 39 weeks, Annie was no longer reliant on her feeding tube and was ready for discharge to her home. At this juncture, we observed Annie's feeding skills and talked with Sarah about what it is like to feed her child.

Prior to the feeding Annie was alert and giving cues of hunger. She sought the nipple when mom stroked her lips and actively opened her mouth and dropped and curled her tongue to receive it. She immediately began sucking but stopped after three sucks. She had not taken any breaths during the sucking burst and continued to pause her breathing even after she stopped. She scanned her environment with a look of worry on her face then took two quick breaths. Sarah moved the nipple in her mouth, placing it deeper, encouraging her to continue to eat. Annie responded and began to suck. Once again, she held her breath during the sucking burst. This time, after approximately five sucks she displayed signs of stress with her eyebrows and forehead raising and her head pulling back and away from the nipple. Milk came forward and drooled out of her lips which now had only a loose hold on the nipple. Sarah asked, "Are you going to stop already?" Annie was still, not breathing and eventually set off her monitor's alarm indicating an oxygen desaturation and a bradycardic event. As soon as her alarms began sounding Sarah removed the nipple, sat Annie upright and stimulated her to breathe. Annie resumed breathing and her oxygen status and heart rate recovered but her arms had dropped to her sides and she appeared to have disengaged from feeding. Despite many attempts, Annie did not root again for the nipple for 6 minutes, at which time she still only showed mild interest in resuming. The feeding continued for another 10 minutes with Annie taking short sucking bursts and showing numerous stress cues, mainly exhibited by her facial muscles, and sounds of tongue clicking, signifying a loose grip on the nipple, and weak sucking. Throughout the feeding, Sarah repeatedly stroked the back of her head and encouraged her to stay awake and finish her bottle. Eventually, Annie fell asleep and quit sucking altogether. She had taken 20 mL of her prescribed 40 mL of breast milk over a 20-minute feeding and appeared exhausted with the effort.

After the feeding was complete and Annie was resting against her mom's chest, Sarah talked with us about how difficult feedings had been and continued to be, how Annie's learning to eat was far more complicated and long in duration than she ever imagined it would be, and how concerned she was that she would be able to help her infant take enough milk to grow once she was home. In addition, Sarah expressed worry about others feeding Annie after discharge, especially since Annie's childcare provider would begin to care for her in 2 weeks. Out of necessity, Sarah would soon be in the role of expert, guiding others to feed her child.

Feeding Challenges

What does this mean for this dyad? Despite impending discharge, we observe an infant who has not fully developed her feeding skills and continues to have physiologic instability during feeding. We observe a mom who is worried and not yet showing skill at "reading" the cues her child is presenting or responding in the most supportive way. Does it all get worked out once they are home? As a neonatal nurse, I assumed infants continued to gain skill and get better at eating after discharge. After all, they were far better eaters the week of discharge than the prior week. I also assumed that their mothers had not yet had the chance to fully get to know their infant since they only were able to observe portions of their day and had not yet had the chance to put together their infant's behavioral patterns. So, would we not expect mothers of preterm infants to follow a similar path as those with full-term healthy infants? Would they not also learn to provide the care their infant needed through repeated experience, focused observation, and a strong drive to learn about their infant?

Evidence tells us we have reason to be concerned about Annie and Sarah and how feeding will unfold in the weeks, months, and years ahead. Compared to full-term, adequately grown infants, preterm infants are three times more likely to have feeding difficulties during infancy that persist into early childhood (Motion, Northstone, Emond, & ALSPAC Study Team, 2001). DeMauro, Patel, Medoff-Cooper, Posencheg, and Abbasi (2011) found that 17% of preterm infants born prior to 34 weeks gestational age required medical services for feeding during their first year. Rommel, De Meyer, Feenstra, & Veereman-Wauters (2003) reported that one third of the preschool-aged children receiving feeding services in their specialty clinic had a history of prematurity.

Infants with low birthweight are at additional risk for long-term feeding problems (Rommel et al., 2003); reportedly they are seven times more likely to have feeding difficulties during infancy that persist into early childhood (Motion et al., 2001). Preterm infants who are small for their gestational age take longer to develop organized sucking patterns, with 46% still demonstrating disorganized sucking with uncoordinated sucking, swallowing, and breathing well past the time of discharge from neonatal care at 48 to 50 weeks PMA (da Costa et al., 2010).

The Meaning of Early Feeding Difficulties

Feeding difficulties in the weeks to months following discharge track to long-standing feeding problems, including delayed feeding skills, difficulty transitioning to complex foods, and food refusal (Hawdon, Beauregard, Slattery, & Kennedy, 2000; Mathisen, Worrall, Masel, Wall, & Shepherd, 1999; Nelson, Chen, Syniar, & Christoffel, 1998; Samara, Johnson, Lamberts, Marlow, & Wolke, 2010). Persistent feeding problems are associated with impaired infant growth and poorer neurodevelopmental and behavioral outcomes (Adams-Chapman, Bann, Vaucher, & Stoll, 2013; Motion et al., 2001; Pridham, Steward, Thoyre, Brown, & Brown, 2007).

Issues Specific to Annie

Annie has several significant risk factors that will continue to constrain her ability to eat after discharge. She was very premature at just under 31 weeks gestational age. She had symmetrical intrauterine growth restriction with weight, height, and head circumference all reduced, indicating significant duration of growth impairment prior to birth. This places her at increased risk for feeding problems, poor growth, and neurodevelopmental abnormalities (Sharma, Farahbakhsh, Shastri, & Sharma, 2016).

She required respiratory support with nasal continuous positive airway pressure for 2 weeks postbirth, and continues to show signs of respiratory impairment. Nearing discharge her respiratory rate is in the 90th centile for an infant her age (Fleming et al., 2011). Pulmonary insufficiency is one of the most significant rate limiters of smooth coordination of sucking, swallowing, and breathing (Mizuno et al., 2007). As an indication of how challenging oral feeding has been for Annie, she has taken longer than usual to achieve full oral feeding (Van Nostrand, Bennett, Coraglio, Guo, & Muraskas, 2015).

During feeding, we observe that Annie continues to demonstrate an unstable cardiorespiratory system. She is not yet integrating breathing within her sucking bursts; instead uncoupling breathing from sucking and swallowing. This tells us she needs to simplify her feeding pattern, and use a less complex suck, swallow, then breathe pattern (Thoyre & Park, 2016). She extends the closure of her airway during swallows, bracketing each swallow with a longer than usual brief apnea (Gewolb & Vice, 2006). Paused breathing during sucking and prolonged apnea during swallowing are indicators of immaturity. Functionally they are protective mechanisms that keep Annie's airway safer from fluid penetration. However, they also place her at risk for insufficient number of breaths during feeding. This can deplete her oxygen stores leading to physical exhaustion and increase her vulnerability to desaturation and bradycardia. The risk for desaturation is highest as feedings begin, especially in the first minute, likely signifying a challenging period of transition for vulnerable infants (Thoyre & Carlson, 2003). Indeed, Annie had at least one significant episode of cardiorespiratory decline early in the feeding. She was not able to sustain engagement in feeding long enough to take in the amount of milk that was prescribed for her. Wang et al. (2010) have demonstrated that the risk for desaturation during feeding can persist to at least 6 months corrected age for very preterm infants.

Mothers describe learning to feed their premature infants as a challenge and report continued difficulties postdischarge. In the hospital, mothers express concern about keeping their infant safe during feeding, specifically, avoiding desaturation, bradycardic, and choking events. They also describe concern for feeding their infants enough milk to grow and knowing when and how to advance the feeding plan once home (Thoyre, 2001). After discharge, mothers report increased awareness of gaps in their knowledge about feeding and trouble interpreting infant feeding cues (Reyna, Pickler, & Thompson, 2006). They worry about providing too much or too little milk and report witnessing worrisome events, including gagging, choking, forgetting to breathe, and reflux (Hawdon et al., 2000; Reyna et al., 2006). One third to one half of mothers of premature infants describe feeling anxious, uncomfortable, and frustrated with feedings during the first year and challenged by coordinating feeding and family life (DeMauro et al., 2011; Torola, Lehtihalmes, Yliherva, & Olsen, 2012). Since infants are perceived to need close monitoring and specific feeding strategies, family help with feeding is offered and accepted less (Reyna et al., 2006). Difficulties with feeding can inadvertently lead to maternal-directed, rather than infant-guided feeding, which in turn may perpetuate feeding difficulties (Estrem, Pados, Park, Knafl, & Thoyre, 2017).

Coming to Know Self as Mother and Their Infants

In the early weeks of life, new mothers are recovering and processing the birth event, and coming to know their infants. In this process, mothers are coming to know themselves as a new mother as well. *Will I be nurturing and will my baby feel my love and the sense of safety I am trying to provide? Can I meet her needs and protect her from stress? Am I being the kind of mother I want to be?* This process unfolds over the early weeks of life through mutual engagement in the other and maternal reflection on how things are going. Being with and reflecting on what worked and did not work to keep the infant safe and satisfied and to feel satisfied with oneself as a new mother drives the development of the maternal–child relationship.

There is disruption in the process of coming-to-know for mothers of children who require neonatal hospitalization. Coughlin (2014) writes about the fundamental trauma experienced by hospitalized infants and their mothers due to the separation they experience from one another. The disruption in coming to know is evident during feeding, particularly when infant skills are at a preterm level of development.

For premature infants, early feeding skills are in an emergent, and therefore unstable, phase of development. They are operating within a biological system that is tenuous in its management of fluid near the airway and in organizing sufficient number and depth of energy-sustaining breaths. This leads to a higher potential for the infant to receive internal cues of threat (Porges, 2007). Infants' responses to cues of threat are subtle, such as eyebrow raise, finger splay, and movement of the head back or to the side. These cues are not intuitive for the new mother to understand and can easily be misinterpreted. For example, an infant who mistimes a swallow and experiences fluid threat may disengage from the feeding in an attempt to reorganize their physiologic and behavioral systems. Mothers may misinterpret this disengagement as loss of interest or arousal; based on this interpretation, they may take action to reinterest or rearouse the infant by encouraging sucking with intraoral stimulation or head stroking. This change in stimulation may reflexively stimulate sucking and thereby provide feedback to the mother that she is successful. However, resuming sucking when rest and recovery is needed can further disorganize the infant. The dyad can become entangled in an asynchronous dance that is progressively dysregulating to the infant and confusing to the mother.

As preterm infants transition from being fed by feeding tube to oral feeding, their mothers typically have limited availability. Breast- or bottle-feeding by the mother may occur once or twice a day with nurses and/or feeding specialists providing the remaining feedings. Mothers of preterms therefore do not receive the same type or amount of feedback from their infants as they are developing their feeding practice as mothers of full-term infants. This loss of feedback collides with atypical feedback from the infant during feeding, such as pauses in breathing, and creates the conditions for maladaptive feeding by both the mother and infant.

Early feeding of infants who are immature with compromised health is not a situation that one can rely on typical developmental processes to work themselves out. It is a time when nurses and feeding specialists need to guide and support both the infant and the mother to learn developmentally functional feeding patterns. The common issues discussed here, along with issues that arise among mothers and infants that are distinct to the individual dyad, form the content of feeding support using GP.

GUIDED PARTICIPATION

Given our understanding of the common feeding issues for very preterm infants and their mothers, neonatal nurses and feeding specialists are positioned to guide mothers as they develop their feeding practice. The motivation of the mother to know and care for her child, the concurrent emergence and, therefore, changing nature of her child's feeding skills, and the frequent and repeated contact with the infant's care providers sets an ideal stage for GP. Informal conversations with mothers about feeding at the infant's bedside are commonplace; however, as Dr. Pridham points out in Chapter 1, GP needs a thoughtful and purposeful approach to be carried out effectively. Since multiple nurses and feeding specialists care for a single child, GP in the hospital setting requires explicit communication among providers about the progress and process of GP as it is unfolding since it inevitably will be provided by more than one guide.

Recently our research team tested the implementation of GP with mothers of very preterm infants in the activity of developing infants' feeding skills and mothers' feeding practices (Thoyre, Hubbard, Park, Pridham, & McKechnie, 2016). Figure 1.1 illustrates the model of GP used to organize the study that can be applied in a hospital setting.

A single nurse guided the mother during five sessions, beginning just prior to the onset of oral feeding. The primary goal of the initial session was to form a relationship with the mother and establish an agreed-upon mindset that the guide and the mother would partner to discover what the infant needed to calmly feed. We developed joint attention to what was to be learned by watching short video clips of other preterm infants learning to feed. We discussed novel cues the infants provided that could be used to guide us in understanding how the feeding was going for the infant. We placed a microphone on the mother's infant and listened together to the infant's pattern of breathing and then listened to infants' breathing on the video clips to see how it changed during feeding. We learned about what the mother had already come to know about her child, what she paid attention to, what meaning she gave to her child's behaviors, and we guided the mother to practice holding her infant in positions that would be used during feeding.

The second session occurred once oral feeding began, either by breast or bottle. For this and subsequent sessions, we again placed a microphone on the infant's neck so the guide and the mother (and if available, the father, nurse, and/or lactation consultant) could listen to the infant's breathing and swallowing sounds throughout the feeding. Bringing attention to nonconscious sensory information during feeding can aid mothers to more fully use their sensory modalities in their feeding practice (Krasnow & Wilmerding, 2015). We videotaped the infant close up during the feeding and sent the amplified feeding sounds from the microphone to the camera so we could review the feeding together after the feeding. We structured the feeding in advance so the mother would know what to expect. We told her she would feed the infant, but we viewed ourselves as feeding the infant together. We would guide her and help to physically support the infant during the feeding if needed. We would help with decisions, like when to start, rest, or stop, thereby attempting to hold responsibility for what she would not yet know. This help would relieve her of the pressure to know what to do and allow her to experience providing a gentle and supportive feeding. What the mother was capable of doing on her own varied by the mother; some had been kangaroo holding and nuzzling at breast and did not need our help to physically support the infant, while others needed more specific strategies like placing hands on the infant to help them receive postural support so the mother could focus on adjustments of the nipple. After the feeding, we talked about what we each had learned, developing a common language to describe the feeding. We made explicit the "gray zones" of feeding—what may not be clear yet, what it made us wonder about and invited the mother to wonder with us. What did she find puzzling, what seemed uncertain? We reviewed the video together paying attention to the questions we each had. For example, the guide might say, "He raises his eyebrows sometimes at the end of a sucking burst. This is considered a sign that he may be getting overwhelmed and needs to take a break or catch some breaths. Let us look at some of the feeding and see if we can figure out what might be going on for him when he does this." As we examined the video together we considered our hypotheses and came up with ideas for what might improve the feeding. The guide may have more ideas to try, but the mother's ideas are also encouraged since she needs to develop skill at reflecting on the feeding and coming up with ways to optimize the feeding. The guide might state, "His eyebrow raises seem to be occurring after his longer sucking bursts. What do you think? [joint viewing of more of the feeding] Perhaps those sucking bursts are feeling too long for him. Sometimes preterm infants will prefer to suck and not know it would be better for them to rest and breathe. Next time let us see if we can help him to keep his sucking bursts shorter, with more frequent pauses to swallow and breathe." At times, we reviewed one of the video clips from another infant to watch how strategies are accomplished, such as maternal pacing/coregulating the breath.

As we reflected on the feeding we also talked about how mom might be feeling. For example, if her infant was taking short sucking bursts and long breathing breaks we might make them explicit and give a language to them and ask her how that is for her: "She is taking short sucking bursts and then resting while she takes extra breaths. She is really good at that—do you see how she is staying so calm? Good for her for figuring out she needs to fit in a lot of breaths. You are amazing at letting her just breathe and rest and not hurrying her along. You figured out so well that she needs you to be calm and help her take those extra breaths. It must be hard sometimes to be so patient, especially when she seems to have a long way to go. Do you find it hard to do?"

Once we reviewed our questions and reflected on the feeding we summarized the plan we had made for the next feeding based on what we had learned.

Early feeding sessions tended to be short since infants often had low endurance. These short feedings provided an opportunity to talk about the energy needed to eat and how quickly it can be spent and how we might protect the infant's energy expenditure prior to and during the feeding. Coregulating the infant's length of the sucking burst was a strategy that was often discussed in relation to infant endurance. If the infant's sucking burst was too long they fatigued quickly. We could guide the infant to take shorter sucking bursts and to rest between bursts.

We learned that mothers' questions changed as they began to learn new strategies and that everything could not be taught all at once. For example, mothers might at first feel unsure about when to provide a rest for their infants or when to cue their infants to stop sucking to breathe. Often long sucking bursts occur in the early minutes of feeding when an infant is most robust. This is prime time for the very preterm infant to spend their limited energy. If they are reducing their respiratory rate due to abbreviated or absent breaths during the sucking burst, their energy is quickly reduced. Often mothers shared they felt hesitant about providing a rest (if at breast) or tipping the bottle down or removing it because it felt like they were interfering with their infant's feeding, especially if they were sucking robustly. This provided an opportunity to connect the idea of coregulating with other coregulatory parenting actions that mothers might more easily relate to. For example, a child may want to cross the street without holding the parent's hand but the parent knows best how to protect their child's safety and may guide the child's agenda. We reframed resting/coregulatory strategies from "interruption" to "protection" of the infant's energy for feeding and acknowledged that mothers can feel unsure about this action since it is novel feeding behavior.

Once mothers began coregulating their infants' breath they might change to feeling unsure of when to resume the feeding once they provided the rest, that is, when is the rest period sufficient, and how will they know. This provided opportunities for us to look together for infant cues of readiness, to listen for easing of the breathing and reorganization of the infant's body, and to make connections with what the mothers already had learned when deciding if their infants were ready to begin the feeding.

As mothers became competent at pacing the feeding and coregulating sufficient breaths new questions arose, such as would their infants always need this? How would they know if they could withdraw this level of support? This provided opportunity to talk about variability in infants' rates of development and the need to observe their own infants for signs that they were changing and developing self-regulated breathing. Ultimately, each mother would need to test whether her infant was ready for a change in coregulatory strategies. We built on this idea and linked it to a discussion of the myriad of other feeding decisions that would be coming in the weeks and months ahead and how a mother could approach them in a similar way. For example, in our nursery, very preterm infants begin feeding in a semielevated side-lying position and use low-flow bottle nipples, if fed by bottle. At some point, the infant is ready for a cradle position and a more normal flow nipple, which typically occurs after discharge, but is often asked about in the nursery. Rather than nurses deciding and informing mothers of their decision, it is better for the mother to experience how this process goes so she can be prepared to do it herself. Feeding a child is not black and white—there are uncertainties and ideas that need to be tested. We can think with the mother how she might try a cradle hold or a faster flow nipple and generate a list with her of what she would observe to tell her if it is time for a change. Mothers need to see our uncertainty; we need to model the ambiguity of some of the decisions we make so mothers see that this is an area of exploration and come to feel capable of testing and evaluating changes in the feeding plan since it is a process she has been guided to participate in.

Mothers set the pace of the timing of the final two sessions. Most mothers who began breastfeeding opted to reserve several sessions for learning how to bottle-feed their infant so they could teach others who would also be participating in feedings. For example, if fathers were going to be offering some bottles while the mother breastfed, the mother, father, and guide participated in the final sessions. In this circumstance, the mother would be positioned as the guide so she could experience and practice this role. Structuring for this transferring of responsibility to the mother allows mothers to increase their sense of competence while the nurse or specialist acting as the guide is available to fill in gaps in her understanding.

One of the important things we learned from this study was the uncertainty mothers experienced when they received conflictual information on how to feed their infant from the guide and from other providers who they were interacting with, many of whom they had also formed trusting relationships with. It became clear to us that all providers who are guiding mothers to become competent feeders need to be working in concert, sharing what they are learning about the infant, using a common language and understanding of infant feeding, not only with the mother but also with each other. Joint attention to the process of GP is required for all of those involved.

GP AS THE FEEDING CULTURE IN THE HOSPITAL SETTING

Guiding mothers to feed infants who need novel approaches in neonatal or pediatric hospital settings can best be accomplished outside the protocol of a research study and instead within the established culture of feeding. It starts at birth and involves every contact we have with new mothers. We begin early with age-appropriate touch, kangaroo care, and joint observation of the infant to prepare mothers to read their infants' communication and come to know how their infant expresses calmness and distress. Once oral feedings have begun, we start with the evolving location of the mother, discovering what she understands about infant feeding and feeding of preterm infants, what she is learning about her own infant, and asking what she is working on so we can smoothly join in. We can listen to infant breathing and swallowing together by laying a stethoscope on the infant's neck. This will help everyone to become more sensitive to the infant's feeding experience. We can use mothers' cell phones to videotape key sections of the feeding that can be reviewed together after the feeding. Mothers can then take this video home with them to look more closely and to share with others. We can plan to reflect on feedings after they are complete with the goal of making the next feeding better for the infant and the mother. Using a common language to describe infant feeding skills and behaviors or sounds that demonstrate challenge keeps everyone on the same page. The Early Feeding Skills Assessment Tool could provide a common language to describe what we are observing during feeding (Thoyre, Park, Pados, & Hubbard, 2013; Thoyre, Shaker, & Pridham, 2005).

CONCLUSION

Content within this chapter has explained the challenges and joys of learning to feed a preterm infant and the important role of GP in developing parent and healthcare team competencies specific to each infant. Understanding the process of GP brings issues, processes, and competences to the foreground so they become part of ongoing discussions within the feeding team. Reflecting on how feedings are going and how they may be improved with all those involved in feeding can become common practice of the hospital's feeding culture. As the infant moves toward discharge, the mother should increasingly become the central person adapting the feeding plan. This will prepare her for caring for her infant after discharge and for communicating with pediatric care providers postdischarge. As guides, we keep in mind the mother–infant feeding system is designed to function well; with thoughtful care using principles of GP it will.

REFERENCES

Adams-Chapman, I., Bann, C. M., Vaucher, Y. E., & Stoll, B. J. (2013). Association between feeding difficulties and language delay in preterm infants using Bayley Scales of Infant Development—Third Edition. *Journal of Pediatrics, 163*(3), 680–685. doi:10.1016/j.jpeds.2013.03.006

Coughlin, M. (2014). *Transformative nursing in the NICU: Trauma-informed age-appropriate care.* New York, NY: Springer Publishing.

da Costa, S. P., van der Schans, C. P., Zweens, M. J., Boelema, S. R., van der Meij, E., Boerman, M. A., & Bos, A. F. (2010). The development of sucking patterns in preterm, small-for-gestational age infants. *Journal of Pediatrics, 157*(4), 603–609, 609, e601–603. doi:10.1016/j.jpeds.2010.04.037

DeMauro, S. B., Patel, P. R., Medoff-Cooper, B., Posencheg, M., & Abbasi, S. (2011). Postdischarge feeding patterns in early- and late-preterm infants. *Clinical Pediatrics, 50*(10), 957–962. doi:10.1177/0009922811409028

Estrem, H. H., Pados, B. F., Park, J., Knafl, K. A., & Thoyre, S. M. (2017). Feeding problems in infancy and early childhood: Evolutionary concept analysis. *Journal of Advanced Nursing, 73*(1), 56–70. doi:10.1111/jan.13140

Fleming, S., Thompson, M., Stevens, R., Heneghan, C., Pluddemann, A., Maconochie, I., ... Mant, D. (2011). Normal ranges of heart rate and respiratory rate in children from birth to 18 years of age: A systematic review of observational studies. *Lancet, 377*(9770), 1011–1018. doi:10.1016/S0140-6736(10)62226-X

Gewolb, I. H., & Vice, F. L. (2006). Maturational changes in the rhythms, patterning, and coordination of respiration and swallow during feeding in preterm and term infants. *Developmental Medicine and Child Neurology, 48*(7), 589–594. doi:10.1111/j.1469-8749.2006.tb01320.x

Hawdon, J. M., Beauregard, N., Slattery, J., & Kennedy, G. (2000). Identification of neonates at risk of developing feeding problems in infancy. *Developmental Medicine and Child Neurology, 42*(4), 235–239.

Krasnow, D., & Wilmerding, M. V. (2015). *Motor learning and control for dance: Principles and practices for performers and teachers.* Champaign, IL: Human Kinetics.

Mathisen, B., Worrall, L., Masel, J., Wall, C., & Shepherd, R. W. (1999). Feeding problems in infants with gastro-oesophageal reflux disease: A controlled study. *Journal of Paediatrics and Child Health, 35*(2), 163–169.

Mizuno, K., Nishida, Y., Taki, M., Hibino, S., Murase, M., Sakurai, M., & Itabashi, K. (2007). Infants with bronchopulmonary dysplasia suckle with weak pressures to maintain breathing during feeding. *Pediatrics, 120*(4), e1035–1042. doi:0.1542/peds.2006-3567

Motion, S., Northstone, K., Emond, A., & ALSPAC Study Team. (2001). Persistent early feeding difficulties and subsequent growth and developmental outcomes. *Ambulatory Child Health, 7,* 231–237.

Nelson, S. P., Chen, E. H., Syniar, G. M., & Christoffel, K. K. (1998). One-year follow-up of symptoms of gastroesophageal reflux during infancy. Pediatric Practice Research Group. *Pediatrics, 102*(6), E67.

Porges, S. W. (2007). The polyvagal perspective. *Biological Psychology, 74*(2), 116–143.

Pridham, K. F., Steward, D., Thoyre, S., Brown, R., & Brown, L. (2007). Feeding skill performance in premature infants during the first year. *Early Human Development, 83*(5), 293–305. doi:10.1016/j.earlhumdev.2006.06.004

Pridham, K. F. (1998). Guided participation and development of care-giving competencies for families of low birth-weight infants. *Journal of Advanced Nursing, 28*(5), 948–958.

Reyna, B. A., Pickler, R. H., & Thompson, A. (2006). A descriptive study of mothers' experiences feeding their preterm infants after discharge. *Advances in Neonatal Care, 6*(6), 333–340. doi:10.1016/j.adnc.2006.08.007

Rommel, N., De Meyer, A. M., Feenstra, L., & Veereman-Wauters, G. (2003). The complexity of feeding problems in 700 infants and young children presenting to a tertiary care institution. *Journal of Pediatric Gastroenterology and Nutrition, 37*(1), 75–84. doi:10.1097/00005176-200307000-00014

Samara, M., Johnson, S., Lamberts, K., Marlow, N., & Wolke, D. (2010). Eating problems at age 6 years in a whole population sample of extremely preterm children. *Developmental Medicine and Child Neurology, 52*(2), e16–e22. doi:10.1111/j.1469-8749.2009.03512.x

Schroeder, M., & Pridham, K. F. (2006). Development of relationship competencies through guided participation for mothers of preterm infants. *Journal of Obstetric, Gynecologic, and Neonatal Nursing, 35*(3), 358–368. doi:10.1111/j.1552-6909.2006.00049.x

Sharma, D., Farahbakhsh, N., Shastri, S., & Sharma, P. (2016). Intrauterine growth restriction—Part 2. *The Journal of Maternal-Fetal & Neonatal Medicine, 29*(24), 4037–4048. doi:10.3109/14767058.2016.1154525

Thoyre, S. (2001). Challenges mothers identify in bottle feeding their preterm infants. *Neonatal Network*, *20*(1), 41–50. doi:10.1891/0730-0832.20.1.45

Thoyre, S., & Carlson, J. (2003). Occurrence of oxygen desaturation events during preterm infant bottle feeding near discharge. *Early Human Development*, *72*(1), 25–36. doi:10.1016/S0378-3782(03)00008-2

Thoyre, S., Hubbard, C., Park, J., Pridham, K. F., & McKechnie, A. (2016). Implementing co-regulated feeding with mothers of preterm infants. *MCN: The American Journal of Maternal/Child Nursing*, *41*(4), 204–211. doi:10.1097/NMC.0000000000000245

Thoyre, S., & Park, J. (2016). *The emergence of complexity in very preterm infant feeding skills: The dynamics of coordinating sucking and breathing across time.* Paper presented at the 2016 Biennial International Congress on Infant Studies, New Orleans, LA.

Thoyre, S., Park, J., Pados, B., & Hubbard, C. (2013). Developing a co-regulated, cue-based feeding practice: The critical role of assessment and reflection. *Journal of Neonatal Nursing*, *19*(4), 139–148. doi:10.1016/j.jnn.2013.01.002

Thoyre, S., Shaker, C. S., & Pridham, K. F. (2005). The early feeding skills assessment for preterm infants. *Neonatal Network*, *24*(3), 7–16. doi:10.1891/0730-0832.24.3.7

Torola, H., Lehtihalmes, M., Yliherva, A., & Olsen, P. (2012). Feeding skill milestones of preterm infants born with extremely low birth weight (ELBW). *Infant Behavior and Development*, *35*(2), 187–194. doi:10.1016/j.infbeh.2012.01.005

Van Nostrand, S. M., Bennett, L. N., Coraglio, V. J., Guo, R., & Muraskas, J. K. (2015). Factors influencing independent oral feeding in preterm infants. *Journal of Neonatal–Perinatal Medicine*, *8*(1), 15–21. doi:10.3233/NPM-15814045

Wang, L. Y., Luo, H. J., Hsieh, W. S., Hsu, C. H., Hsu, H. C., Chen, P. S., … Jeng, S. F. (2010). Severity of bronchopulmonary dysplasia and increased risk of feeding desaturation and growth delay in very low birth weight preterm infants. *Pediatric Pulmonology*, *45*(2), 165–173. doi:10.1002/ppul.21171

6

Caregiving for Extremely Premature Infants

Karen Kavanaugh and Terry Griffin

Caregiving for extremely premature infants (born between 22 and 25 weeks gestation) carries with it the need for complex skills in partnering with clinicians in the NICU to develop their rightful role as caregivers, historians, and stewards of safety. Ideally, beginning in the prenatal period, parents develop meaningful and essential partnerships with staff to achieve competence in communication and participation in decision making, which extends to including caregiving in the NICU. These partnerships often entail the guided participation (GP) strategy of cocreating, meaning parents and staff work together for the betterment of the baby's health, safety, and relationships. During the neonatal period, the parents must simultaneously develop their parenting role while wrestling with concurrent feelings of guilt, fear, and hope.

BACKGROUND INFORMATION

Despite improvements in care, infants born at this gestation continue to have high mortality, particularly at the lower spectrum of gestational age. Mortality rates vary from 91% at 22 weeks gestation to 19% at 25 weeks gestation (Stoll et al., 2015). Therefore, parents live with much uncertainty that begins antenatally when expectant mothers experience complications during the pregnancy. When this occurs, the mother and father are confronted with an often unexpected hospitalization of the mother which disrupts the parents' lives, especially when there are younger children in the family. Hospitalization of the mother during this time can be as short as hours before birth or can extend to weeks. During this time, parents are quickly faced with making life-support treatment decisions for their infant, such as whether to attempt resuscitation at the time of birth.

When infants are admitted to the NICU, parents must develop their rightful role in the context of physical and emotional challenges. Mothers are recovering from childbirth and medical complications of pregnancy. Their partners may also be physically and emotionally exhausted from struggling with competing responsibilities at home, work, and supporting the mother while struggling with their own overwhelming feelings about having a preterm infant. Parents must define and perfect their role in caregiving and decision making through the development of essential and meaningful partnerships with the medical and nursing staff who serve as gatekeepers to their infant. Nurses are particularly suited to share the infant's care and guide parents throughout the infant's hospitalization.

Nearly 30 years have passed since attention was given to the special challenges of supporting parents of extremely premature infants (Kavanaugh, 1988). Despite an evolution of practice guidelines which calls for more attention to parent involvement in decision making (American College of Obstetricians and Gynecologists and the Society for Maternal–Fetal Medicine et al., 2016; Batton & Committee on Fetus and Newborn, 2009; Cummings & the Committee on the Fetus and Newborn, 2015), challenges remain when providing care that is individualized to the infant and family. Experts advocate for involving parents in life-support treatment decisions prenatally because of the potential of high mortality and morbidity for extremely premature infants, and because parents bear the consequences to the infant and their family (Bohnhorst, Ahl, Peter, & Pirr, 2015; Lemyre et al., 2016; Tomlinson, Kaempf, Ferguson, & Stewartm, 2010). Clinicians should elicit parent information needs and their values and preferences during decision making (Boss, Hutton, Sulpar, West, & Donohue, 2008; Dupont-Thibodeau, Barrington, Farlow, & Janvier, 2014; Janvier, Lorenz, & Lantos, 2012; Janvier et al., 2014), particularly because of prognostic uncertainty; this recommendation has been supported by research on parent perspectives of their experiences with decision making (Kavanaugh et al., 2015). However, the research on parent involvement in life-support decisions for infants demonstrates that parents and clinicians are not always involved in a collaborative decision-making process that focuses on parent needs and values (Kavanaugh et al., 2015). Furthermore, parents and healthcare professionals often have differing views on how their attitudes toward disability impact decision making (Kavanaugh et al., 2015; Lam et al., 2009).

Collaboration is critical because parents and clinicians bring different perspectives on what is important to consider. For example, the importance of hope is critical for parents but has different meanings for parents and clinicians (Roscigno et al., 2012). Parents rely on hope to sustain them through their difficult experience, whereas many clinicians worry about giving false hope and misleading the parents from the truth (Roscigno et al., 2012). Also, parents differ in their desired role in decision making, but clinicians do not always elicit their preferred role or honor their preferences. The meaning of shared decision making is unclear and needs clarification (Haward, Kirshenbaum, & Campbell, 2011). Knowing parent preferences for their involvement in decision making is important because the impact of different types of parent involvement in decision types has long-term effects on the parents. Parents who perceive that they have had the opportunity for shared decision making have lower grief scores in comparison to other parents with other decision types, such as one that is physician controlled (Caeymaex et al., 2012). These data provide additional support for the use of cocreation, with parents and their baby's care providers joining together to make decisions about many aspects of the baby's life and care.

Parents desire honest and detailed information about their infant's condition and balanced information with the full range of potential outcomes when making life-support decisions (Branchett & Stretton, 2012; Grobman, Kavanaugh, Moro, Regnier, & Savage, 2010; Miquel-Verges et al., 2009). Parents also want the information presented with compassion, emotional support, and realistic hope (Grobman et al., 2010). Clinicians should communicate information needs in a supportive way that conveys concern and an attempt to understand what matters to parents (Kavanaugh et al., 2015; Roscigno et al., 2012). Currently, however, counseling is often done with a focus on relaying prognostic information on morbidity and mortality without attention to the individual information needs of the parents (Janvier, Lorenz, & Lantos, 2012). Also, counseling practices are largely dependent on institutional practices (Edmonds, McKenzie, Farrow, Raglan, & Schulkin, 2015) and clinicians' characteristics (McKenzie, Robinson, & Edmonds, 2016).

Various individuals can play a critical role in supporting parents during decision making antenatally and extending into the experience in the NICU. Nurses support parents during decision making as they provide emotional support, relay a hopeful attitude, clarify information, and meet physical care needs (Kavanaugh, Moro, & Savage, 2010). When making end-of-life decisions for their infant, parents have described the importance of support from their family in addition to a trusting relationship with clinicians and a hopeful attitude (Moro et al., 2011). Even when parents do not seek the advice of extended family for treatment decisions, they do seek emotional support and help with understanding information (Kavanaugh, Nantais-Smith, Savage, Schim, & Natarajan, 2014). It is vital to remember that sources of support for some mothers may be burdensome for others (Smith, Steelfisher, Salhi, & Shen, 2012). Others have suggested that contact with parents who have gone through similar experiences might be as valuable as providing factual information (Lam et al., 2009).

GUIDED PARTICIPATION

Anna, a 30-year-old, who was pregnant with her first baby, was admitted to the antepartum unit several days before delivery secondary to pregnancy-induced hypertension, which required the prompt delivery of her infant girl, Ava. Ava was born at 25 weeks gestation and weighed 780 g; she was admitted directly to the NICU from the delivery room. The neonatologist was able to meet with Anna prior to delivery to share expected management of her preterm infant. A NICU nurse and neonatal nurse practitioner (NNP) met with her to reinforce the doctors' information and explain the important role she would play in helping Ava. The NNP shared that there was every reason to be hopeful about Ava's outcome. After delivery, Ava was quickly taken to the NICU, which was located on a different floor. Anna's physical condition required her extended stay in the labor and delivery unit where she was administered medication to control her blood pressure.

During that time, Anna was unable to journey to the NICU to see her infant, or meet the nurses and physicians helping to care for her infant. The neonatologist, the NNP, and the staff nurse all went to her room to update her on Ava's medical condition, appearance, and personality. More than 24 hours later, when Anna was transported by wheelchair, she resisted entering Ava's room. Anna sat in her wheelchair stationed in the hall, and with her head bowed, staring quietly, while fighting back tears, stating that she did not want to see Ava because she did not want to become attached to her. The NNP and nurse who had previously met with her were able to encourage her to see and touch her infant.

Parental Competency of Communicating and Engaging With Others

Parents need to be competent in communicating and engaging with others, namely clinicians and extended family members, in order to nurture and protect their infant during the mother's antenatal and infant's neonatal hospitalization. During Anna's hospitalization, she is likely to encounter many different clinicians, including obstetrical nurses and maternal–fetal medicine specialists. These clinicians are new to the parents and do not know them as their primary care clinicians have come to know them during prenatal care. Thus, Anna and clinicians have to quickly establish a relationship so that open communication can occur.

Strategies for Communicating and Engaging With Others

The parental competency of communicating and engaging with others requires trust. This compentency is especially relevant in cases when there is an imminent delivery and obstetric and neonatal staff must build trust in emergent situations. Conversations can be brief but powerful as in: "You and your infant are in good hands. This is what we do every day. But we understand that all of this is new and scary for you. I wonder what I could do for you right now that would help you feel more certain and have more hope." Consider "wondering" what is on the parent's mind by doing these three things: (a) be mindful of your own anxiety and perhaps even doubt. Pause. Take a long, deep breath while focusing on the breath going in and out of your body; (b) sit to be in physical proximity with the parent; and (c) demonstrate your own engagement (the competency you identified as the one that will help the parent or parents build trust, confidence, and hope) by careful listening and smiling or showing warmth. Imagine that the mother says to you as tears fill her eyes, "I am so afraid my baby won't be okay." Recognize that she has become more competent in expressing emotion. You might say, "That is a hard thing to say and think. Yes, a lot can happen, but there is every reason to be hopeful that everything will be okay. That is why we do what we do. We will help you through this. I will be right here and whenever I can I will quietly explain what is happening. Will that help?"

Antenatal consultation for the anticipated birth of an extremely premature infant with the neonatologist is important for parents so that they can participate in decision making for their infant and ideally meet the doctor who will be responsible for their infant's care. Ideally, the NICU nurse meets with the parents antenatally, as what occurred with Anna, to build the foundation for their long-term relationship in the NICU, which includes sharing care of the infant. There are times, however, when the primary care clinicians might not have an opportunity to meet the parents until just before the birth of the infant.

Parents may also find that this is the first time that they are engaging in conversations of this nature with family members and may hear, for the first time, of others in the family who have given birth to a preterm infant. These family members, and those with a background in obstetrical or neonatal care, can be a tremendous source of support for information and advice for families (Kavanaugh et al., 2014). Another strategy for helping Anna communicate and engage with others would be to ask "Is there anyone in your family, or do you have a friend, who has experienced something similar or is a professional who cares for premature infants?" Followed by "Is that person someone you might want to talk to for support or advice?"

GP Processes

As part of GP, the process of building bridges and making connections is an important initial process to building parent competency surrounding communicating (effective communications) with others. This process is achieved by establishing a trusting relationship with parents beginning in the antenatal period. Relationships that begin in the antenatal period are critical for open communication and eventually shared decision making to occur and extend into the neonatal period (Bohnhorst et al., 2015). Healthcare professionals need to convey that the parents' and infant's well-being are of utmost importance and that they value them as individuals and not as a medical diagnosis. Although providing this type of care may be part of routine practice for professionals, this experience is by no means routine for parents. As we began to explain in the example presented earlier, much respect, individual attention, and patience are required.

Healthcare professionals show respect by referring to parents by their preferred name, not "Mom" or "Dad," and speaking to both parents and not just the mother who gave birth (parents may be the same sex and/or may have used a surrogate), which often occurs when these conversations are arranged solely around the clinician's schedule, such as during medical rounds. Clinicians also show respect by acknowledging the infant's place in the family as a son or daughter and referring to the infant by name or "your infant" and not a medical diagnosis (Staub et al., 2014), such as a "23 weeker." Examples of giving individual attention and being patient include sitting whenever a conversation occurs with the parent, avoiding any interruptions during the conversation, holding discussions over more than one session, allowing for privacy, and providing comfort. Allowing for privacy means that conversations do not occur when others, such as other professionals, family members, or friends, are present without the expressed permission of the parent. One way to approach this situation is to first find out the names and importance of family and friends who are in the room and then to say to the parents "I have some personal health information to talk to you about. Normally I do not talk when anyone else is present. Should we proceed that way or do you prefer to have your family/friends stay?" Ideally, this conversation occurs in advance of family and friends being present. Providing comfort allows the parents to be in an optimal physical state to participate in what might be an emotion-laden discussion. Nurses are in a unique position to provide comfort due to their extensive physical presence with the parents. Examples of providing comfort are making sure that the mother does not have unnecessary interruptions during sleep and that the father has adequate nourishment.

Once the relationship is established, healthcare professionals engage in the GP process of joining attention, which is being focused on a mutual goal. But first there needs to be a shared understanding, or being on the same page and using the same language. It is helpful to let the parents lead the conversation. An initial question could be "So many different physicians and nurses must have come in already to talk to you. Can you tell me what you remember they told you about your condition and how we are caring for you and your infant?" This question enables the clinicians to see how the parents view the situation and gives insight into the type of language to use when providing information to her. Then parents should be welcomed to tell their story without interruption, making sure that the father (or other parent) has the opportunity to share his perspectives. Other valuable questions to ask early on are "Before you came to the hospital to be cared for, what did you know about premature babies?" or "Had you known anyone who went through anything similar or gave birth to a premature infant? What was their experience like?" Using this approach, GP is structured in a way that enables parents to connect with what they already know (bridging). Responses to this question could be a good entry into explaining types of potential treatment options. It can also be used to clarify any misinformation, dispel any fears, and also offer hope.

Parents need clear, honest, and balanced information in order to engage in decision making. To avoid overloading the parents with information, it is important to pace discussions and provide information that parents desire, not a detailed description of mortality and morbidity for every possible gestational age. Adequate time should be given to allow the parents time to process the information and go at their pace and readiness for more information. It is important to return after an initial meeting to make sure that parents understood the information and also give them time to ask questions. Verbal information should be supplemented with written information and recommended websites. Parents should also be advised to write down information or have someone with them to write down information. Parents might want a trusted family member present for this purpose.

Nurses can also serve as interpreters of the medical information that parents receive as well as messengers of hope, as illustrated with Anna. Therefore, it is important to make sure that nurses know when other clinicians are talking with parents so that the nurse caring for the parents can be present. Nurses can also provide question prompts regarding the types of questions to ask the different medical specialists. This strategy is particularly important because most parents have had no prior experience with premature infants or, given their age, little to no experience with making treatment decisions for serious conditions in extended family members. A tour of the NICU should be offered for parents as it can decrease the parent's stress (Griffin, Kavanaugh, Soto, & White, 1997; Staniszewska et al., 2012). If Anna was not able to travel to the NICU, her partner could be accompanied to the NICU, and Anna could be offered a virtual tour. This is equally important in other situations when babies are transferred to another hospital, as mothers are comforted knowing where their infant will receive care.

While the role of the obstetrician and neonatologist is to guide the medical care, nurses play an important role in offering support antenatally and promoting the parenting role (Kratovil & Julion, 2017). Because nurses and parents share caregiving in the NICU, developing a relationship with the nurse is paramount. Once the antenatal neonatal consultation is completed, the NICU nurse should meet with the mother on a regular basis, as the nurse did with Anna, to build the necessary partnership and share information about supporting and developing the parents' role in caregiving and decision making. At the very least, the parents should be able to witness firsthand the care and compassion exuded by the NICU nurse which will be extended to their infant.

Peer-to-peer support is an important strategy which can benefit parents in role development and coping (Hall, Ryan, Beatty, & Grubbs, 2015; Rossman, Greene, & Meier, 2015). Parent support can be face to face, individualized, group, or via technology, and it is important to recognize that different formats are needed (Hurst, 2006).

Clinicians must update the parents during the initial stabilization phase of the infant around the time of birth. Ideally, clinicians welcome the father to his infant's bedside and the mother is given verbal updates as she cannot necessarily see her infant. Reassuring words to Anna could be "Anna, your baby is okay. You do not hear her crying because she has a breathing tube in place. But she has a good color and (a strong) heart beat." If possible, before leaving the delivery room, the mother should see and touch the infant (Shields-Poe & Pinelli, 1997). At the very least, the father can take pictures during the stabilization and can share them with the mother. The primary care clinicians must update the mother about the infant prior to leaving the delivery room. The father should be welcomed to join the staff on the journey and admission of the infant to the NICU. Parents must have unrestricted access to their infants in the delivery room and NICU from admission to discharge, including during procedures and resuscitation (Eichner & Johnson, 2012; Gooding et al., 2011; Griffin, 2006, 2013; Tinsley et al., 2008).

Parental Competency of Problem Solving and Decision Making

Although most parents prefer shared decision making, a small number will prefer that the decisions be made by the clinicians or exclusively by the parents. Therefore, it is important to clarify the parent's preferred role and desire to include others in the process. Questions that could be asked of Anna at this point are "What is helpful for me to know about how you want to be involved in making treatment decisions?" "Is there anyone close to you who can help you as you think about the treatment decisions?" It is important to know that even those parents who desire a shared approach vary in their interpretation of the meaning of shared. For some, shared means that the clinician makes a recommendation and seeks the parents' approval. For others, shared means that the clinician seeks an understanding of parents' values and preferences and then decides the treatment. This approach is also cocreated, as the healthcare provider is learning about how the parents make decisions, what is comfortable for them, and finally, the healthcare provider can make things happen according to the parents' wishes. This is one form of cocreation because all parties are involved and each is listening to the other. Cocreating solutions in this way also work toward the goal of "doing the task," an important competency for parents of an extremely premature baby with whom their decision making is more limited than if the baby was full term.

GP Processes

The guided process of structuring the task and the learning will assist the clinician to assist the parents through the decision-making process. The clinician needs to determine the parents' preferences and values. In other words, finding out what matters to parents is especially important for those parents who are relying on the clinicians for a very active role in decision making. If there came a time when decisions had to be made concerning life support, one question to ask Anna is "What concerns you the most as you hear all of this information I have given you?" "What are you hoping for?" At no time should the clinicians impose guilt or pressure or allow their values and beliefs to impact on the information given to parents or decisions that are made. Also, clinicians should avoid assumptions about what might matter to parents. For example, having a child with a disability does not have the same meaning for all parents (Dupont-Thibodeau et al., 2014; Kavanaugh et al., 2015; Lam et al. 2009).

The final GP process of transferring responsibility of decision maker to the parents involves respecting parent choices, even when those choices are not in agreement with the clinician's choices. For example, a parent of an infant at a lower gestational age than Anna's, and which is unlikely to survive, might request that a full resuscitation be attempted for her infant. The clinicians can commit to this while sharing the challenges to making this successful. "If she is not breathing when she is born, we will try to insert a breathing tube to help her. But, if this is not possible because of her size, knowing there isn't anything else to help her, we recommend stopping so she can be held and loved by you."

Parental Competencies of Being With the Child and Giving Care to the Child

An extremely premature infant typically requires a lengthy hospitalization, and during this time parents experience stress from alteration in their role (Wigert, Johansson, Berg, & Hellstrom, 2006). With the delivery of a preterm infant, the mother and father become parents, but their role expectations are adversely affected with an NICU hospitalization (Watson, 2010). Mothers desire a collaborative relationship and partnership with the staff (Fegran & Helseth, 2009; Hurst, 2001a, 2001b; Schenk & Kelley, 2010) and desire to participate in their infant's care (Lilo, Shaw, Corcoran, Storfer-Isser, & Horwitz, 2016; McAllister & Dionne, 2006; Shin & White-Traut, 2007; Smith, Steelfisher, Salhi, & Shen, 2012).

When premature infants are admitted to the NICU, parents are forced to trust the staff to provide the needed care for their infant. Trust between Anna and the NICU clinicians will be enhanced because antenatal connections were made with both the medical and nursing staff who encouraged Anna to be with her infant. Sharing information antenatally can empower parents and enhance confidence in clinicians (Kratovil & Julion, 2017).

GP Processes

The process of building bridges and making connections that began antenatally lays the foundation for relationships between parents and clinicians in the NICU. Nurses are in a unique position to enhance these relationships and support the parents' role as they are the gatekeepers to their infant (Griffin, 1990). Early on in the NICU, nurses should encourage mothers, like Anna, to tell their stories beginning with the description of their high-risk pregnancy, as this is important to being the mother (Schenk & Kelley, 2010). Discussions about previous experiences are important because they can affect the mothers' reaction to having an infant in the NICU (Holditch-Davis & Miles, 2000).

Nurses can show respect for the parents' role by welcoming them to be with their infant 24 hours per day and acknowledging that parents are essential partners with the rest of the NICU team (Hall, Phillips, & Hynan, 2016; McAllister & Dionne, 2006; Schenk & Kelley, 2010) and valued in improving short- and long-term outcomes (Craig et al., 2015). Doing so builds staff competencies in being with the parents and knowing them as persons, central competencies for trust and compassion. When parents are respected as partners in care, feelings of the infant belonging to the mother emerge (Heerman, Wilson, & Wilhelm, 2005) and maternal confidence is enhanced during the infant's hospitalization and extend after discharge (Wataker, Meberg, & Nestaas, 2012).

A key component of welcoming parents as partners in the care of their infant is acknowledging and modifying the NICU culture, because organizational factors can adversely affect partnerships (Asai, 2011; Griffin, 2013). Parents want a welcoming environment and policies that are supportive of their roles as collaborative partners, which includes 24 hours per day access to their infant (Craig et al., 2015; Griffin, 2006; Lilo et al., 2016; Schenk & Kelley, 2010; Staniszewska et al., 2012; Warre, O'Brien, & Lee, 2014).

Relationships between clinicians and parents can be enhanced by choosing the right language (Griffin & Celenza, 2014; McAllister & Dionne, 2006). It is imperative to acknowledge the power of language when communicating and to use the language of "partnership" rather than the language of "power." Traditionally, nurses have used words of "power" such as "allow," "permit," and "require," which do not support partnerships between parents and staff. Instead words such as "welcome" and "encourage" can cement the value of parents in their infant's life. Even antenatally, the NICU nurse can reinforce this message by saying "Parents are our partners in helping babies get better. There are things that only we can do and things that only you can do, and together we will partner to do all we can to help your baby get better." Avoiding words such as "visit" and "visitor" are important as they connote that the parents are inconsequential in care and outcomes. Nurses must insist "You are never visitors. You are his/her mom/other parent and important in his/her life." "We do not have visiting hours, because you are not a visitor. You are welcome to be with here 24 hours a day. We will work together to help her get better" (Griffin & Celenza, 2014).

Nurses must encourage parents to be with and connect with their babies in the presence of the parents' physical and emotional challenges, including the fear that the infant will not survive (Watson, 2010). Nurses may reinforce parents' reluctance to see their infant and even discourage them from participating in care because the infant is "too sick" or "too small" (Heermann, Wilson, & Wilhelm, 2005). This can exacerbate the parents' feeling of powerlessness (Watson, 2010). Parents want to help their babies (Hurst, 2011a, 2011b), and even the most preterm and critically ill require care that the parents can provide. The most critical babies are the most likely to die and this can be the only time the parents can help them. Caregiving includes nurturing, protecting, and socializing (Limbo & Lathrop, 2014; Schroeder & Pridham, 2006). Acts of caregiving can include temperature taking, skin care, diaper changes, positioning, and comfort. Once Anna is emotionally and physically ready, nurses can teach, guide, and support her in further developing her parenting role to include softly singing, reading a book through the incubator's porthole, and socializing by taking photos that are shared with family and friends whose love for the baby is boundless.

Nurses' roles change from solely focusing on the tasks of the infant's care to sharing care with the parents and supporting their role. Nurses structure the task and the learning of caregiving by mentoring them (Reis, Rempel, Scott, Brady-Fryer, & Van Aerder, 2010; Schenk & Kelley, 2010; Warre, et al., 2014). The development of partnerships with parents that support and encourage their rightful role as decision makers and caregivers (Craig et al., 2015; Griffin, 2006), even in the face of a terminal illness (Carter, Brown, Brown, & Meyer, 2012), are necessary. The goal is to change from the discharge teaching model to parent participation in care throughout hospitalization and eventual transfer of responsibility (Griffin & Abraham, 2006; Schroeder & Pridham, 2006; Warre et al., 2014).

In addition to providing direct care, parents have a unique and important perspective as historians and stewards of safety (Hurst, 2001a, 2001b). Medical rounds and nurse handoffs should be conducted with the parents as they can offer their assessments and dispel misinformation in addition to receiving information and participating in decision making (Abdel-Latif, Boswell, Broom, Smith, & Davis, 2015; Craig, Phillips, Hall, Smith, & Browne, 2015; Griffin, 2010; Hall, Phillips, Hynan, 2016; McAllister & Dionne, 2006). Nurses may need to guide Anna in this role, as the processes in an NICU can be overwhelming. Anna should be encouraged to speak up if she is worried about her infant. This can be achieved if nurses directly ask and support her to share any worries and concerns about her infant.

Parents must be invited to plan and participate in milestone caregiving activities in addition to participation caregiving and decision making. For example, Ava's first oral feeding should be at the breast if Anna plans to nurse, and the first bottle-feeding should be offered by Anna or the baby's other parent. When Ava can be dressed, Anna should be encouraged to bring clothing from home, and if Anna is unable to provide clothing, she should be given the opportunity to select from a pool of donated clothes. Anna should identify and direct the celebration of holidays important to the family. Often nurses determine how and which holidays are celebrated. While this may be born of kindness, it undermines the parent's ability to decide which and how holidays are celebrated. Nurses can invite Anna's participation simply by asking, "Christmas is coming. Is this a holiday you wish to celebrate? Typically, Santa Claus comes to see the babies and we take pictures. Would this be okay? Would you like to be here?" Such questions offer the staff the opportunity to collaborate with the parents to ensure that their wishes are respected.

CONCLUSION

Parents of extremely premature infants are often faced with assuming new roles as parents in unfamiliar areas. The lengthy hospitalization of these infants provides ample opportunity for nurses to assist parents in assuming their new roles. GP is an approach that can be used to prepare parents to carry out their roles in participating in treatment decisions for their infant and caregiving in the NICU.

REFERENCES

Abdel-Latif, M. E., Boswell, D., Broom, M., Smith, J., & Davis, D. (2015). Parental presence on neonatal intensive care unit clinical bedside rounds: Randomized trial and focus group discussion. *Archives of Disease in Childhood. Fetal Neonatal Edition, 0*, F1–F7.

American College of Obstetricians and Gynecologists and the Society for Maternal–Fetal Medicine, Ecker, J. L., Kaimal, A., Mercer, B. M., Blackwell, S. C., deRegnier, R. A., . . . Sciscione, A. C. (2016). Periviable birth: Interim update. *American Journal of Obstetrics and Gynecology, 215*, B2–B12.e1.

Asai, H. (2011). Predictors of nurses' family-centered care practices in the neonatal intensive care unit. *Japan Journal of Nursing Science, 8*(1), 57–65.

Batton, D. G., & Committee on Fetus and Newborn. (2009). Clinical report—Antenatal counseling regarding resuscitation at an extremely low gestation. *Pediatrics, 124*, 422–427.

Bohnhorst, B., Ahl, T., Peter, C., & Pirr, S. (2015). Parents' prenatal, onward, and postdischarge experiences in case of extreme prematurity: When to set the course for a trusting relationship between parents and medical staff. *American Journal of Perinatology, 32*, 1191–1197. doi:10.1055/s-0035-1551672

Boss, R. D., Hutton, N., Sulpar, L. J., West, A. M., & Donohue, P. K. (2008). Values parents apply to decision-making regarding delivery room resuscitation for high-risk newborns. *Pediatrics, 122*, 583–589.

Branchett, K., & Stretton, J. (2012). Neonatal palliative and end of life care: What parents want from professionals. *Journal of Neonatal Nursing, 18*, 40–44.

Caeymaex, L., Jousselme, C., Vasilescu, C., Danan, C., Falissard, B., Bourrat, M. M., . . . Speranza, M. (2013). Perceived role in end-of-life decision making in the NICU affects long-term parental grief response. *Archives of Disease in Childhood. Fetal Neonatal Edition, 98*, F26–F31.

Carter, B. S, Brown, J. B., Brown, S., & Meyer, E. C. (2012). Four wishes for Aubrey. *Journal of Perinatology, 32*, 10–14.

Craig, J. W., Glick, C., Phillips, R., Hall, S. L., Smith, J., & Browne, J. (2015). Recommendations for involving the family in developmental care of the NICU infant. *Journal of Perinatology, 35*, S5–S8.

Cummings, J., & the Committee on the Fetus and Newborn. (2015). Antenatal counseling regarding resuscitation and intensive care before 25 weeks of gestation. *Pediatrics, 136*, 588–595.

Dupont-Thibodeau, A., Barrington, K. J., Farlow, B., & Janvier, A. (2014). End-of-life decisions for extremely low-gestational-age infants: Why simple rules for complicated decisions should be avoided. *Seminars in Perinatology, 38*, 31–37.

Edmonds, B., McKenzie, F., Farrow, V., Raglan, G., & Schulkin, J. (2015). A national survey of obstetricians' attitudes toward and practice of periviable intervention. *Journal of Perinatology, 35*, 338–343.

Eichner, J., & Johnson, B. F. (2012). Patient and family-centered care and the pediatrician's role. *Pediatrics, 129*, 394–404.

Fegran, L., & Helseth, L. (2009). The parent-nurse relationship in the neonatal intensive care unit context-closeness and emotional involvement. *Scandanavian Journal of Caring Sciences, 23*, 667–673.

Gooding, J. S., Cooper, L. G., Blaine, A. I., Franck, L. S., Howse, J. L., & Berns, S. D. (2011). Family support and family-centered care in the neonatal intensive care unit: Origins, advances, impact. *Seminars in Perinatology, 35*, 20–28.

Griffin, T. (1990). Nurse barriers to parenting in the special care nursery. *Journal of Perinatal and Neonatal Nursing, 4,* 56–67.

Griffin, T. (2006). Family-centered care in the NICU. *Journal of Perinatal and Neonatal Nursing, 20,* 98–102.

Griffin, T. (2010). Bringing change-of-shift report to the bedside: A patient- and family-centered approach. *Journal of Perinatal and Neonatal Nursing, 24,* 348–353.

Griffin, T. (2013). A family-centered "visitation" policy in the neonatal intensive care unit that welcomes parents as partners. *Journal of Perinatal and Neonatal Nursing, 27,* 160–165.

Griffin, T., & Abraham, M. (2006). Transition to home from the newborn intensive care unit: Applying the principles of family-centered care to the discharge process. *Journal of Perinatal and Neonatal Nursing, 20*(3), 243–249.

Griffin, T., & Celenza, J. (2014). *Family-centered care for the newborn.* New York, NY: Springer Publishing.

Griffin, T., Kavanaugh, K., Soto, C. F., & White, M. (1997). Parental evaluation of a tour of the neonatal intensive care unit during a high-risk pregnancy. *Journal of Obstetric, Gynecologic, and Neonatal Nursing, 26,* 59–65.

Grobman, W. A., Kavanaugh, K., Moro, T., Regnier, R., & Savage, T. (2010). Providing advice to parents for women at acutely high risk of periviable delivery. *Obstetrics and Gynecology, 115,* 904–909. PMCID: PMC3735348

Hall, S. L., Phillips, R., & Hynan, M. T. (2016). Transforming NICU care to provide comprehensive family support. *Newborn & Infant Nursing Reviews, 16,* 69–73.

Hall, S. L., Ryan, D. J., Beatty, J., & Grubbs, L. (2015). Recommendations for peer-to-peer support for NICU parents. *Journal of Perinatology, 35,* S9–S13.

Haward, M. E., Kirshenbaum, N. W., & Campbell, D. E. (2011). Care at the edge of viability: Medical and ethical issues. *Clinics in Perinatology, 38,* 471–492.

Heermann, J. A., Wilson, M. E., & Wilhelm, P. A. (2005). Mothers in the NICU: Outsider to partner. *Pediatric Nursing, 31,* 176–181, 200.

Holditch-Davis, D., & Miles, M. (2000). Mothers' stories about their experiences in the neonatal intensive care unit. *Neonatal Network: The Journal of Neonatal Nursing, 1,* 13–21.

Hurst, I. (2001a). Mothers' strategies to meet their needs in the newborn intensive care nursery. *Journal of Perinatal and Neonatal Nursing, 15,* 65–82.

Hurst, I. (2001b). Vigilant watching over: Mothers' actions to safeguard their premature babies in the newborn intensive care nursery. *Journal of Perinatal and Neonatal Nursing, 15,* 39–57.

Hurst, I. (2006). One size does not fit all parents' evaluations of a support program in a newborn intensive care nursery. *Journal of Perinatal and Neonatal Nursing, 20,* 252–261.

Janvier, A., Barrington, K. J., Aziz, K., Bancalari, E., Batton, D., Bellieni, C., . . . Verhagen, E. (2014). CPS position statement for prenatal counselling before a premature birth: Simple rules for complicated decisions. *Paediatrics and Child Health, 19,* 22–24, F26–F31.

Janvier, A., Lorenz, J. M., & Lantos, J. D. (2012). Antenatal counseling for parents facing an extremely preterm birth: Limitations of the medical evidence. *Acta Pediatrica, 101,* 800–804.

Kavanaugh, K. (1988). Infants weighing less than 500 grams at birth: Providing parental support. *Journal of Perinatal and Neonatal Nursing, 2,* 58–66.

Kavanaugh, K., Moro, T., & Savage, T. (2010). How nurses assist parents during decision making regarding life support decisions for extremely premature infants. *Journal of Obstetric, Gynecologic, and Neonatal Nursing, 39,* 147–158. PMCID: PMC2859457

Kavanaugh, K., Nantais-Smith, L. M., Savage, T. A., Schim, S. M., & Natarajan, G. (2014). The role of extended family in supporting parents faced with life support decisions for extremely premature infants. *Neonatal Network: The Journal of Neonatal Nursing, 33,* 255–262.

Kavanaugh, K., Roscigno, C. I., Swanson, K. M., Savage, T. A., Kimura, R. E., & Kilpatrick, S. J. (2015). Perinatal palliative care: Parent perceptions of caring in interactions surrounding counseling for risk of delivering an extremely premature infant. *Palliative and Supportive Care, 13,* 145–155.

Kratovil, A. L., & Julion, W. A. (2017). Health-care clinician's communication with expectant parents during a prenatal diagnosis: An integrative review. *Journal of Perinatology, 37,* 2–12.

Lam, H. S., Wong, S. P. S., Liu, F. Y. B., Wong, H. L., Fok, T. F., & Ng, P. C. (2009). MD attitudes toward neonatal intensive care treatment of preterm infants with a high risk of developing long-term disabilities. *Pediatrics, 123,* 1501–1508.

Lemyre, B., Daboval, T., Dunn, S., Kekewich, M., Jones, G., Wang, D., ... Moore, G. P. (2016). Shared decision making for infants born at the threshold of viability: A prognosis-based guideline. *Journal of Perinatology, 36,* 503–509.

Lilo, E. A., Shaw, R. J., Corcoran, J., Storfer-Isser, A., & Horwitz, S. M. (2016). Does she think she is supported? Maternal perceptions of their experiences in the neonatal intensive care unit. *Patient Experience Journal, 3,* 15–24.

Limbo, R., & Lathrop, A. (2014). Caregiving in mothers' narrative of perinatal hospice. *Illness, Crisis & Loss, 22*(1), 43–65.

McAllister, M., & Dionne, K. (2006). Partnering with parents: Establishing effective long-term relationships with parents in the NICU. *Neonatal Network, 25*, 329–337.

McKenzie, F., Robinson, B. K., & Edmonds, B. T. (2016). Do maternal characteristics influence maternal–fetal medicine physicians' willingness to intervene when managing periviable deliveries? *Journal of Perinatology, 36*, 522–528.

Miquel-Verges, F., Woods, S. L., Aucott, S. W., Boss, R. D., Sulpar, L. J., & Donohue, P. K. (2009). Prenatal consultation with a neonatologist for congenital anomalies: Parental perceptions. *Pediatrics, 124*(4), e573–e579. doi:10.1542/peds.2008-2865

Moro, T., Kavanaugh, K., Savage, T., Reyes, M., Kimura, R., & Bhat, R. (2011). Parent decision making for life support decisions for extremely premature infants: From the prenatal through end-of-life period. *Journal of Perinatal and Neonatal Nursing, 25*, 52–60. PMCID: PMC3085847

Reis, M. D., Rempel, G. R., Scott, S. D., Brady-Fryer, A., & Van Aerde, J. (2010). Developing nurse/parent relationships in the NICU through negotiated partnership. *Journal of Obstetric, Gynecologic, and Neonatal Nursing, 39*, 675–683.

Roscigno, C. I., Savage, T. A., Kavanaugh, K., Moro, T. T., Kilpatrick. S. J., Grobman, W. J., . . . Kimura, R. (2012) Divergent views of hope influencing communications between parents and hospital clinicians. *Qualitative Health Research, 22*, 1232–1246. PMCID: PMC3572714

Rossman, B., Greene, M. M., & Meier, P. P. (2015). The role of peer support in the development of maternal identity for "NICU moms." *Journal of Obstetric, Gynecologic, and Neonatal Nursing, 44*, 3–16.

Schenk, L. K., & Kelley, J. H. (2010). Mothering an extremely low birth-weight infant. *Advances in Neonatal Care, 10*, 88–97.

Schroeder, M., & Pridham, K. F. (2006). Development of relationship competencies through guided participation for mothers of preterm infants. *Journal of Obstetric, Gynecologic, and Neonatal Nursing, 35*, 358–368.

Shields-Poe, D., & Pinelli, J. (1997). Variables associated with parental stress in neonatal intensive care units. *Neonatal Network, 16*(1), 29–37.

Shin, H., & White-Traut, R. (2007). The conceptual structure of transition to motherhood in the neonatal intensive care unit. *Journal of Advanced Nursing, 58*, 90–98.

Smith, V. C., Steelfisher, G. K., Salhi, C., & Shen, L. Y. (2012). Coping with the neonatal intensive care experience. *Journal of Perinatal and Neonatal Nursing, 26*, 343–352.

Staniszewska, S., Brett, J., Redshaw, M., Hamilton, K., Newburn, M., Jones, N., & Taylor, L. (2012). The POPPY study: Developing a model of family-centered care for neonatal units. *Worldviews on Evidence-Based Nursing, 9*, 243–255.

Staub, K., Baardsnes, J., Hebert, N., Hebert, M., Newell, S., & Pearce, R. (2014). Our child is not just a gestational age: A first-hand account of what parents want and need to know before premature birth. *Acta Paediatrica, 103*, 1035–1038.

Stoll, B., Hansen, N. I., Bell, E. F., Walsh, M. C., Carlo, W. A., Shankaran, S., . . . Higgins, R. D. (2015). Trends in care practices, morbidity, and mortality of extremely preterm neonates, 1993–2012. *Journal of the American Medical Association, 314*, 1039–1051.

Tinsley, C., Hill, B., Shah, J., Zimmerman, G., Wilson, M., Freier, K., & Abd-Allah, S. (2008). Experience of families during cardiopulmonary resuscitation in a pediatric intensive care unit. *Pediatrics, 122*, e799–e804.

Tomlinson, M. W., Kaempf, J. W., Ferguson, L. A., & Stewartm, V. T. (2010). Caring for the pregnant woman presenting at periviable gestation: Acknowledging the ambiguity and uncertainty. *American Journal of Obstetrics and Gynecology, 202*, 529, E1–E6.

Warre, R., O'Brien, K., & Lee, S. K. (2014). Parents as primary caregivers for their infant in the NICU: Benefits of challenges. *NeoReviews, 15*, e472–e477.

Wataker, H., Meberg, A., & Nestaas, E. (2012). Neonatal family care for 24 hours per day: Effects on maternal confidence and breast-feeding. *Journal of Perinatal and Neonatal Nursing, 26*, 336–342.

Watson, G. (2010). Parental liminality: A way of understanding the early experiences of parents who have a very preterm infant. *Journal of Clinical Nursing, 20*, 1462–1471.

Wigert, H., Johansson, R., Berg, M., & Hellstrom, A. L. (2006). Mothers' experience of having their newborn child in a neonatal intensive care unit. *Scandinavian Journal of Caring Sciences, 20*, 35–41.

7

Caregiving During the First Year of a Very Premature Infant's Life

Deborah Steward, Tondi M. Harrison, and Hallie Straka

Prematurity is a significant global health problem. Approximately 15 million infants are born premature worldwide, and prematurity is the leading cause of death in children younger than the age of 5 (World Health Organization, 2016). In the United States, the issue of prematurity is just as significant. In 2015, 381,321 infants were born premature, accounting for 9.63% of all live births (Hamilton, Martin, & Osterman, 2016). The result is that approximately one in 10 infants is born premature. The prematurity rate demonstrated an encouraging and steady decline in the United States from 2007 to 2014, with rates dropping from a high of 12.8% of all live births to 9.57%. Unfortunately, the rate of premature births increased in 2015 for the first time in 8 years (March of Dimes, 2016), with an increase from 9.57% to 9.63% (Hamilton et al., 2016).

Across the breadth of prematurity, gestational age provides some guidance in considering rates of survival and short- and long-term outcomes (Manuck et al., 2016). There is an inverse relationship between gestational age at birth and mortality, development of comorbidities, and neurodevelopmental alterations. Survival rates for premature infants, especially those born extremely premature, continue to improve with each additional week of gestation increasing the probability of survival (Manuck et al., 2016). However, paralleling the declining mortality rates is the increasing numbers of infants confronting comorbidities that are unique to the premature population, including respiratory distress syndrome, necrotizing enterocolitis, intraventricular hemorrhage, and patent ductus arteriosus (Manuck et al., 2016; Stoll et al., 2015). Management of these unique illnesses and the subsequent sequelae that can develop, such as broncho-pulmonary dysplasia, is associated with various degrees of alterations in neurodevelopment (de Kieviet, Zoetebier, van Elburg, Vermeulen, & Oosterlaan, 2012; Lax et al., 2013; Richards, Drews-Botsch, Sales, Flanders, & Kramer, 2016). The purpose of this chapter is to describe the complex needs of very premature infants and their families using the relational model of guided participation (GP).

CAREGIVING COMPETENCIES USING GP

Due to improving survival rates, increasing numbers of premature infants, especially extremely premature infants, are discharged from the NICU requiring advanced caregiving skills in the home environment. Responsibility for performance of these advanced skills is most often assumed by the mother, who is the usual primary caretaker. One of the most important and time-consuming caregiving activities in the home environment is supporting the feeding experiences of infants. Because of their developmental immaturity, a large percentage of premature infants are discharged from the NICU with feeding issues that can persist throughout infancy. Of concern are the increasing numbers of premature infants, especially extremely premature infants, at risk for experiencing feeding difficulties.

Managing feeding issues in the home environment is an important source of maternal stress. When feeding issues are present at discharge, mothers question whether their infants are truly ready for discharge (Phillips-Pula, Pickler, McGrath, Brown, & Dusing, 2013). This is critical since managing their infant's nutrition at home is one of the most important topics identified by mothers to be included in discharge teaching (Burnham, Feeley, & Sherrard, 2013) and, yet, mothers report inadequate discharge preparation for managing their infant's feeding experiences at home (Boykova, 2016; Stevens, Gazza, & Pickler, 2014). Inadequate preparation has been linked to numerous feeding issues during the first few weeks at home (Smith, Dukhovny, Zupancic, Gates, & Pursley, 2012). Importantly, the feeding experience is the primary mechanism through which the mother–infant partnership evolves since the majority of interactive time during the infant's first few months of life is focused on infant feeding. Thus, strategies are needed to support the developing feeding competencies of mothers and infants, with the goal of supporting the evolving mother–infant relationship. GP facilitates the mothers' development of competencies in the care of their premature infant through mutual partnership and goal setting between a nurse guide and the learner parent (Pridham, Limbo, Schroeder, Thoyre, & Van Riper, 1998).

ACHIEVING FEEDING MILESTONES IN THE NICU

Feeding-related developmental milestones, including readiness for oral feeding, initiation of oral feeding, and successful transition to full oral feedings, are the most important milestones for premature infants to achieve while in the NICU (Briere, McGrath, Cong, & Cusson, 2014; Dodrill, Donovan, Cleghorn, McMahon, & Davies, 2008). Premature infants initially rely on enteral feedings due to anatomic, physiologic, and neurobehavioral immaturity of critical organ systems (Silberstein et al., 2009a). The transition from enteral to oral feeding proceeds when the necessary systems needed for oral feeding are deemed developmentally ready.

Successful transition to full oral feedings necessitates that premature infants manage sensory input while maintaining an alert state, an appropriate level of energy, and postural and oral-motor tone throughout the length of the feeding (Browne & Ross, 2011). The immature physiology of the premature infant is often overwhelmed by the complex nature of the oral feeding process. Consequentially, oral feedings can become stressful to premature infants because of their inability to regulate autonomic function and behavioral organization (Delaney & Arvedson, 2008). Delays in achieving full oral feeding are most often attributed to cardiorespiratory instability or ineffective mechanisms to protect the airway and esophagus (Jadcherla, Wang, Vijayapal, & Leuthner, 2010). The result is that significant numbers of premature infants continue to exhibit immature coordination of the suck–swallow–breathe reflexes even when full oral feedings are achieved (Dodrill, 2011). As two mothers commented on their premature infants at 1 month corrected age:

> "... and the suck, swallow, and breathe at the same time is really hard for her even yet ..."

> "But he can't coordinate everything in his mouth and swallow."

Gestational age, the infant's illness trajectory, and the culture of the NICU can be hindrances to timely acquisition of oral-motor skills (Browne & Ross, 2011). There is an inverse relationship between gestational age and time to full oral feeding and the presence of comorbidities and time to full oral feeding (Giannì et al., 2015; Jadcherla et al., 2010). Earlier gestational age and the presence of comorbidities impacts the progression from initiating enteral feeding to achieving full oral feeding, delaying the achievement of expected feeding milestones and, ultimately, discharge from the NICU (Dodrill et al., 2008; Park, Knafl, Thoyre, & Brandon, 2015; Ross & Browne, 2013; Van Nostrand, Bennett, Coraglio, Guo, & Muraskas, 2015).

In addition, specific interventions for illness management such as endotracheal intubation, nasogastric (NG)/orogastric tube placement, and suctioning of the nasopharynx or oropharynx provide noxious stimuli to the oral/perioral area resulting in oral hypersensitivity and subsequent heightened sensitivity to further oral-motor stimulation (Gennattasio, Perri,

Baranek, & Rohan, 2015). The presence of oral hypersensitivity delays the acquisition of oral-motor skills. Use of NG tubes for enteral feeding present unique challenges to achievement of oral feedings. The prolonged reliance on enteral feedings increases oral hypersensitivity and oral defensive behaviors that may persist after discharge from the NICU (Browne & Ross, 2011).

TRANSITION HOME FROM THE NICU

Discharge from the NICU is contingent upon the ability of the premature infant to safely consume all feedings orally without cardiorespiratory compromise while maintaining normal body temperature and demonstrating a sustained pattern of growth (American Academy of Pediatrics Committee of Fetus and Newborn, 2008), independent of the presence of comorbidities and/ or neurodevelopmental alterations. The time required to transition to full oral feedings delays discharge from the NICU, especially for extremely premature infants. While readiness to feed guides the progression of oral feeding experiences, pressure mounts to facilitate hospital discharge when full oral feeding is the only factor preventing discharge (Raiten et al., 2016). Mothers are keenly aware of the goal to achieve full oral feeding and often employ strategies to assist their infant in accomplishing this goal (Brown, Griffin, Reyna, & Lewis, 2013). The result is that determination of oral feeding success for discharge is often volume-driven without full consideration of achievement of oral-motor competencies (Pickler, Reyna, Griffin, Lewis, & Thompson, 2012; Shaker, 2013). The risk is that premature infants are discharged with oral-motor skills that are developmentally immature. A significant number of premature infants exhibit disorganized or dysfunctional oral feeding ability at discharge (Crapnell, Rogers, Neil, Inder, Woodward, & Pineda, 2013) despite consuming all nutritional intakes via the oral route. For a subset of premature infants, achievement of full oral feedings does not occur and they are discharged home requiring a combination of oral and enteral feedings (Jadcherla et al., 2010).

In the immediate period following discharge, the focus on feedings at home remains goal oriented with the expectation the premature infant will consume a prescribed amount of calories at each feeding that will support a positive pattern of growth. The mother is now charged with accomplishing these goals for her infant without the ready support of the NICU staff. While mothers embrace these goals (Brown et al., 2013), consequentially, feeding becomes the focus for mothers as they comprehend the complex and time-consuming nature of the feeding process (González & Espitia, 2014; Lutz, 2012; Reyna, Pickler, & Thompson, 2006). Mothers report numerous challenges with feeding their premature infant following discharge (Boykova, 2016). As one mother reported:

> "I get really worried because she's had a lot of spells with that where her breathing and stuff is all out of whack and that take a lot out of her when she starts choking and she's using all her energy to get it either up or down. So I get really worried when she starts choking like that."

These challenges add to mothers' stress in caring for their premature infant as mothers often equate feeding success with infant well-being (Delaney & Arvedson, 2008).

The feeding process during the early weeks at home may not allow for the development of a supportive reciprocal process between mother and infant because of the focus on caloric intake and growth. As expressed by one mother:

> "Basically just to get nutrition into them, it's not a bonding time because [she's] more interested in everything else ... so it's just to get her nutritional intake."

For many mothers, stress and concern surrounding the feeding is a persistent undercurrent during feeding interactions with their infants (Lutz, 2012). Further, the focus on intake and growth does not necessarily allow for consideration of the infant's individual feeding competency (Pickler et al., 2012). As a result, mothers may be less responsive to their infant's feeding cues and more controlling of the feeding process because of their focus on accomplishing the nutritional goals prescribed for their premature infant (Black & Aboud, 2011).

NUTRITION MANAGEMENT IN THE HOME ENVIRONMENT

Nutritional management in the home is critical for the growth and development of premature infants because of the relationship between growth and neurodevelopmental outcomes (Nzegwu & Ehrenkranz, 2014). Postdischarge nutritional needs are influenced by accrued growth deficits, presence of comorbidities, prescribed medications, and composition of the feeding (Raiten et al., 2016). The result is that premature infants may have increased nutrient requirements, that is, calories or proteins. Premature infants are often discharged from the NICU with complex prescriptions for nutritional management and directions for advancing the infant's nutritional intake. Nutritional management may include feedings with increased nutritional density or additional nutrient fortification, off-label use of nutrient products, combinations of breast and bottle-feeding, and fluid volume restriction (Raiten et al., 2016). The complexity of the nutritional plan can be a source of stress and misunderstanding for mothers. In addition, mothers are confused when interpreting such discharge instructions as "advance as tolerated" or "feed ad lib" (Reyna et al., 2006). Without a clear understanding of their infant's nutritional plan, mothers are at risk for overfeeding or underfeeding their premature infant (Raiten et al., 2016).

MATERNAL LEARNING: THE PROCESS OF FEEDING THE PREMATURE INFANT

Because of its critical importance, feeding is one of the most important tasks to be mastered by the mother and premature infant (Silberstein et al., 2009b). Successfully feeding the premature infant requires a different set of psychomotor and observation skills on the part of the mother than those required to feed a full-term infant. The complexity of skills to be employed are influenced by the gestational age and presence of any comorbidities. Learning to manage oral feedings starts in the NICU where both the infant and mother begin to develop the necessary feeding competencies. Mastery of feeding competencies continues into the home environment where responsibility for the feeding experience is transferred to the mother (Swanson et al., 2012). Thus, it becomes the mother's responsibility to facilitate the continuing development of her and her infant's feeding competencies. Through experience, mothers learn which psychomotor and observation skills are effective in supporting their infant's developing feeding competencies (Brown et al., 2013).

Mothers report the importance of focusing on the technical aspects of feeding their premature infant, such as recognition of infant behavioral state and providing chin support and postural control, and learning what strategies are effective in safely feeding their infant and maintaining physiologic control (Stevens et al., 2014). As one mother explained what was going on during the feeding:

> "That's why my fingers are under his chin; he smacks. His mouth is going up and down, but he's not sucking."

Importantly, because feeding can be a stressful experience for premature infants, mothers must be observant of various parameters during the feeding to ensure that their infant is safely tolerating the feeding and does not experience physiologic instability. Another mother described the situation as follows:

> "If he's like, if he's real panicked and going—like every three gulps, I'll pull it out of his mouth, just because I know if I let him go to five, he's going to all of a sudden choke on me."

These parameters include coordination of suck–swallow–breathe, state of arousal, respiratory rate, color, and body temperature (Shaker, 2013; Stevens et al., 2014).

To successfully feed their infant, mothers must learn to interpret infant feeding readiness, hunger, and satiation cues (Reyna et al., 2006) as the premature infant's behavior is the primary channel of communication (Shaker, 2013). Unfortunately, infant cues may be subtle and difficult to interpret, especially during the first few weeks following discharge. Without the guidance of the NICU nursing staff, mothers report difficulties in understanding their infant's feeding cues and a lack of congruence with what was taught in the NICU (González & Espitia, 2014). The risk is that infant feeding becomes less infant regulated and more parent driven, thus impacting the social interaction associated with feeding (Crapnell, Woodward, Rogers, Inder, & Pineda, 2015). However, mothers agree that success in interpreting their premature infant's feeding cues evolves across time as the mother–infant dyad participates in multiple feeding experiences (Brown et al., 2013) and increases mutual enjoyment during feeding interactions.

Prevalence of Feeding Issues Across the First Year of Life

Oral feeding is one of the most complex activities that premature infants engage in during the first year of life (Pineda, 2016). It is during this time period that oral-motor skills increase in complexity allowing the infant to progress from a liquid diet to a diet that contains foods with various tastes and textures (van der Heul, Lindeboom, & Haverkort, 2015). The process of feeding encompasses the oral phase of eating as well as interactions between mother and infant during the process (Delaney & Arvedson, 2008). The first few weeks following discharge are a pivotal time in the infant's continued mastery of the feeding process. It is during this time that immature oral-motor skills continue to mature in the home environment under the guidance of the mother (Browne & Ross, 2011). However, feeding challenges are one of the most prominent maternal concerns during the early postdischarge period (Boykova, 2016; Griffin & Pickler, 2011). Maternal reports of feeding difficulties during this pivotal time demonstrate that the maturation process does not necessarily occur as a linear process. The prevalence of feeding issues is not unexpected as the performance of oral-motor skills by premature infants may have been sufficient enough to achieve discharge goals but the continued performance of these skills may not yet be developmentally proficient (Browne & Ross, 2011; Thoyre, 2007).

A significant number of premature infants are discharged from the NICU with documented disorganized or dysfunctional oral feeding skills (Crapnell et al., 2013; Törölä, Lehtihalmes, Yliherva, & Olsén, 2012). This is supported by Jonsson, Van Doorn, and Van Den Berg (2013) who found that 48% of the mothers in their study reported feeding difficulties in their infant at the time of discharge from the NICU. These feeding difficulties have the potential to give rise to further issues with feeding. Pickler et al. (2012) demonstrated that oral-motor skills present at discharge from the NICU were predictive of oral-motor skills 2 weeks after discharge. Thus, premature infants with inefficient oral-motor skills at discharge will continue to exhibit inefficiency. This is validated by mothers who reported that their premature infants experienced difficulties with regulating the feeding experience due to issues with coordinating suck–swallow–breath cycles and maintaining a state of arousal (Kmita, Urma ska, Kiepura, & Polak, 2011). As one mother described her infant's difficulty with maintaining interest:

> "Sometimes I put it [nipple] in his mouth and he goes—eh. He just wants to sleep. He just won't eat."

Several of the most commonly reported feeding issues during the first few weeks after discharge include choking, spitting/vomiting, difficulties with coordination of suck–swallow–breathe, latching on, reluctance to feed, and prolonged feeding (DeMauro, Patel, Medoff-Cooper, Posencheg, & Abbasi, 2011; Jonsson et al., 2013; Lutz, 2012). One mother described her concern with choking:

> "Only thing that bothers us is when he chokes or when he gets real panicked. That's difficult. It's difficult because you don't want to see your child choking and you don't want [to] see him getting to the point where he's so frustrated that he's panicked."

Premature infants are at risk for exhibiting feeding issues throughout the first year of life, especially during periods of nutritional transition that require developmentally advanced oral-motor skills necessary for the introduction of solids and varying textures. A significant number of mothers report that feeding issues continue throughout the first year of life (Cerro, Zeunert, Simmer, & Daniels, 2002; DeMauro et al., 2011; Horner et al., 2014; Howe, Sheu, Wang, & Hsu, 2014; Jonsson et al., 2013) and often surround the introduction of solid foods and varying food textures (Kmita et al., 2011; Sanchez, Spittle, Slattery, & Morgan, 2016). Maternal concerns were validated by Törölä et al. (2012) who demonstrated that premature infants who exhibited disorganized or dysfunctional oral feeding skills at 40 weeks postmenstrual age (PMA) were more likely to have feeding issues later in infancy. Feeding issues observed during later infancy include arching with meals, apparent discomfort during the feeding, choking, gagging, spitting/vomiting, holding food in the mouth, and avoidance of some food textures (Chung, Lee, Spinazzola, Rosen, & Milanaik, 2014; DeMauro et al., 2011; den Boer & Schipper, 2013; Horner et al., 2014; Jonsson et al., 2013). Feeding issues in the first year of life are described by these two mothers:

> "Seems like he, I don't want to say drools a lot, but his tongue really forces forward when he eats, I've noticed. That was one thing that was really hard when he started eating with a spoon. His tongue was right there and it would not let that spoon in. But it still forces the food a lot forward."

> "We just introduced the third or fourth stage, the stuff with chunks in it. He tries to get used to that. He doesn't know what to do with it in his mouth. If he should swallow them or what to do."

Behavioral feeding difficulties include struggling for control, low food consumption, picky eating, unorganized and distractible feeding habits, and little independent and efficient feeding (Silberstein et al., 2009a).

One of the most important contributing factors to later feeding difficulties in premature infants is a lack of recognition for the developmental maturation of the infant resulting in the achieved age of the infant underpinning maternal decision making. Reliance on "correction for gestational age" as a proxy for developmental readiness does not take into consideration the infant's developmental maturation and achieved feeding competencies.

Premature infants are at increased risk for developing avoidant feeding behaviors when they are not developmentally ready for the introduction of feeding experiences that require advanced oral-motor skills (Chung et al., 2014). Avoidant feeding behaviors in premature infants prolong the learning process for managing solid foods and various food textures (Törölä et al., 2012). When age is corrected for gestational age, premature infants continue to exhibit developmentally immature oral-motor skills that lag behind those expected for a specific age (Pridham et al., 2005; Ross & Browne, 2013). Thus, corrected age and overall developmental status need to be considered when making decisions to advance feeding experiences (Delaney & Arvedson, 2008).

When age is the sole consideration for feeding decisions, the result is the early introduction of solids and texturized foods. Concerns over slow infant weight gain are a contributing factor to the early introduction of solid foods (Törölä et al., 2012). Mothers reported introducing solids at an average corrected age of 3 to 3.5 months (Cerro et al., 2002; Jonsson et al., 2013; van der Heul et al., 2015). Braid, Harvey, Bernstein, and Matoba (2015) demonstrated that two-thirds of premature infants in their study were introduced to solid foods before 4 months corrected age. However, maternal actions are greatly influenced by information provided by the infant's pediatrician. Unfortunately, pediatrician recommendations are highly variable. Pediatricians were found to recommend introduction of solids at an average corrected age of 3.9 ± 2.1 months (Chung et al., 2014) while others made recommendations based solely on chronological age (D'Agostino et al., 2013). The result is the introduction of solids before the premature infant is developmentally ready. Given concerns over the growth of premature infants, early introduction of solid foods is to the detriment of receiving the maximum nutritional benefit afforded through breast milk or infant formula, especially if fortified with specific nutrients (D'Agostino et al., 2013).

From a developmental perspective, the increasingly complex oral-motor skills that manifest during later infancy facilitate the infant's ability to become a more independent participant during the feeding process. This time period is characterized by the transition from a predominantly caregiver-regulated feeding to feeding patterns determined by the self-regulated behaviors of the infant (Silberstein et al., 2009a). The American Academy of Pediatrics Committee on Fetus and Newborn (2008) recommends that developmental readiness be assessed prior to introducing solid foods to premature infants. Consideration of adjusting for gestational age and developmental readiness should be considered for the first 24 months of age (Delaney & Arvedson, 2008). Importantly, even when a premature infant is assessed to be developmentally ready to transition to more complex oral-motor skills, the infant may require an extended period of time to demonstrate mastery of the skill (Törölä et al., 2012).

Without foundational knowledge of developmental readiness, maternal expectations for infant feeding behaviors will influence decision making. Mothers report uncertainty with advancing nutritional foods when informational needs for nutrition and growth are not addressed (Boykova, 2016). Chung et al. (2014) found that mothers who received anticipatory guidance in relation to advancing nutrition were more likely to have premature infants who were developmentally ready for the introduction of solids. However, premature infants who were not developmentally ready when solids were introduced exhibited avoidant feeding behaviors such as pushing food away, gagging with meals, holding food in the mouth, and crying (Chung et al., 2014). Jonsson et al. (2013) demonstrated similar findings including vomiting, refusal to accept certain food textures, and gagging with meals.

Progression of oral-motor skills is contingent upon the provision of feeding experiences that promote achievement of developmentally mature complex oral skills (Pineda, 2016). Feeding issues may arise during later infancy due to a lack of opportunity to attempt new feeding experiences when the premature infant exhibits signs of developmental readiness. Mothers may respond to concerns over earlier feeding issues by a hesitancy to introduce more advanced feeding skill opportunities, even when their premature infant exhibits developmental readiness, or may initially introduce advanced feeding opportunities but limit these opportunities in response to any signs of feeding difficulties. As one mother explained in response to providing her 12-month-old infant with a baby pretzel:

"I don't really like giving that to her because she doesn't chew it up well."

Pridham, Steward, Thoyre, Brown, and Brown (2007) found for a minority of infants a lack of opportunity to engage in feeding skills associated with new foods or new feeding modalities. The continued reliance on breast or bottle feeding further takes away from opportunities to develop maturing oral-motor skills and is associated with feeding issues during later infancy (van der Heul et al., 2015).

Evolving Mother–Infant Relationship

Caregiving activities provide the platform for the development of a synchronous, reciprocal relationship between a mother and her infant. Because of the central role of nutritional intake to an infant's growth and development during the first year of life, the quality and frequency of feeding experiences play a critical role in the development of the mother–infant interaction (Silberstein et al., 2009b). Successful mother–infant interaction during feeding is contingent upon a reciprocal relationship that is mutually responsive based on the behaviors of both participants (Delaney & Arvedson, 2008). Maternal sensitivity when responding, coupled with the ability of the infant to clearly communicate interactive and hunger/satiety cues, fosters the developing mother–infant relationship (Gueron-Sela, Atzaba-Poria, Meiri, & Yerushalmi, 2011). Reciprocal mother–infant interactions during feeding will translate into mutually enjoyable interactions during nonfeeding opportunities.

The context for caregiving and, specifically, feeding activities is qualitatively different for mothers of premature infants when compared to those for full-term infants. A premature infant's specific healthcare needs, goals for nutritional intake and growth, and neurodevelopment will shape the interactive exchanges between mother and infant. Because of the premature infant's developmental immaturity, the infant is not capable of exhibiting interactive cues that are robust and easily interpreted. Mothers report that it takes time to come to know their infants and recognize their unique behavioral cues (Brown et al., 2013) and realize that coming to know their infant will continue following discharge (Swift & Scholten, 2009). Because of the developmentally evolving interactive behaviors of their premature infants, mothers have to expend greater energy to engage with their infants than mothers of full-term infants (Howe et al., 2014).

For mothers of premature infants, the unexpected delivery of their infant necessitates that development of the maternal role begins within the confines of the NICU environment and is significantly influenced by the illness trajectory of their infant and concerns over survival and long-term outcomes. Mothers often experience a delayed sense of motherhood as they navigate within an NICU culture that does not necessarily allow for autonomous maternal decision making surrounding their infant's care (Adama, Bayes, & Sundin, 2016; Boykova, 2016; González & Espitia, 2014). To successfully navigate the NICU environment and participate in infant caregiving activities, mothers must learn a new vocabulary and perform technical skills, such as enteral tube feedings, for which they most likely have had no previous experience (Swanson et al., 2012). Further, development of the maternal role and fledgling attempts at participatory caregiving occur under the observant, and potentially intrusive watchfulness, of the NICU staff.

An important mediator of maternal role attainment is the elevated stress that characteristically accompanies admission to the NICU. Although occurring in parallel, mothers must not only employ effective coping strategies to manage the stress but also come to know their infant through increasing participation in caregiving activities. Ineffective stress management will allow maternal stress to escalate subsequently interfering with maternal role attainment and the developing relationship with her infant (Holditch-Davis et al., 2015; Purdy, Craig, & Zeanah, 2015; Spinelli, Poehlmann, & Bolt, 2013). Maternal role development is facilitated through implementation of family-centered care principles. The developing mother–infant relationship is nurtured when mothers are invited to be active participants in their infant's care (Giannì et al., 2016; Raiskila, Axelin, Rapeli, Vasko, & Lehtonen, 2014).

Maternal caregiving of a premature infant in the home environment provides new challenges that can escalate the stress that accompanies the bringing of a new infant home. Mothers are responsible for monitoring their infant's progress in ways that mothers of healthy infants do not experience. Many premature infants are discharged home with lingering medical issues that require continued treatments and pharmacologic management. After a prolonged period of NICU healthcare providers in charge of their infant's care, mothers are now thrust into the unfamiliar role of full-time caregiver for a premature infant at a time that their own role as a mother continues to evolve (Dellenmark-Blom & Wigert, 2014; Griffin & Pickler, 2011). Mothers experience a tension between wanting to have their infant home and recognizing they are now the primary caregiver (Adama et al., 2016; Boykova, 2016; Griffin & Pickler, 2011; Swanson et al., 2012).

Mothers must not only come to know their infant as a unique individual but are expected to perform advanced assessment and caregiving skills that support the growth and development of their vulnerable premature infant. Responsibility for and performance of these advanced skills increases maternal apprehension and stress (Murdoch & Franck, 2012; Phillips-Pula et al., 2013; Spinelli et al., 2013) as they fear that something detrimental to their infant's well-being will occur under their care (Adama et al., 2016; González & Espitia, 2014). Importantly, the focus on the special healthcare needs of their infant and the performance of advanced assessment and caregiving responsibilities become components of "mothering" behaviors (Boykova, 2016). However, mothers do perceive that directed attention on their infant's healthcare needs and completion of the associated advanced skills places demands on their role as a mother (Spinelli et al., 2013). The risk is that the performance of advanced caregiving skills results in maternal caregiving becoming task oriented and less focused on developing a reciprocal interactive relationship with their infant that is mutually satisfying.

The previous discussion of caloric intake and growth has the potential to specifically alter maternal role attainment beginning during the NICU hospitalization and continuing throughout infancy. With the emphasis on transitioning to full oral feedings and sustained weight gain in order to be discharged, the focus shifts from supporting the developing mother–infant interaction to supporting the feeding competency of the infant (Brown et al., 2013; Swift & Scholten, 2009). This has the potential to increase the maternal stress associated with feeding her infant. For infants who experience difficulties in making the transition to full oral feedings, mothers may employ intrusive behaviors with the goal of increasing the volume obtained with each feeding (Silberstein et al., 2009b). Because, as previously described, a significant number of premature infants are discharged while still experiencing immature and inefficient feeding behaviors, the risk is that mothers will continue to employ these intrusive feeding behaviors during feeding interactions in the home environment. In a longitudinal study, maternal interactive behaviors during feeding present at the time of discharge from the NICU were predictive of feeding interactive behaviors at 1 year of age (Silberstein et al., 2009a).

Because of the continued focus on nutritional intake and growth in the home environment, the feeding experience is the primary means by which mothers and premature infants interact (Parker, Rybin, Heeren, Thoyre, &

Corwin, 2016). Thus, the necessary focus on nutritional intake and the amount of time surrounding the feeding process may be to the detriment of other interactive opportunities with the infant (Lutz, 2012). One mother described the situation as follows:

> "But her feedings sometimes take up to an hour cause she takes these little breaks, but she's not finished yet."

Researchers demonstrated that early interactive difficulties during feeding and nonfeeding experiences were still present at 1 year of age (Silberstein et al., 2009a). Thus, the focus on nutritional intake prevents mothers from appreciating the critical importance of infant–mother interactions during feeding to the developing synchrony between the infant and mother (Reyna, Brown, Pickler, Myers, & Younger, 2012). Mothers who are concerned about their infant not growing appropriately are at higher risk of developing negative feeding interactions with their infant as their focus on nutritional intake heightens (Gueron-Sela et al., 2011). Unfortunately, early concerns about growth often persist throughout infancy (Kmita et al., 2011) and may result in mothers attempting to regulate their infant's nutritional intake independent of the infant's hunger and satiety cues (Cerro et al., 2002). Researchers have demonstrated an inverse relationship between maternal control during feeding of solid foods and infant weight gain (Farrow & Blissett, 2006). These concerns are expressed by this mother:

> "I don't want her to skip meals or not have meals, she doesn't have extra fat on her."

Mothers are at risk for evaluating their own maternal competence within the context of their premature infant's feeding success and subsequent growth (Black & Aboud, 2011; Browne & Ross, 2011; González & Espitia, 2014), with maternal confidence diminishing in response to infant feeding difficulties (Swift & Scholten, 2009). Maternal confidence also fluctuates in response to the infant's pattern of growth (Murdoch & Franck, 2012). Difficulties with feeding that impact growth can result in a negative feedback loop where the presence of feeding difficulties increases maternal focus on feeding, decreases her focus on the development of other maternal role competencies, decreases her confidence as a mother, and increases her anxiety and stress related to meeting nutritional intake and growth goals. As anxiety increases, mothers may no longer view the feeding experience as a rewarding interaction with their infant. Mothers of infants who exhibit feeding difficulties report increased stress during feeding times (Chung et al., 2014; DeMauro et al., 2011; Howe et al., 2014; Törölä et al., 2012). Importantly, given the focus on maintaining adequate growth, mothers who perceive their infants are experiencing feeding issues are less satisfied with their infant's growth (Chung et al., 2014).

The presence of feeding issues and slow growth heighten maternal perceptions of infant vulnerability and influence their approach to feeding interactions with her infant (González & Espitia, 2014; Hill, 2015). As two mothers explained:

> "He's still gaining weight nicely, if he had stopped or slowed way down and was starting to lose weight, I would get concerned."

> "I'm not concerned about her weight yet, when she starts losing, then I'll be really concerned as to how much she takes. But she's really stabilized in her weight."

Maternal concern over nutritional intake and growth, coupled with the stress surrounding infant feeding issues, could result in an increase in the use of intrusive and controlling maternal behaviors while feeding their infant with the goal of increasing their infant's intake. Maternal intrusive behaviors are characterized by maternal overriding behavior that disregards the infant's signals and interrupts the infant's behavior and are driven by the mother's agenda rather than that of the infant (Silberstein et al., 2009a). Mothers may not appreciate the consequential impact of these behaviors on the developing mother–infant interaction during feeding and nonfeeding interactions. In the short term, these behaviors may have a positive effect on intake, but implementation of these behaviors is not without consequences. Positive effects reinforce the use of these behaviors during subsequent feedings.

However, continued reliance on intrusive and controlling behaviors can become counterproductive, resulting in worsening of nutritional intake and growth (Farrow & Blissett, 2006). For example, intrusive behaviors have been associated with less robust infant feeding behavior and inefficient infant sucking behaviors during bottle feeding (Silberstein et al., 2009b). This, in turn, can lead to further discomfort and asynchrony during the feeding interaction. More importantly, this narrow focus during feeding prevents mothers from appreciating the important opportunity that the feeding process provides for interacting with their infants (Reyna et al., 2012). Silberstein et al. (2009a) demonstrated that by 1 year of age, mothers of premature infants with feeding difficulties were more intrusive and less adaptable during feeding interactions and the infants were less involved and more withdrawn. Importantly, nonsupportive maternal behaviors during the feeding interactions were also found to be present during nonfeeding interactions (Silberstein et al., 2009a). Thus, negative maternal affective behaviors that develop in response to concerns over their infant's feeding behaviors permeate other interactive opportunities.

Summary of Potential Feeding Issues and Their Consequences

Feeding issues are present among premature infants during the first year of life, especially for those infants who were extremely immature at birth or confronted numerous morbidities during their NICU hospitalization. The presence of feeding issues are not without consequences for both the infant and mother. Feeding issues present during infancy can persist into toddlerhood and beyond (Crapnell et al., 2015; Johnson et al., 2016).

Continued feeding difficulties undermine the potential for enjoyable feeding experiences and can result in persistent concerns related to growth. Importantly, a significant relationship has been demonstrated between feeding issues and later alterations in neurodevelopmental outcomes (Adams-Chapman, Bann, Vaucher, & Stoll, 2013; Parker et al., 2016). This relationship has ramifications for the long-term growth and development throughout childhood.

Mothers play a critical role in supporting the long-term development of their infant. Because of the persistence of feeding issues and later alterations in neurodevelopmental outcomes, it has been hypothesized that the quality of the mother–infant interaction during feeding is a modifiable factor that can support the infant's neurodevelopment (Parker et al., 2016). However, researchers have demonstrated that interactional conflicts associated with infant feedings can persist into early toddlerhood (Salvatori, Andrei, Neri, Chirico, & Trombini, 2015). Thus, it is imperative that strategies are implemented that support the developing mother–infant feeding interaction, beginning during hospitalization in the NICU and continuing throughout the first year of life. A reciprocal, mutually satisfying mother–infant interaction will maximize the infant's long-term neurodevelopment.

USING GP IN THE CONTEXT OF FEEDING VULNERABLE PREMATURE INFANTS

GP provides a useful technique for supporting mothers as they take on the caregiving role, particularly the critical task of feeding that not only ensures adequate caloric intake and growth, but also serves as the context for development of the social relationship between mother and infant. Learning to feed their infant is one of the primary caregiving tasks a parent must learn. As discussed, feeding a prematurely born infant is technically and qualitatively different from feeding a term infant. The goals and approach underpinning the feeding of premature infants are complex and directed at supporting nutritional intake, growth, feeding competencies, and social development of the premature infant.

Given these differences, even mothers who have previously and successfully fed their full-term infants will be learners, along with first-time parents, in feeding their prematurely born infant (Swanson et al., 2012). The opportunity for a nurse guide to work together with learner parents to feed the infant in the home environment presents itself during the early discharge period and extends as needed throughout infancy. Whatever intervention is used to support the mother's success in feeding her infant, the nurse will be assessing the mother's feeding competencies and developing a plan for enhancing them that are responsive to issues and concerns that are present in the moment. We argue that GP provides the framework for best accomplishing this critical nursing responsibility. The use of GP can bridge the gap between the security of the NICU and increasing maternal competence in the home environment (Dellenmark-Blom & Wigert, 2014).

There are six critical processes associated with providing a GP intervention. The process of intervening using GP begins with the nurse guide *developing a relationship* with the mother. Ideally, the guide(s) will be nurses who are either in the NICU Follow-Up Clinic or are making visits to the home. The developing relationship will be strengthened by consistency in the nurses with whom the mother will interact. The evolving trusting relationship will subsequently foster the development of maternal competency in feeding her premature infant. Mothers feel empowered to care for their premature infant when supported and reassured by nurses in the home environment (Adama et al., 2016; Boykova, 2016). This will be key since mothers report that effectively feeding their premature infant is one of the most important concerns following discharge.

As this relationship develops, the purpose of the connection as it relates to supporting caregiving is identified through *reaching and maintaining joint attention* to a particular issue, (e.g., feeding the premature infant at home). This connection is critical since many premature infants experience feeding issues at the time of discharge (Crapnell et al., 2013) that are a source of significant maternal concern during the first few weeks at home (Lutz, 2012). During this process, the nurse guide is learning about feeding this particular infant, what competencies the mother brings to this task, and what additional competencies may be needed to support infant feeding success. The mother may communicate concerns about feeding her infant by tone of voice, reluctance to be present at feedings, reporting of previous difficulties with feeding, or frustration at infant response (or lack of) during feeding. The nurse may also elicit these concerns as part of routine assessment. A critical component of this assessment will include focused questions to the mother in order to elicit the mother's internal working model (IWM) of feeding this vulnerable infant. The mother's motivations for feeding the infant (i.e., goals), what she expects of herself and others, and the actions she intends to pursue are critical pieces of information to inform the nurse guide's approach to intervention.

The nurse guide's foundational GP goal is to assist the mother in developing an IWM that is open, flexible, and realistic and with understanding of the effects of current behavior on future development and relationship (Pridham et al., 1998). For a premature infant with feeding issues, a "healthy" maternal IWM may involve setting realistic goals that are based on an accurate assessment of the infant's feeding behaviors and oral-motor skills with the intent of supporting developmental maturation of the infant's feeding ability, while recognizing that realistic goals are not necessarily guided by the infant's corrected age but where the infant is developmentally. The IWM may also articulate how the nurse guide can support the mother in implementing infant feeding strategies that are infant driven and not driven by unrealistic maternal expectations.

Within the guide–learner relationship, as the participants develop a meaningful trust relationship and focus on a mutually agreed upon issue, they discuss and refine each other's understanding of what the situation is and what the goals are, what may work or not work to address the situation, and how it affects them emotionally and behaviorally. This process, *creating a shared understanding* of the issue, enables the nurse guide, using knowledge of the mother's motivations, expectations, and intentions, to respond appropriately or to initiate or suggest focused activities as well as to correct or reinterpret potential misconceptions related to infant feeding. Maternal concern over infant feeding issues may result in the mother's reliance on intrusive or controlling behaviors during feeding that she believes are beneficial to the infant's feeding experience (Black & Aboud, 2011; Silberstein et al., 2009a). GP includes an equal focus on the mother's and infant's emotional and behavioral responses as well as planning ahead for potential difficulties or unexpected events.

Simply learning or teaching specific behavioral techniques does not address the meaning that the infant's behavior has for the mother that can influence her emotional and behavioral response (Pridham et al., 1998). In addition, the infant's early interaction/experience with the mother becomes the basis on which the IWM of the mother develops and subsequently affects the future relationship. Importantly, the nurse guide recognizes that feeding a vulnerable premature infant is an emotional experience for the mother and the infant and that the mother often equates her ability to effectively feed her infant with her developing competence as a mother.

A fourth critical process of GP is *building bridges* between what is known and what is unknown, including cognitive, emotional, and behavioral factors. Within the work of the GP intervention, the guide and learner will work together to identify areas where more knowledge and experience are needed. Mothers report informational needs following infant discharge from the NICU and often seek informational resources to answer their questions (Boykova, 2016). The focus on feeding a vulnerable premature infant is necessarily or often geared toward physical feeding techniques (e.g., how to hold the bottle, what position to place the infant in, how much to feed, and when and how to burp). Although these needs are perhaps most clearly understood and frequently practiced using specific feeding techniques, cognitive and emotional gaps also need to be identified. A learner mother may have unrealistic expectations of her prematurely born infant or she may be struggling emotionally with feelings of disappointment or failure. Because premature infants often do not exhibit robust behavioral cues, interpretation of these cues may be inaccurate resulting in maternal actions that are stress producing for both interactive partners (Brown et al., 2013; González & Espitia, 2014). The gaps between what exists and what is desired in these cognitive and emotional issues are no less important to identify and address as a learner–guide team.

Building bridges between these gaps requires collaboratively *structuring the tasks or learning* that need to take place. Maternal recognition of their knowledge needs is important, as mothers often have unanswered questions related to feeding their premature infant but do not necessarily have the foundation to articulate their knowledge deficits (Reyna et al., 2006). Using a GP approach, the nurse guide and the learner may decide that videotaping a feeding may help them work together on identifying potential areas of adjustment of feeding technique. Or they may decide that having the learner observe the nurse guide during feeding will be most useful—or a combination of both techniques. Both of these approaches will entail nonjudgmental and supportive reflection from the guide. A useful technique using video is to "wonder" with the learner mother about specific events upon replay, for example, facial expressions of mother or infant, behaviors with bottle and nipple, or decision to end the feeding. Structuring learning related to emotional or cognitive needs may entail pulling in additional resources, such as written materials or videos or arranging talks with experienced mothers of premature infants with a similar background to provide emotional support and reinforcement of typical or expected trajectories of the evolving mother–infant feeding interaction.

One of the mutually derived goals of the GP intervention will be for the guide and learner to develop a process for *transferring responsibility* of the feeding task to the mother. Because of the mother's initial apprehension with feeding her premature infant in the home, there is a risk that the mother will heavily rely on the nurse guide and her perspective on infant feeding and not assume full ownership for her infant's developing feeding competency. In transferring responsibility, it will be imperative that the nurse guide support the mother's developing competencies and knowledge related to feeding her infant, with the goal of increasing maternal confidence and independence. In turn, the mother will gain confidence in managing other aspects of her premature infant's care.

The need for intervention is not over at the time of hospital discharge as mothers are stressed by assuming primary responsibility for their infant's feeding experiences in the home environment. Issues and concerns identified by the nurse guide and learner mother will change over time in response to the premature infant's evolving feeding competencies throughout infancy. How the nurse guide and learner mother build their trusting relationship, identify gaps in maternal knowledge and set realistic goals, and implement strategies to support developing competencies has important ramifications for mother–infant feeding interactions throughout infancy. When mothers do not possess the necessary knowledge and set unrealistic feeding goals for their infant, feeding issues may either persist or arise in later infancy. Premature infants are more successful mastering developmentally complex oral-motor skills and feeding behaviors when mothers have the necessary knowledge to support their infant's feeding experiences (Chung et al., 2014).

Case Example 7.1

Michael is 6½ months old (uncorrected age) and is being seen today for the first time by a home health nurse. Michael was referred by his pediatrician due to concerns related to Michael's weight gain and reported feeding difficulties. In reviewing Michael's history, the nurse learns that Michael was born extremely premature at 24 5/7 weeks gestation with a birthweight of 608 g. He had a difficult NICU course that included ligation of a patent ductus arteriosus, medical management of necrotizing enterocolitis, treatment for late-onset sepsis, and development of bronchopulmonary dysplasia following prolonged ventilatory management and a continued oxygen requirement. Michael was discharged from the NICU at 5½ months of age with instructions that included 0.1 L of oxygen per bi-nasal cannula, infant formula 94 mL every 3 hours, and infant vitamins 1 mL/d.

At this initial visit, Michael's mother, Claudia, expresses concern that Michael is not easy to feed and at times seems disinterested in his feeding and spits out his food. She is also concerned about his weight gain because she knows that if Michael does not gain weight he may be hospitalized and she is worried the NICU staff will think she is not a good mother. Since discharge, Michael has only gained 250 g. Claudia, who is a single mother, expresses her frustration at how difficult it is to care for Michael and at the lack of sleep she is getting.

Because of Claudia's distress and Michael's weight loss, the home health nurse will be most effective if she begins to establish a trusting relationship with Claudia. Acknowledging Claudia's concerns and assuring her that she and Claudia will work together to develop a plan for Michael will provide a foundation for building this relationship. Mothers feel empowered to care for their premature infant when supported and reassured by nurses in the home environment (Adama et al., 2016; Boykova, 2016). Recognizing the linkage between Michael's nutrition and weight gain, the joint attention to Michael's nutritional needs and growth facilitates the home health nurse and Claudia in identifying and focusing on the issues impacting Michael's feeding experience. During this process, the home health nurse is learning about Claudia's experiences in feeding Michael and what competencies and knowledge that Claudia brings to this experience. The home health nurse is also afforded the opportunity to determine what additional competencies and knowledge that Claudia may be need to successfully manage Michael's nutrition.

Claudia tells the home health nurse that it can take Michael about 30 minutes to finish a feeding and expresses concern over his increased respiratory effort while feeding. Through continued discussion the home health nurse learns that Claudia is also frustrated because the formula comes as a powder and she feels like she is wasting formula because she has to mix more volume then needed (per instructions) to provide the prescribed 94 mL. The home health nurse assures Claudia that her frustration is common as mothers of premature infants often find their infant's nutrition plan complex and a source of stress (Reyna et al., 2006).

As the home health nurse continues to guide Claudia in sharing information about Michael's nutrition, she learns that Claudia has been feeding Michael 90 mL per feeding instead of 94 mL because of her concerns about wasting formula. She has been doing this for about 2 weeks.

Because Claudia has expressed concerns about Michael's weight gain, the home health nurse probes this issue further to understand Claudia's perceptions, especially in light of the reduced nutritional intake, and learns that Claudia has been feeding Michael 1 tbsp of rice cereal mixed with formula three times a day and is feeding him with a spoon. She thought Michael was old enough to eat from a spoon since he is 6½ months old and she thought "food" would help him gain weight. The home health nurse learns that, when Claudia talked earlier of Michael spitting out his feeding, she was referring to the rice cereal.

The home health nurse and Claudia review Michael's feeding issues as described by Claudia and develop a shared understanding of these feeding issues. Claudia's knowledge of Michael's feeding issues can be enhanced by the home health nurse clarifying misconceptions of infant nutrition through building bridges between what Claudia knows and what she needs to know. Claudia's recognition of her knowledge deficits will allow the home health nurse to structure her approach to teaching Claudia the new information. Maternal recognition of their knowledge needs is important as mothers often have unanswered questions related to feeding their premature infant but do not necessarily have the foundation to articulate their knowledge deficits (Reyna et al., 2006). However, in order to support the developing relationship, the home health nurse should positively acknowledge the rationale that Claudia provides for her decision making and continuing to remind her that mothers of premature infants often make these same decisions. The home health nurse explains that slow weight gain is often a reason that mothers introduce solid foods (Törölä et al., 2012) and the age of her infant often guides the decision to introduce solid foods (van der Heul et al., 2015). She further explains that it is important to be sure that Michael is developmentally ready to accept food solids from a spoon and this cannot be based on his age alone (Delaney & Arvedson, 2008).

Finally, the home health nurse, in a nonaccusatory and supportive approach, needs to help Claudia understand the relationship between Michael's weight gain and the apparent decrease in nutritional intake. The home health nurse can explain that, even though the difference between 94 mL and 90 mL may seem small, the cumulative effects of this difference on weight gain can be significant in a premature infant who has high nutritional needs. She will also need to explain that infant rice cereal does not have the same caloric and nutrient value as the infant formula and provides less nutrition to Michael.

Enhancing Claudia's knowledge will allow the two to work together to set goals for Michael's nutrition. Together, they agree on the following plan:

- Provide Michael the prescribed infant formula of 94 mL every 3 hours.
- Do not provide rice cereal to Michael at this time.
- Monitor whether Michael sleeps better because his nutritional intake has increased and he may be more satisfied.

- The home health nurse will contact the pediatrician to develop a less wasteful approach to mixing Michael's formula.
- The home health nurse will return in 1 week:
  - To assess Michael's weight gain.
  - To provide instruction on formula preparation based on the pediatrician's recommendation.
  - To observe a feeding between Claudia and Michael in order to offer strategies to enhance the feeding interaction.

Using the process of GP as a framework will allow the home health nurse to assist Claudia in developing the competencies needed to manage Michael's current nutrition and growth needs. Importantly, this framework will allow the home health nurse to continue to assist Claudia with nutrition and growth issues as they arise. This is critical since premature infants confront numerous obstacles as they achieve mastery of oral-motor skills and maintain a positive growth trajectory during the first year of life.

CONCLUSION

Very premature infants account for approximately 10% of births in the United States each year. Due to developmental immaturity, these infants need specialized caregiving, especially involving feeding and growth. A central aspect of caregiving for all mothers is nurturing that is often demonstrated through successful feeding. The caregiving relationship may bring disappointment and guilt when complex feeding skills are needed. This chapter has outlined ways that the healthcare team can use the practice of GP to help parents and infants be together in loving and nurturing ways during feeding, resulting in new learning, self-confidence, and heightened relationship skills.

REFERENCES

Adama, E. A., Bayes, S., & Sundin, D. (2016). Parents' experiences of caring for preterm infants after discharge from neonatal intensive care unit: A meta-synthesis of the literature. *Journal of Neonatal Nursing, 22,* 27–51. doi:10.1016/j.jnn.2015.07.006

Adams-Chapman, I., Bann, C. M., Vaucher, Y. E., & Stoll, B. J. (2013). Association between feeding difficulties and language delay in preterm infants using *Bayley Scales of Infant Development-Third Edition. Journal of Pediatrics, 163,* 680–685. doi:10.1016/j.jpeds.2013.03.006

American Academy of Pediatrics Committee of Fetus and Newborn. (2008). Hospital discharge of the high-risk neonate. *Pediatrics, 122,* 1119–1126. doi:10.1542/peds.2008-2174

Black, M. M., & Aboud, F. E. (2011). Responsive feeding is embedded in a theoretical framework of responsive parenting. *Journal of Nutrition, 141,* 490–494. doi:0.3945/jn.110.129973

Boykova, M. (2016). Life after discharge: What parents of preterm infants say about their transition to home. *Newborn & Infant Nursing Reviews, 16,* 58–65. doi:10.1053/J.NAINR.2016.03.002

Braid, S., Harvey, E. M., Bernstein, J., & Matoba, N. (2015). Early introduction of complementary foods in preterm infants. *Journal of Pediatric Gastroenterology and Nutrition, 60,* 811–818. doi:10.1097/MPG.0000000000000695

Briere, C. E., McGrath, J., Cong, X., & Cusson, R. (2014). State of the science: A contemporary review of feeding readiness in the preterm infant. *Journal of Perinatal & Neonatal Nursing, 28,* 51–58. doi:10.1097/JPN.0000000000000011

Brown, L. F., Griffin, J., Reyna, B., & Lewis, M. (2013). The development of a mother's internal working model of feeding. *Journal for Specialists in Pediatric Nursing, 18,* 54–64. doi:10.1111/jspn.12011

Browne, J. V., & Ross, E. S. (2011). Eating as a neurodevelopmental process for high-risk newborns. *Clinics of Perinatology, 38,* 731–743. doi:10.1016/j.clp.2011.08.004

Burnham, N., Feeley, N., & Sherrard, K. (2013). Parents' perceptions regarding readiness for their infant's discharge from the NICU. *Neonatal Network, 32,* 324–334. doi:10.1891/0730-0832.32.5.324

Cerro, N., Zeunert, S., Simmer, K. N., & Daniels, L. A. (2002). Eating behaviour of children 1.5–3.5 years born preterm: Parents' perceptions. *Journal of Paediatrics and Child's Health, 38,* 72–78. Retrieved from https://www.ncbi.nlm.nih.gov/pubmed/?term=cerro+Zeunert+simmer

Chung, J., Lee, J., Spinazzola, R., Rosen, L., & Milanaik, R. (2014). Parental perception of premature infant growth and feeding behaviors: Use of gestation-adjusted age and assessing for developmental readiness during solid food introduction. *Clinical Pediatrics, 53,* 1271–1277. doi:10.1177/0009922814540039

Crapnell, T. L., Rogers, C. E., Neil, J. J., Inder, T. E., Woodward, L. J., & Pineda, R. G. (2013). Factors associated with feeding difficulties in the very preterm infant. *Acta Paediatrica, 102,* e539–e545. doi:10.1111/apa.12393

Crapnell, T. L., Woodward, L. J., Rogers, C. E., Inder, T. E., & Pineda, R. G. (2015). Neurodevelopmental profile, growth, and psychosocial environment of preterm infants with difficult feeding behaviors at age 2 years. *Journal of Pediatrics, 167,* 1347–1353. doi:10.1016/j.jpeds.2015.09.022

D'Agostino, J. A., Gerdes, M., Hoffman, C., Manning, M. L., Phalen, A., & Bernbaum, J. (2013). Provider use of corrected age during health supervision visits for premature infants. *Journal of Pediatric Health Care, 27,* 172–179. doi:10.1016/j.pedhc.2011.09.001

de Kieviet, J. F., Zoetebier, L., van Elburg, R. M., Vermeulen, R. J., & Oosterlaan, J. (2012). Brain development of very preterm and very low-birthweight children in childhood and adolescence: A meta-analysis. *Developmental Medicine and Child Neurology, 54,* 313–323. doi:10.1111/j.1469-8749.2011.04216.x

Delaney, A. L., & Arvedson, J. C. (2008). Development of swallowing and feeding: Prenatal through first year of life. *Developmental Disabilities Research Reviews, 14,* 105–117. doi:10.1002/ddrr.16

Dellenmark-Blom, M., & Wigert, H. (2014). Parents' experiences with neonatal home care following initial care in the neonatal intensive care unit: A phenomenological hermeneutical interview study. *Journal of Advanced Nursing, 70,* 575–586. doi:10.1111/jan.12218

DeMauro, S. B., Patel, P. R., Medoff-Cooper, B., Posencheg, M., & Abbasi, S. (2011). Postdischarge feeding patterns in early- and late-preterm infants. *Clinical Pediatrics, 50,* 957–962. doi:10.1177/0009922811409028

den Boer, S., & Schipper, J. A. (2013). Feeding and drinking skills in preterm and low birth weight infants compared to full term infants at a corrected age of nine months. *Early Human Development, 89,* 445–447. doi:10.1016/j.earlhumdev.2012.12.004

Dodrill, P. (2011). Feeding difficulties in preterm infants. *ICAN: Infant, Child, & Adolescent Nutrition, 3,* 324–331. doi:10.1177/1941406411421003

Dodrill, P., Donovan, T., Cleghorn, G., McMahon, S., & Davies, P. S. W. (2008). Attainment of early feeding milestones in preterm neonates. *Journal of Perinatology, 28,* 549–555. doi:10.1038/jp.2008.56

Farrow, C., & Blissett, J. (2006). Does maternal control during feeding moderate early infant weight gain? *Pediatrics, 118,* e293–e298. doi:10.1542/peds.2005-2919

Gennattasio, A., Perri, E. A., Baranek, D., & Rohan, A. (2015). Oral feeding readiness assessment in premature infants. *MCN. The American Journal of Maternal Child Nursing, 40,* 96–104. doi:10.1097/NMC.0000000000000115

Giannì, M. L., Sannino, P., Bezze, E., Comito, C., Plevani, L., Roggero, P., ... Mosca, F. (2016). Does parental involvement affect the development of feeding skills in preterm infants? A prospective study. *Early Human Development, 103,* 123–128. doi:10.1016/j.earlhumdev.2016.08.006

Giannì, M. L., Sannino, P., Bezze, E., Plevani, L., di Cugno, N., Roggero, P., ... Mosca, F. (2015). Effect of co-morbidities on the development of oral feeding ability in pre-term infants: A retrospective study. *Scientific Reports, 5*(16603), 1–8. doi:10.1038/srep16603

González, M. P. O., & Espitia, E. C. (2014). Caring for a premature child at home: From fear and doubt to trust. *Texto & Contexto Enfermagem, 23,* 828–835. doi:10.1590/0104-07072014003280013

Griffin, J. B., & Pickler, R. H. (2011). Hospital-to-home: Transition of mothers of preterm infants. *MCN. The American Journal of Maternal Child Nursing, 36,* 252–257. doi:10.1097/NMC.0b013e31821770b8

Gueron-Sela, N., Atzaba-Poria, N., Meiri, G., & Yerushalmi, B. (2011). Maternal worries about child underweight mediate and moderate the relationship between child feeding disorders and mother–child feeding interactions. *Journal of Pediatric Psychology, 36,* 827–836. doi:10.1093/jpepsy/jsr001

Hamilton, B. E., Martin, J. A., & Osterman, M. J. K. (2016). Births: Preliminary data for 2015. *National Vital Statistics Reports, 65*(3), 1–15.

Hill, A. S. (2015). Mothers' perceptions of child vulnerability in previous preterm infants. *ABNF Journal, 26*, 11–16. Retrieved from https://www.ncbi.nlm.nih.gov/pubmed/27386663

Holditch-Davis, D., Santos, H., Levy, J., White-Traut, R., O'Shea, M., Geraldo, V., & David, R. (2015). Patterns of psychological distress in mothers of preterm infants. *Infant Behavior and Development, 41*, 154–163. doi:10.1016/j.infbeh.2015.10.004

Horner, S., Simonelli, A. M., Schmidt, H., Cichowski, K., Hancko, M., Zhang, G., & Ross, E. S. (2014). Setting the stage for successful oral feeding: The impact of implementing the SOFFI feeding program with medically fragile NICU infants. *Journal of Perinatal & Neonatal Nursing, 28*, 59–68. doi:10.1097/JPN.0000000000000003

Howe, T. H., Sheu, C. F., Wang, T. N., & Hsu, Y. W. (2014). Parenting stress in families with very low birth weight preterm infants in early infancy. *Research in Developmental Disabilities, 35*, 1748–1756. doi:10.1016/j.ridd.2014.02.015

Jadcherla, S. R., Wang, M., Vijayapal, A. S., & Leuthner, S. R. (2010). Impact of prematurity and co-morbidities on feeding milestones in neonates: A retrospective study. *Journal of Perinatology, 30*, 201–208. doi:10.1038/jp.2009.149

Johnson, S., Matthews, R., Draper, E. S., Field, D. J., Manktelow, B. N., Marlow, N., … Boyle, E. M. (2016). Eating difficulties in children born late and moderately preterm at 2 y of age: A prospective population-based cohort study. *American Journal of Clinical Nutrition, 103*, 406–414. doi:10.3945/ajcn.115.121061

Jonsson, M., Van Doorn, J., & Van Den Berg, J. (2013). Parents' perceptions of eating skills of pre-term vs full-term infants from birth to 3 years. *International Journal of Speech-Language Pathology, 15*, 604–612. doi:10.3109/17549507.2013.808699

Kmita, G., Urma ska, W., Kiepura, E., & Polak, K. (2011). Feeding behaviour problems in infants born preterm: A psychological perspective. Preliminary report. *Medycyna Wieku Rozwojowego, 15*, 216–223. Retrieved from https://www.ncbi.nlm.nih.gov/pubmed/22006476; http://www.medwiekurozwoj.pl/articles/2011-3-1-2.html

Lax, I. D., Duerden, E. G., Lin, S. Y., Chakravarty, M. M., Donner, E. J., Lerch, J. P., & Taylor, M. J. (2013). Neuroanatomical consequences of very preterm birth in middle childhood. *Brain Structure and Function, 218*, 575–585. doi:10.1007/s00429-012-0417-2

Lutz, K. F. (2012). Feeding problems of neonatal intensive care unit and pediatric intensive care unit graduates: Perceptions of parents and providers. *Newborn and Infant Nursing Reviews, 12*, 207–213. doi:10.1053/j.nainr.2012.09.008

Manuck, T. A., Rice, M. M., Bailit, J. L., Grobman, W. A., Reddy, U. M., Wapner, R. J., … Tolosa, J. E. (2016). Preterm neonatal morbidity and mortality by gestational age: A contemporary cohort. *American Journal of Obstetrics and Gynecology, 215*, 103.e1–103.e14. doi:10.1016/j.ajog.2016.01.004

March of Dimes. (2016). 2016 Premature birth report cards. Retrieved from http://www.marchofdimes.org/mission/prematurity-reportcard.aspx

Murdoch, M. R., & Franck, L. S. (2012). Gaining confidence and perspective: A lived phenomenological study of mothers' lived experiences caring for infants at home after neonatal unit discharge. *Journal of Advanced Nursing, 68*, 2008–2020. doi:10.1111/j.1365-2648.2011.05891.x

Nzegwu, N. I., & Ehrenkranz, R. A. (2014). Post-discharge nutrition and the VLBW infant: To supplement or not supplement? *Clinics in Perinatology, 41*, 463–474. doi:10.1016/j.clp.2014.02.008

Park, J., Knafl, G., Thoyre, S., & Brandon, D. (2015). Factors associated with feeding progression in extremely preterm infants. *Nursing Research, 64*, 159–167. doi:10.1097/NNR.0000000000000093

Parker, M. G. K., Rybin, D. V., Heeren, T. C., Thoyre, S. M., & Corwin, M. J. (2016). Postdischarge feeding interactions and neurodevelopmental outcome at 1-year corrected gestational age. *Journal of Pediatrics, 174*, 104–110. doi:10.1016/j.jpeds.2016.03.074

Phillips-Pula, L., Pickler, R., McGrath, J. M., Brown, L. F., & Dusing, S. C. (2013). Caring for a preterm infant at home: A mother's perspective. *Journal of Perinatal & Neonatal Nursing, 27*, 335–344. doi:10.1097/JPN.0b013e3182a983be

Pickler, R. H., Reyna, B. A., Griffin, J. B., Lewis, M., & Thompson, A. M. (2012). Changes in oral feeding in preterm infants 2 weeks after discharge. *Newborn & Infant Nursing Reviews, 12*, 202–206. doi:10.1053/j.nainr.2012.09.012

Pineda, R. G. (2016). Feeding: An important, complex skill that impacts nutritional, social, motor and sensory experiences. *Acta Pædiatrica, 105*, e458. doi:10.1111/apa.13535

Pridham, K. F., Brown, R., Clark, R., Limbo, R. K., Schroeder, M., Henriques, J., & Bohne, E. (2005). Effect of guided participation on feeding competencies of mothers and premature infants. *Research in Nursing & Health, 28*, 252–267. doi:10.1002/nur.20073

Pridham, K. F., Limbo, R., Schroeder, M., Thoyre, S., & Van Riper, M. (1998). Guided participation and development of care-giving competencies for families of low birth-weight infants. *Journal of Advanced Nursing, 28,* 948–958. doi:10.1046/j.1365-2648.1998.00814.x

Pridham, K. F., Steward, D., Thoyre, S., Brown, R., & Brown, L. (2007). Feeding skill performance in premature infants during the first year. *Early Human Development, 83,* 293–305. doi:10.1016/j.earlhumdev.2006.06.004

Purdy, I. B., Craig, J. W., & Zeanah, P. (2015). NICU discharge planning and beyond: Recommendations for parent psychosocial support. *Journal of Perinatology, 35*(Suppl. 1), S24–S28. doi:10.1038/jp.2015.146

Raiskila, S., Axelin, A., Rapeli, S., Vasko, I., & Lehtonen, L. (2014). Trends in care practices reflecting parental involvement in neonatal care. *Early Human Development, 90,* 863–867. doi:10.1016/j.earlhumdev.2014.08.010

Raiten, D. J., Steiber, A. L., Carlson, S. E., Griffin, I., Anderson, D., Hay, W. W., … Pre-B Consultative Working Groups. (2016). Working group reports: Evaluation of the evidence to support practice guidelines for nutritional care of preterm infants—The Pre-B Project. *American Journal of Clinical Nutrition, 103*(2), 648S–678S. doi:10.3945/ajcn.115.117309

Reyna, B. A., Brown, L. F., Pickler, R. H., Myers, B. J., & Younger, J. B. (2012). Mother–infant synchrony during infant feeding. *Infant Behavior & Development, 35,* 669–677. doi:10.1016/j.infbeh.2012.06.003

Reyna, B. A., Pickler, R. H., & Thompson, A. (2006). A descriptive study of mothers' experiences feeding their preterm infants after discharge. *Advances in Neonatal Care, 6,* 333–340. doi:10.1016/j.adnc.2006.08.007

Richards, J. L., Drews-Botsch, C., Sales, J. M., Flanders, W. D., & Kramer, M. R. (2016). Describing the shape of the relationship between gestational age at birth and cognitive development in a nationally representative U.S. birth cohort. *Paediatric and Perinatal Epidemiology, 30,* 571–582. doi:10.1111/ppe.12319

Ross, E. S., & Browne, J. V. (2013). Feeding outcomes in preterm infants after discharge from the neonatal intensive care unit (NICU): A systematic review. *Newborn and Infant Nursing Reviews, 13,* 87–93. doi:10.1053/J.NAINR.2013.04.003

Salvatori, P., Andrei, F., Neri, E., Chirico, I., & Trombini, E. (2015). Pattern of mother–child feeding interactions in preterm and term dyads at 18 and 24 months. *Frontiers in Psychology, 6,* 1–10. doi:10.3389/fpsyg.2015.01245

Sanchez, K., Spittle, A. J., Slattery, J. M., & Morgan, A. T. (2016). Oromotor feeding in children born before 30 weeks' gestation and term-born peers at 12 months corrected age. *Journal of Pediatrics, 178,* 113–118. doi:10.1016/j.jpeds.2016.07.044

Shaker, C. S. (2013). Cue-based feeding in the NICU: Using the infant's communication as a guide. *Neonatal Network, 32,* 404–408. doi:10.1891/0730-0832.32.6.404

Silberstein, D., Feldman, R., Gardner, J. M., Karmel, B. Z., Kuint, J., & Geva, R. (2009a). The mother–infant feeding relationship across the first year and the development of feeding difficulties in low-risk premature infants. *Infancy, 14,* 501–525. doi:10.1080/15250000903144173

Silberstein, D., Geva, R., Feldman, R., Gardner, J. M., Karmel, B. Z., Rozen, H., & Kuint, J. (2009b). The transition to oral feeding in low-risk premature infants: Relation to infant neurobehavioral functioning and mother–infant feeding interaction. *Early Human Development, 85,* 157–162. doi:10.1016/j.earlhumdev.2008.07.006

Smith, V. C., Dukhovny, D., Zupancic, J. A. F., Gates, H. B., & Pursley, D. M. (2012). Neonatal intensive care unit discharge preparedness: Primary care implications. *Clinical Pediatrics, 51,* 454–461. doi:10.1177/0009922811433036

Spinelli, M., Poehlmann, J., & Bolt, D. (2013). Predictors of parenting stress trajectories in premature infant–mother dyads. *Journal of Family Psychology, 27,* 873–883. doi:10.1037/a0034652

Stevens, E. E., Gazza, E., & Pickler, R. (2014). Parental experience learning to feed their preterm infants. *Advances in Neonatal Care, 14,* 354–361. doi:10.1097/ANC.0000000000000105

Stoll, B. J., Hansen, N. I., Bell, E. F., Walsh, M. C., Carlo, W. A., Shankaran, S., … Higgins, R. D. (2015). Trends in care practices, morbidity, and mortality of extremely preterm neonates, 1993–2012. *JAMA, 314,* 1039–1051. doi:10.1001/jama.2015.10244

Swanson, V., Nicol, H., McInnes, R., Cheyne, H., Mactier, H., & Callander, E. (2012). Developing maternal self-efficacy for feeding preterm babies in the neonatal unit. *Qualitative Health Research, 22,* 1369–1382. doi:10.1177/1049732312451872

Swift, M. C., & Scholten, I. (2009). Not feeding, not coming home: Parental experiences of infant feeding difficulties and family relationships in a neonatal unit. *Journal of Clinical Nursing, 19,* 249–258. doi:10.1111/j.1365-2702.2009.02822.x

Thoyre, S. (2007). Feeding outcomes of extremely premature infants after neonatal care. *Journal of Obstetric, Gynecologic, and Neonatal Nursing, 36*, 366–376. doi:10.1111/j.1552-6909.2007.00158.x

Törölä, H., Lehtihalmes, M., Yliherva, A., & Olsén, P. (2012). Feeding skill milestones of preterm infants born with extremely low birth weight (ELBW). *Infant Behavior & Development, 35*, 187–194. doi:10.1016/j.infbeh.2012.01.005

van der Heul, M., Lindeboom, R., & Haverkort, E. (2015). Screening solid foods infants 1 (SSFI-1) development of a screening tool to detect problems in the transition from milk to solid food in infants from six to nine months of age. *Infant Behavior and Development, 40*, 259–269. doi:10.1016/j. infbeh.2015.06.006

Van Nostrand, S. M., Bennett, L. N., Coraglio, V. J., Guo, R., & Muraskas, J. K. (2015). Factors influencing independent oral feeding in preterm infants. *Journal of Neonatal–Perinatal Medicine, 8*, 15–21. doi:10.3233/NPM-15814045

World Health Organization. (2016). Preterm birth. Retrieved from http://www.who.int/mediacentre/ factsheets/fs363/en/

Section III

GUIDED
PARTICIPATION
IN CARING
FOR CHILDREN
WITH ACUTE
AND CHRONIC
CONDITIONS

8

Supporting Families When a Child Has a Complex Chronic Condition

Stephanie Hosley, Rosie Zeno, Tondi M. Harrison, and Deborah Steward

The presence of multiple chronic conditions (MCC) in children is a growing concern in the United States as increasing numbers of children confront MCC. An estimated 15.1% of children in the United States (11.2 million) have special healthcare needs and 40.5% of the children have at least two or more chronic conditions (USDHHS, Health Resources and Services Administration, Maternal and Child Health Bureau, 2013). Children with MCC represent the most fragile subcategory of children with special healthcare needs, and they also have the highest resource utilization (Liberman, Song, Radbill, Pham, & Derrington, 2016). Advances in the management of neonatal and pediatric illness have reduced mortality and increased survival rates for acutely/critically ill children who confront such issues as birth asphyxia, prematurity, congenital anomalies, trauma, child abuse, and metabolic, genetic, oncologic, and hematologic disorders (Agrawal, 2015; Cohen et al., 2011). An important outcome is the parallel increase in the number of children who develop chronic health conditions, characterized by increasing medical complexity (Cohen et al., 2011) as a result of the initial illness (Burke & Alverson, 2010; Burns et al., 2010). Although a heterogeneous group, a significant number of these children have multisystem health problems, including neurodevelopmental disabilities, gastrointestinal illnesses, pulmonary complications, musculoskeletal abnormalities, and nutritional deficits that require the use of assisted medical technology, such as a tracheostomy or gastrostomy tube, and a need for multiple medications (Cohen et al., 2012; Elias, Murphy, & Council on Children with Disabilities, 2012). Importantly, limitations in cognitive and/or physical functioning resulting from these chronic illnesses increase the medical complexity confronted by children and their families (Berry, Hall, Cohen, O'Neill, & Feudtner, 2015).

CHILDREN WITH MCC: HEALTHCARE UTILIZATION

The increasing numbers of children with MCC are placing newer and greater demands on healthcare resources, requiring members of the healthcare team to refocus their efforts in order to provide well-coordinated care that is comprehensive and maximizes the child's developmental potential (Burke & Alverson, 2010). The chronicity and complexity of their health status has resulted in a parallel increase in the number of healthcare services utilized by these children, including the need for medical management by multiple subspecialists (Boyle et al., 2011). Parents report that their child sees an average of five subspecialists in addition to their primary care provider (Kuo et al., 2013). The complex relationships among the child's health status, functional limitations, and healthcare needs directly contribute to increased utilization of healthcare resources by these children (Berry et al., 2015).

Children with MCC account for a significant number of inpatient hospital days and use of hospital resources for management of comorbidities (Berry et al., 2013; Burns et al., 2010). Approximately 20% of all admissions to pediatric hospitals are attributed to these children (Berry, Bloom, Foley, & Palfrey, 2010; Simon et al., 2010), reflecting the increasing medical complexity associated with pediatric MCC (Cohen et al., 2011). A significant number of these hospital days are the result of repeated hospital admissions with a positive relationship between the medical complexity of the child's chronic illness and the number of rehospitalizations. In addition, reliance on indwelling devices, numbers of medications, and neuromuscular diagnoses are predictive of increased number of hospital days and probability for rehospitalization (Amin, Ford, Ghazarian, Love, & Cheng, 2016; Berry et al., 2011; Braddock, Leutgeb, Zhang, & Koop, 2015). Increasing complexity and dependence upon technology is associated with increased referral to home healthcare upon discharge (Berry et al., 2016).

Fragmentation of healthcare services, prolonged period of time waiting for specialist appointments, and inadequate communication among healthcare clinicians exacerbates the resource usage and costs associated with MCC (Hellander & Bhargavan, 2012). Disparities in healthcare quality and access to community-based services are associated with increasing complexity of the child's health status (Cheak-Zamora & Thullen, 2017; Rosen-Reynoso et al., 2016). Parents report either difficulty or delay in receiving needed services for their child (USDHHS, 2013). Importantly, as medical complexity increases there is a parallel increase in the number of unmet healthcare needs (Houtrow, Okumura, Hilton, & Rehm, 2011; Kuo et al., 2014).

This is concerning because parents report that their child's condition changes frequently, often necessitating healthcare intervention (Houtrow et al., 2011). Adding to the frustration associated with unmet healthcare needs, parents also experience dissatisfaction with the healthcare provided to their child (Kuo et al., 2015) as well as inadequate care coordination among healthcare clinicians (Golden & Nageswaran, 2012; Houtrow et al., 2011).

Children with MCC are typically discharged into the care of pediatric primary care clinicians (Burke & Alverson, 2010). However, there is growing concern that families will struggle to find a primary care provider since fewer pediatricians are willing to accept these children into their practice (Agrawal et al., 2013). When children with MCC become ill, an estimated 25% of these children are treated in a clinic, health center, or emergency department instead of by a primary care provider (USDHHS, 2013), thereby increasing the fragmentation of their care. Frequently children are referred to a subspecialist following an acute illness visit. However, parents report difficulties in making an appointment with a subspecialist when a referral is made (Amin et al., 2016; Bethell et al., 2011). Maximizing the health of children with MCC is predicated upon equal and ready access to needed healthcare services as well as continuity of care. Unfortunately, for many of these children access to these services is difficult because of geographic barriers, limited availability of services, health insurance coverage, and turnover in healthcare clinicians (Bethell et al., 2011).

Summary

Children with MCC require the coordination of numerous healthcare services for effective management of their chronic health needs. However, increasing complexity is an important determinant in receiving much needed healthcare services (Kuo et al., 2014). Maintaining the child in the home environment necessitates meeting healthcare needs, optimally managing acute illness, and minimizing exacerbation of their chronic illness through coordinated outpatient care (Berry et al., 2011). Unmet healthcare needs, coupled with a lack of care coordination, impacts the health and quality of life of children with MCC, resulting in hospitalization/rehospitalization.

GOAL SETTING WITH PARENTS

Parents are the primary caregivers for children with MCC who are cared for in the home environment and, thus, are responsible for decisions related to their child's care. Parents acknowledge that managing their child in the home necessitates a reenvisioning of the parental role and assuming a variety of roles (Woodgate, Edwards, Ripat, Borton, & Rempel, 2015). These roles require a different set of parental competencies that are complex and differ from those for a normally developing child (Burkhard, 2013; Manhas & Mitchell, 2012). They spend a significant amount of time each week participating in advanced healthcare activities (e.g., suctioning a tracheostomy) that are critical to their child's survival (McDonald, McKinlay, Keeling, & Levack, 2015; Romley et al., 2017). Successful management of their child's complex care is contingent upon parental knowledge and confidence in their ability to provide the necessary care. Parents report that they do not always receive effective education (Amin et al., 2016) and the education is often not individualized to their child (McDonald, McKinlay, Keeling, & Levack, 2016). The lack of individualized education may be a reflection of the healthcare provider's limited knowledge related to the child's MCC or not giving serious consideration to child-related information provided by parents (Drainoni et al., 2006).

An initial, but critical, step is to engage in collaborative goal setting with the parents as the planned goals for the child will lay the foundation for the knowledge parents will need to effectively care for their child. Parental confidence in managing their child's care is enhanced when they participate in mutual goal setting (Lindblad, Rasmussen, & Sandman, 2005). Parents perceive that effective goal setting for their child involves sharing their goal ideas, participating in developing short- and long-term goals, and ensuring that all involved in their child's care have a shared vision (Terwiel et al., 2017). Importantly, as the child's medical complexity increases, the number of decisions to be made and goals to be set increases (Hubner, Feldman, & Huffman, 2016). Goal setting and acquisition of knowledge will be a fluid process in response to the child's dynamic health status. Parents appreciate that goal setting is a process that will require prioritization, reassessment, and revision of goals in order to meet their child's complex needs (Forsingdal, St. John, Miller, Harvey, & Wearne, 2013).

Unfortunately, parents report a lack of consistency in being included as a partner in decisions related to their child's management plan. This exclusion is partially attributed to the complexity of their child's care (Butler, Elkins, Kowalkowski, & Raphael, 2015; Cheak-Zamora & Thullen, 2017; Hubner et al., 2016) and contributes to the dissatisfaction parents express related to the management of their child's healthcare (Hayles, Harvey, Plummer, & Jones, 2015). Parents want healthcare clinicians to take a holistic view of their child and that includes having a thorough knowledge of the child (Miller et al., 2009) and viewing parents as important partners (Forsingdal et al., 2013; Golden & Nageswaran, 2012; Terwiel et al., 2017). Embracing the philosophy of collaborative goal setting has been associated with positive outcomes for the child (Brewer, Pollock, & Wright, 2014). In addition, hospitalizations, emergency department visits, and office visits are decreased when parents share in decision making related to their child's complex care (Fiks, Mayne, Localio, Alessandrini, & Guevara, 2012).

Healthcare clinicians need a working understanding of the goals parents envision for their child and for the knowledge they perceive is needed to effectively care for their child. Healthcare clinicians also need to understand how parents perceive the chronicity and complexity of their child's health status (Berry et al., 2015) as parents are keenly aware of the interdependent challenges associated with their child's care (Kuo & Houtrow, 2016). Effective goal setting will occur if healthcare clinicians appreciate that the extensiveness and unrelenting nature of parental caregiving and responsibilities are the context in which parental goal setting occurs (Carnevale, Rehm, Kirk, & McKeever, 2008). However, healthcare clinicians should also appreciate that, while parents desire to be involved in collaborative goal setting, the extent of their involvement may vary in response to the dynamic nature of their child's health status (Wiart, Ray, Darrah, & Magill-Evans, 2010) and that collaborative expectations are individualized to account for parental desire to participate (Forsingdal et al., 2013).

Collaborative goal setting and strategies to accomplish these goals must take into account the individuality of the child (Dodds & Rempel, 2016) and should be guided by the philosophy of maximizing the child's quality of life and developmental outcomes (Agrawal, 2015). However, consideration must take into account the family context and home environment in which the child resides since incorporation of the child's complex care requirements into the home challenging and may be restrictive for ideal therapies (Elias et al., 2012). Parents express concern when the management plan is not contextualized to the child's home environment (McDonald et al., 2016). Goal setting and planned interventions are most effective when perceived as realistic and achievable (Forsingdal et al., 2013; Øien, Fallang, & Østensjo, 2009) and designed within the context of the child's home environment (Brewer et al., 2014).

Dealing With Uncertainty

The reality for parents is that the chronicity and complexity of their child's health will most likely be lifelong and, in some instances, life limiting. For many children, the physical care requirements will not diminish and will increase as the child ages (Burkhard, 2013). Parents report that their child's healthcare needs are dynamic and continually evolving in response to the child's changing physiology and functional abilities (Hayles et al., 2015). Parental goal setting within the context of their child's MCC is impacted by the perceived uncertainty that surrounds the daily and long-term care of their child. Uncertainty is a multidimensional construct that occurs in response to situations perceived to be "ambiguous, complex, unpredictable, or probabilistic; when information is unavailable or inconsistent; and when people feel insecure in their own state of knowledge or the state of knowledge in general" (Brashers, 2001, p. 478).

Parental uncertainty is multifaceted and includes such factors as knowledge of the child's MCC and associated therapies and equipment needs, variable health/illness trajectory, recognition and management of acute exacerbations, navigating the complex healthcare environment, reframing expectations for "normal" child development and family life, unpredictability of the future, and transition from pediatric healthcare clinicians to adult healthcare clinicians. Importantly, there is a significant relationship between parental uncertainty and parental perceptions of caregiving demands (Chaney et al., 2016). The appraisal of these multiple factors will affect the level of uncertainty that parents experience. Because these multiple factors are interrelated, uncertainty associated with one factor cannot exist in isolation but exists in connection to other uncertainties (Babrow, 2001; Kerr & Haas, 2014). The uncertainty surrounding their child's health status is unsettling for parents and can be further heightened due to a lack of information and the inability to obtain definitive answers to address their concerns (Al-Yateem, Docherty, Altawil, Al-Tamimi, & Ahmad, 2017; Burkhard, 2013; Kerr & Haas, 2014; Manhas & Mitchell, 2012).

The complex nature of their child's health status results in uncertainty being integrated into the daily life of parents and, because uncertainty is chronic, necessitates that parents develop strategies to effectively adapt to this ever-present uncertainty (Kerr & Haas, 2014). How parents deal with uncertainty will impact their decision making and the management of their child's complex health needs (Al-Yateem et al., 2017). Researchers have demonstrated a relationship between parental uncertainty related to their child's chronic illness and self-reported psychological functioning with higher levels of uncertainty related to lower psychological functioning, while negative parental coping styles were associated with greater uncertainty (Szulczewski, Mullins, Bidwell, Eddington, & Pai, 2017). Thus, coping strategies employed to manage the uncertainty associated with their child's chronic health status become critical as lower psychological functioning may impact their child's well-being.

Navigating the Healthcare System

For parents of children with MCC, navigating the healthcare system is an enormous responsibility that impacts many aspects of their lives and influences parental goal setting. Children with MCC often require the care of a primary care provider; multiple medical and surgical subspecialists; home healthcare; rehabilitative and developmental therapists; specialized community-based services; multiple pharmaceutical therapies; nutritional and growth support; ongoing laboratory and diagnostic imaging services; and durable medical equipment to maintain optimal wellness and function (Cohen et al., 2011). The burden of navigating a complex network of care on families of children with MCC is depicted in the care map (Figure 8.1). Coordinating care and services for their children is further complicated by the dynamic nature of their child's growth, development, and medical conditions that constantly change the needs of families over time.

The Agency for Healthcare Research and Quality (AHRQ, 2014) defines care coordination as "the deliberate organization of patient care activities between two or more participants involved in a patient's care to facilitate the appropriate delivery of healthcare services . . . and is often managed by the exchange of information among participants responsible for different aspects of care." Parents of children with MCC report a median of

2 hours per week spent coordinating care for their children (Kuo, Cohen, Agrawal, Berry & Casey, 2011). Time spent coordinating care increases with the number and complexity of a child's MCC and the number of clinicians and services they require. Parents report that they struggle to ensure and maintain continuity and coordination among the varied and unique service clinicians, as they must serve as the conduit between different healthcare clinicians, institutions, and community-based services for the planning and provision of services (Miller et al., 2009). Part of navigating the healthcare system is dealing with variability in the quality of care provided by the various clinicians and agencies that deliver services, supplies, and equipment; and furthermore, navigating the system means persistently advocating with care clinicians and agencies (including insurance companies) for their children to receive the medical, psychosocial, and educational services they need (Golden & Nageswaran, 2012).

The difficulty in navigating services is further illustrated by the fact that families of children with MCC are more likely to have multiple unmet medical service needs (Kuo et al., 2011). Communicating with and across multiple healthcare clinicians is a pervasive stressor in the lives of parents of children with MCC. Parents report frustration from trying to obtain information from and share information with the many clinicians involved in the care of their children, resulting in delayed, or missed, care and adding to the stress of caregiving (Golden & Nageswaran, 2012). Parents feel that communication is an integral feature of positive experiences in ensuring continuity of care and relationship building throughout the complex network of care they must navigate (Miller et al., 2009).

Transition Into a School Setting

The Individuals With Disabilities Education Act (IDEA) mandates that children with disabilities have the right to a public education in the least restrictive environment possible (U.S. Department of Education, 2017). While parents want their child to attend school, much uncertainty surrounds this goal, necessitating the need for coordinated planning and decision making between all involved. Based upon their child's capabilities, parents must decide whether their child should be mainstreamed into a regular classroom, placed in a special education classroom, or attend a school specifically designed for children with a variety of disabilities (Mesman, Kuo, Carroll, & Ward, 2013). Once the decision is made, parents want to be active partners, as specified in the IDEA (Halfon, Houtrow, Larson, & Newacheck, 2012), in designing the educational plan and goals for their child (MacLeod, Causton, Radel, & Radel, 2017).

The transition from the home to the school setting requires coordination among the family, school faculty and support staff, home nursing, and the healthcare clinicians. Optimal communication among all involved can prevent breaks in the system and ensure continuity of care between the home and school, thus facilitating positive child outcomes (Rosen-Reynoso et al.,

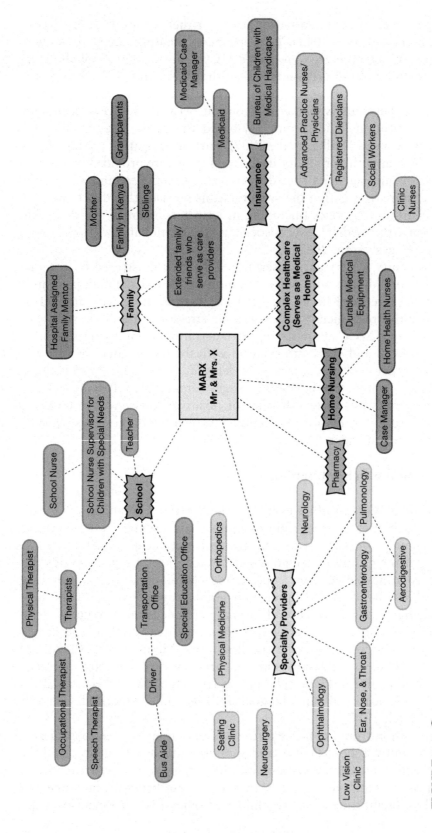

FIGURE 8.1 Care map.

2016). Parents have reported the importance of school personnel having knowledge of their child in order to effectively relate to their child in safe and supportive interactions. This knowledge comes from not only quality written communication but also through developing a relationship with the child and family that allows for understanding the unique behavioral and physiologic responses of the child (Miller et al., 2009).

Children with MCC enter school with complex healthcare needs requiring school staff to be proficient in managing the child's care requirements, such as medication administration, enteral feedings, and respiratory equipment. Individual variation in care requirements across children with MCC presents a challenge for the school nurse and other school staff and requires that school personnel are appropriately trained to manage the child's care (Singer, 2012). School nurses are concerned about having a sufficient amount of time to provide the necessary care to the child along with meeting the needs of other children (Singer, 2012). To address these concerns, the healthcare needs of the child should be incorporated into the education plan for the child so that the child can participate fully in school activities and school staff can arrange to have the necessary resources available to meet the child's needs (Elias et al., 2012).

COMPLEXITIES OF MANAGING THE CHILD AT HOME

The philosophy is that children with MCC are cared for in the home environment. The growth and development of these children is maximized when cared for in a loving and supportive home environment (Friedman & Norwood, 2016). However, adapting the home to accommodate their child's complex care needs, including functional and mobility issues, and managing their child's daily healthcare needs and activities of daily living presents multiple challenges. Daily life for families of children with MCC is fraught with significant physical, psychological, social–emotional, and financial burdens (Carnevale et al., 2008). Time is also an important consideration in managing the child's complex care in the home. Parents and healthcare clinicians need to be cognizant that, despite the parents' best intentions, the cumulative stressors that accompany caring for their child have the potential to impact the emotional climate of the home environment and, thus, the child's well-being (Goudie, Narcisse, Hall, & Kuo, 2014).

Demands on Parental Time

The time required to manage the various aspects of their child's care is significantly greater than the usual demands on parenting time. The complexity of the child's care impacts the amount of time required (Zan & Scharff, 2015) and parents have to be ready to provide additional care at any time (Woodgate et al., 2015). Parents report that a significant amount of time each day is devoted to the physical care of their child that includes hygiene, dressing, toileting, and feeding (McCann, Bull, & Winzenberg, 2012). The dependent nature of their child, including the need to complete various therapies and manage medical equipment, also increases the demand on their time (Romley et al., 2017; Whiting, 2014b). In addition, a substantial amount of hours are devoted to preparing their child for transportation, transporting their child to various appointments, and coordinating their child's care through communication with multiple healthcare and service clinicians. Parents often rely on a structured daily routine to manage the time demands (Davey, Imms, & Fossey, 2015). Importantly, the time spent caring for the child with MCC is time that could be devoted to other family responsibilities and social activities (Romley et al., 2017; Walter, DeCamp, Warrier, Murphy, & Keefer, 2013). Healthcare clinicians may find that parents are resistant to some of the goals for their child's in-home therapy because the parents do not possess the time capital to complete the therapies (Forsingdal et al., 2013). Parents and healthcare clinicians will need to collaborate on setting realistic goals for their child's care that is mindful of the parents' time requirements.

Adapting the Home

When the MCCs initially manifest, the immediate challenge is adapting the home environment. This is not a benign process for families. Numerous factors have to be considered including space needs, need for privacy, bathing and toileting, flow from room to room, mobility of the child, and storage of supplies and equipment. If the decision is made to structurally alter the home to accommodate the child's evolving growth and developmental needs, consideration must be given to how these needs will continue to evolve across time (Pierce, 2013; Roy, Rousseau, Allard, Feldman, & Majnemer, 2008).

Critical steps in adapting the home are to understand what meaning the concept of home has for the family, recognize that it is more than a physical space, and determine what the necessary adaptations mean for the siblings and family life (Chase, 2012; Morgan, Boniface, & Reagon, 2016). The space in the home and how it is to be used or modified is of concern to parents (Mayes, Cant, & Clemson, 2011). Initially, parents may not be ready to make too many adaptations, especially permanent ones, until they have experienced the child in the home environment and have a better understanding of how the child's care and mobility needs impact the home. This is important since effective adaptations can reduce the physical demands of caring for their child (Roy et al., 2008). It is important to note that families who reside in rental properties may not be able to make adaptations or may have to relocate in order to obtain the necessary adaptations (Morgan et al., 2016).

Medical supplies and equipment are ever-present in the home. Approximately 70% of children require medical equipment for survival and activities of daily living (Kuo et al., 2013). Parents have to consider how to position equipment within the home that allows the child to be a part of the social nature of the family but does not hinder family activities (Davey et al., 2015).

Just as important is that the home looks "normal." Families implement strategies to normalize the home as much as possible so that the environment does not look "medicalized" (Mayes et al., 2011; Morgan et al., 2016). This includes how their child's supplies and equipment are stored so that they are not readily visible (Carnevale, Alexander, Davis, Rennick, and Troini, 2006).

Physical Demands

Providing care to a child with MCC is physically demanding for caregivers and the burden increases as the child grows and functional and mobility capabilities decrease. Increasing the physical demands is the dependency of the child upon the parent to carry out those activities of daily living that a child of the same developmental age would be able to accomplish (Kuo & Houtrow, 2016). Parents are challenged by the unrelenting nature of the physical demands (Burkhard, 2013) and the need to be vigilant of their child's needs especially when the child is asleep (McCann, Bull, & Winzenberg, 2015).

Parents are often not afforded the opportunity to gain respite from the physically demanding care. Depending upon the child's needs, aspects of care continue around the clock. Children who have the highest care needs during the day also have the highest care needs at night (Bourke-Taylor, Pallant, Law, & Howie, 2013). The result is that parents experience interruptions in their nighttime sleep patterns, poor sleep quality, and less total sleep time (McBean & Schlosnagle, 2016; McDonald et al., 2016). The lack of sleep takes a toll on the parents and can impact parental physical and emotional health (Bourke-Taylor et al., 2013; McBean & Schlosnagle, 2016; Meltzer, Sanchez-Ortuno, Edinger, & Avis, 2015; Woodgate et al., 2015). Researchers have demonstrated an inverse relationship between psychological functioning (i.e., anxiety, depression, and stress) and quality of sleep in mothers of children with developmental disabilities (Chu & Richdale, 2009; Wayte, McCaughey, Holley, Annaz, & Hill, 2012). The impact of inadequate sleep on parental physical and emotional health can perpetuate a negative feedback loop where the difficulties in all three arenas continue to persist (McCann et al., 2015).

Emotional Roller Coaster

Providing care to a child with MCC is a stressful experience. Parental stress is heightened by chronic fatigue (McCann et al., 2015) and impacted by the functional and mobility capabilities of their child (Almogbel, Goyal, & Sansgiry, 2017). The uncertainty surrounding their child's MCC, coupled with the stressful nature of the caregiving demands associated with their child's condition, places parents on an emotional roller coaster. Parents report experiencing distress at their child's complex situation as well as report rewarding experiences (Carnevale et al., 2006). Ever-present for parents is the worry that their child can become acutely ill and die (Øien et al., 2009).

More importantly, parents live in fear that they may cause harm to their child from the therapies they perform or will miss the signs that their child is becoming acutely ill (Kerr & Haas, 2014). Contributing to their emotional journey, parents perform procedures on a regular basis that are distressing to the child and elicit a variety of emotions in the parents. Parents have to remain emotionally neutral during the procedure so they can perform it effectively and then manage the emotions they experience (McDonald et al., 2016).

Adding to the emotional journey of parents is confronting the dilemma of whether they can continue to care for their child at home. Families may come to a point where caring for their child at home is no longer safe or sustainable (Friedman & Norwood, 2016). Parents have to consider numerous factors in making the decision. The most common reasons that families cite for eventually placing their children in long-term, out-of-home residential care include around-the-clock caregiving, increasing complexity of care, lack of community and family resources, lack of financial resources, and emotional depletion of the family (Bruns, 2000; Llewellyn, Dunn, Fante, Turnbull, & Grace, 1999). Once the decision is made, parents experience conflicted emotions including guilt, sadness, and relief (Bruns, 2000).

Social Isolation

The social aspect of family life is impacted by the child with MCC. The unrelenting responsibilities of caregiving cause families to forfeit recreational time and other vital social functions. The risk is that families may become socially isolated. To consider a social outing, parents have to take into account transportation needs, the child's health status, critical supply and equipment needs, and potential architectural or structural barriers (Carnevale et al., 2008). Families cannot be spontaneous in taking advantage of social opportunities because of the detailed planning that goes into taking their child on a social outing (Davey et al., 2015; Woodgate et al., 2015). Families may find all of the necessary planning a deterrent to participating in social activities outside of the home, increasing the likelihood of social isolation. For families who do seek social opportunities, they have to ensure that the outings they choose accommodate the child's mobility, nutrition, and toileting needs (Davey et al., 2015).

Potentially contributing to social isolation is the appearance of the house. Families may not be comfortable with members of their social circle seeing the adaptations made to the home. Parents perceive that home adaptations make their child's MCC visible to visitors to the home (Roy et al., 2008). In addition, the mobility devices, especially a wheelchair, used by the child can leave marks on or damage to walls, doorways, floors, and furniture. Families may install protective devices, but they increase the visibility of their child's MCC (Mayes et al., 2011).

Respite care provides parents with an opportunity to take a break from caring for their child and participate in social activities. Taking advantage of periods of respite care decreases the stress and fatigue associated with caring for their child (Tétreault et al., 2014). However, obtaining respite care is a challenge due to the complex medical needs of their children. Parents report that obtaining respite care is a significant area of unmet need (Whiting, 2014a). They cannot rely on usual childcare alternatives because of the knowledge and psychomotor skills needed to effectively care for their child. Thus, parents often must locate and train their own respite care clinicians in order to participate in social activities and overcome feelings of social isolation (Mesman et al., 2013).

In considering social isolation, one has to also consider the impact on the individual child with MCC. Multiple avenues for social interaction, separate from the immediate family, have important ramifications for maximizing the child's development. However, the child's care requirements often limit opportunities for social interaction outside of the home environment (Mesman et al., 2013). The school setting provides an excellent opportunity for social interactions. However, children with MCC experience numerous school absences due to illness, medical appointments, and hospitalization (Zan & Scharff, 2015).

Financial Challenges

The family of a child with MCC confront several financial challenges. The stress from these challenges impacts the emotional health of parents (Goudie et al., 2014). Healthcare costs are significantly higher for children with MCC when compared to healthy children (Kuo et al., 2015; Zan & Scharff, 2015). The child's insurance coverage is often not sufficient to cover all expenses and places a financial burden on the family. In addition, there may be lifetime limits imposed by the insurance company (Walter et al., 2013). Parents report financial strain from multiple out-of-pocket medical expenses increasing their healthcare expenditures (Kuo et al., 2011). Continued parental employment becomes precarious. Parents of children with MCC report high rates of unemployment/underemployment. Oftentimes a parent, most often the mother, has to stop working or significantly reduce work hours in order to care for the child, thus adding to the financial burden (Kuo et al., 2011; Romley et al., 2017). This greatly limits the family's financial resources. In addition, the limited financial resources may prevent families from making the desired adaptations to the home or securing necessary equipment (Davey et al., 2015), resulting in families constructing their own adaptations, such as a wheelchair ramp, that may violate safety standards (Roy et al., 2008).

Summary

Parents strive to provide a supportive home environment for their child that maximizes their child's growth and development. However, caring for children with MCC presents numerous challenges for parents.

Accompanying these challenges are the uncertainties that surround their child's daily and long-term care. For parents, the unrelenting nature of their child's complex care is ever-present and adds to their caregiving burden (Bourke-Taylor et al., 2013). Guided participation provides a mechanism for mutual goal setting and assisting families with managing the complexities of the journey that they are on with their child.

Case Example 8.1

Marx is a 12-year-old who presents to the clinic with his uncle Mr. X to establish a primary care provider. He was referred by the emergency department following evaluation for seizure activity. Marx is new to this specific healthcare system and the diagnoses listed in the electronic medical record are seizure disorder and global developmental delay. Marx was born in Washington, DC, after an uncomplicated pregnancy to a healthy mother and was discharged home with his mother. At about 2 weeks of age, Marx was admitted for seizure activity and was discharged home on phenobarbital after a 2-week hospital stay. He and his mother moved to her home in Kenya approximately 1 month later. Marx was relocated to the United States from Kenya 1 month prior to this visit to live with his aunt and uncle, Mr. and Mrs. X, who are now his legal guardians. They stated the healthcare system in his home country was less than adequate and there were no rehabilitative or educational services available to meet Marx's needs.

There have been no changes to Marx's plan of care since moving to Kenya. He remains on phenobarbital, and the dose has been adjusted with age. He has never attended school or received any therapies. Marx has not achieved any developmental milestones beyond rolling over and modified army crawl. He takes all food orally. His uncle reports that they cut Marx's food into small pieces but it is an extremely slow process. He drinks from an open cup with assistance but does better with a straw. Marx experiences intermittent episodes of vomiting with and without cough. Mr. X reports the wheelchair they are currently using was given to them secondhand. Marx did not have a wheelchair or any other medical equipment in Kenya. Phenobarbital is his only medication. Mr. X verbalizes frustration with trying to obtain healthcare for Marx. He states that it is not easy to access services and this is what led to the emergency room visit. Mr. X has not yet received a medical card for Marx and has not been able to take him to a healthcare provider. He ran out of Marx's phenobarbital.

Marx is nonambulatory and nonverbal. He is slouched in a donated wheelchair that is too large and has no restraint mechanisms or footrests. He requires frequent repositioning. Marx expresses pain through facial grimacing and/or crying and kicks the floor or wall to communicate that he is hungry or wet. Mr. X interprets Marx's frequent moving as attempts to reposition himself to reach a surface to kick. He is thin and has minimal subcutaneous tissue, and his weight is at less than the tenth percentile.

Marx has contractures at the hips, knees, ankles, elbows, and wrists and nonpurposeful movement of all four extremities. There is also some spasticity of the lower extremities. He has generalized hypotonia with poor head control and truncal tone and is unable to sit unsupported. He smiles intermittently when his uncle is talking, but does not make eye contact. Marx had an abnormal EEG in the emergency department and was given a refill on his phenobarbital. A referral had been sent to neurology and an appointment made.

Mr. X also shared his frustration with Marx's poor sleep habits that has resulted in significant loss of sleep for himself as well. Marx is staying with another family member when there is a gap in care between Mr. X and his wife, and sometimes falls asleep while waiting for Mr. or Mrs. X to pick him up. Mr. X is enrolled in school during the day and works in the evening, and Mrs. X works evenings. The family caregiver is now expressing concern about continuing to care for him because of the level of attention he needs and is especially concerned about his seizure activity.

During this initial visit, the advanced practice nurse guide began the process of developing a relationship with this family. A fundamental level of trust was developed as the nurse guide efficiently and professionally initiated the appropriate treatments and referrals to address the immediate needs based on the initial interview and identified by the family and the nurse together. Because of the complexity of this child's health needs, he and his family would experience interactions with multiple health, social, and educational services (see Figure 8.1). Following considerable discussion, the guide and family determined that Marx needed the following services immediately:

1. MRI of his brain to assess for causes for his underlying condition
2. Video swallow study (VSS) to assess for dysphagia
3. Dual-energy x-ray absorptiometry (DEXA) scan to assess bone density secondary to his nonambulatory status
4. Referral to physical, occupational, and speech therapies
5. Referral to physical medicine to address contractures, need for orthotics
6. Referral to the seating clinic for an appropriate wheelchair
7. Social work to assist in determining status of medical card so that the previously listed services can be obtained
8. Discussion with dietician regarding appropriate dietary supplements until VSS can be obtained
9. Immunizations and tuberculosis (TB) test

Although the sleep issue was a major concern for this family, both Mr. X and Marx were fatigued with this relatively long initial appointment. The nurse guide worked on creating a shared understanding by talking briefly with Mr. X about the common occurrence of sleep disturbance in children with neurodevelopmental disorders such as Marx's (Robinson-Shelton & Malow, 2016; Sandella, O'Brien, Shank, & Warschausky, 2011), and that there were options that may improve Marx's current sleep pattern. The nurse guide encouraged them to return soon to work together on improving sleep for the family. This process of maintaining joint attention and creating a shared understanding strengthened the growing relationship between Mr. X and the guide and supported the family's efforts to care for Marx.

Mr. X and Marx returned 1 month later with continued complaints of poor sleep with resultant fatigue for Mr. X that was affecting his academic and work performance. The nurse guide elicited a thorough history related to the sleep issue in order to build a bridge between what was currently occurring and what type of interventions might be needed. Mr. X reported sleeping on a bed in Marx's room or on the couch in the living room. Mr. X is unable to leave Marx unattended in the bed because he moves frequently and has fallen out of the bed. Marx will only sleep if someone is beside him, and he does not have a consistent bedtime. Marx sleeps frequently during the day and wakes repeatedly at night. A major problem is that Marx is often sleeping when Mr. X picks him up at the family caregiver's home near midnight when he finishes his shift at work. Marx awakens and has difficulty going back to sleep after arriving home.

After making sure there was a shared understanding of the issue, the guide talked with Mr. X about sleep hygiene, which refers to routine parent and child behaviors or habits that occur before bedtime and are modifiable to promote quality sleep (Mindell, Meltzer, Carskadon, & Chervin, 2009). The information was provided in an engaging, informal manner with multiple opportunities and invitations for questions and comments by Mr. X. This approach allowed additional bridging of previous habits with routines shown to improve sleep. In this case, the guide needed to focus on modifications of traditional sleep hygiene concepts to ensure their appropriateness for children with neurodevelopmental disorders (Blackmer & Feinstein, 2016). As each idea was suggested by the guide, such as establishing a routine for activity during the day and sleep rituals at night, she encouraged Mr. X to think about and share how this may be accomplished given their particular circumstances and what barriers might exist. This joint problem solving enabled Mr. X to work out alterations in the plan and receive immediate feedback on the potential impact on this child's sleep hygiene. In this way, several recommendations were discussed including exposure to natural light during the day, staying out of bed during the day, and creating a quiet environment in the bedroom with special attention to remove blue light sources in the bedroom that may disrupt sleep. In addition to these behavioral changes, the nurse guide initiated discussion about using melatonin to help Marx fall asleep more easily, a recommended treatment for sleep issues in children with neurodevelopmental disabilities (Schwichtenberg & Malow, 2015). The guide carefully explained how melatonin was used and optimal times for administering it, which is about an hour before bedtime.

The guide and Mr. X then talked about how to best use melatonin given the frequency of bedtime occurring when Marx was with the family caregiver. This discussion brought up the larger issue of how Mr. X could support the family caregiver who was caring for Marx several days a week at bedtime when Mr. and Mrs. X were working. Mr. X expressed concern about asking too much of this family caregiver and not wanting to burden her more. The guide validated his concerns, and together they brain-stormed as to how this could be managed. Two primary plans of action resulted. One was to ask the family caregiver to come in with Mr. X and Marx to discuss the sleep issue with the guide. Although this appointment may be seen as a burden for the family caregiver, it also provides the opportunity for the family caregiver to share her own perceptions and ideas about how to address the sleep problem, with the nurse guiding and supporting both of them with this discussion. The second plan of action was for the nurse guide to investigate the potential for in-home nursing services to provide much-needed respite for this family. At the end of the visit, Mr. X stated he felt more hopeful that the sleep issue could be improved, yet also verbalized recognition that this would be a process and change may not be seen quickly. The guide offered positive feedback for Mr. X's care of Marx and confirmed he knew how best to reach her for additional questions and concerns. They arranged to have a follow-up appointment in 4 weeks.

CONCLUSION

The guide anticipated that several follow-up visits would be needed and possibly telephone contact between visits to continue developing the relationship, bridging what was known and unknown, continued teaching about possible interventions to improve sleep and helping the family structure these tasks, and gradually transferring responsibility for managing the sleep issue to Mr. and Mrs. X. Working through the process of guided participation may not only help Mr. and Mrs. X develop competency in improving sleep but may also serve as a template for work on other issues that will now come to the forefront for this child with very complex health and developmental needs.

REFERENCES

Agency for Health Care Research and Quality (AHRQ). (2014). *Chapter 2: What is care coordination?* Rockville, MD: Author. Retrieved from http://www.ahrq.gov/professionals/prevention-chronic-care/improve/coordination/atlas2014/chapter2.html

Agrawal, R. (2015). Complex care in pediatrics: Great progress, great challenges. *Journal of Pediatric Rehabilitation Medicine, 8*, 71–74. doi:10.3233/PRM-150331

Agrawal, R., Shah, P., Zebracki, K., Sanabria, K., Kohrman, C., & Kohrman, A. F. (2013). The capacity of primary care pediatricians to care for children with special health care needs. *Clinical Pediatrics, 52*, 310–314. doi:10.1177/0009922813476572

Almogbel, Y., Goyal, R., & Sansgiry, S. (2017). Association between parenting stress and functional impairment among children diagnosed with neurodevelopmental disorders. *Community Mental Health Journal, 53*, 405–414. doi:10.1007/s10597-017-0096-9

Al-Yateem, N., Docherty, C., Altawil, H., Al-Tamimi, M., & Ahmad, A. (2017). The quality of information received by parents of children with chronic ill health attending hospitals as indicated by measures of illness uncertainty. *Scandinavian Journal of Caring Sciences*, Advance online publication. doi:10.1111/scs.12405

Amin, D., Ford, R., Ghazarian, S. R., Love, B., & Cheng, T. L. (2016). Parent and physician perceptions regarding preventability of pediatric readmissions. *Hospital Pediatrics, 6*, 80–87. doi:10.1542/hpeds.2015-0059

Babrow, A. S. (2001). Uncertainty, value, communication, and problematic integration. *Journal of Communication, 51*, 553–573. doi:10.1111/j.1460-2466.2001.tb02896.x

Berry, J. G., Bloom, S., Foley, S., & Palfrey, J. S. (2010). Health inequity in children and youth with chronic health conditions. *Pediatrics, 126*(Suppl. 3), 111–119. doi:10.1542/peds.2010-1466D

Berry, J. G., Hall, M., Cohen, E., O'Neill, M., & Feudtner, C. (2015). Ways to identify children with medical complexity and the importance of why. *Journal of Pediatrics, 167*, 229–237. doi:10.1016/j.peds.2015.04.068

Berry, J. G., Hall, M., Dumas, H., Simpser, E., Whitford, K., Wilson, K. M., . . . O'Brien, J. (2016). Pediatric hospital discharges to home health and postacute facility care: A national study. *JAMA Pediatrics, 170*, 326–333. doi:10.1001/jamapediatrics.2015.4836

Berry, J. G., Hall, M., Hall, D. E., Kuo, D. Z., Cohen, E., Agrawal, R., . . . Neff, J. (2013). Inpatient growth and resource use in 28 children's hospitals: A longitudinal, multi-institutional study. *JAMA Pediatrics, 167*, 170–177. doi:10.1001/jamapediatrics.2013.432

Berry, J. G., Hall, D. E., Kuo, D. Z., Cohen, E., Agrawal, R., ... Neff, J. (2011). Hospital utilization and characteristics of patients experiencing recurrent readmissions within children's hospitals. *JAMA, 305*, 682–690. doi:10.1001/jamapediatrics.2011.122

Bethell, C. D., Kogan, M. D., Strickland, B. B., Schor, E. L., Robertson, J., & Newacheck, P. W. (2011). A national and state profile of leading health problems and health care quality for U.S. children: Key insurance disparities and across-state variations. *Academic Pediatrics, 11*, S22–S33. doi:10.1016/j.acap.2010.08.011

Blackmer, A. B., & Feinstein, J. A. (2016). Management of sleep disorders in children with neurodevelopmental disorders: A review. *Pharmacotherapy, 36*, 84–98. doi:10.1002/phar.1686

Bourke-Taylor, H., Pallant, J. F., Law, M., & Howie, L. (2013). Relationships between sleep disruptions, health and care responsibilities among mothers of school-aged children with disabilities. *Journal of Paediatrics and Child Health, 49*, 775–782. doi:10.1111/jpc.12254

Boyle, C. A., Boulet, S., Schieve, L. A., Cohen, R. A., Blumberg, S. J., Yeargin-Allsopp, M., . . . Kogan, M. D. (2011). Trends in the prevalence of developmental disabilities in U.S. children, 1997-2008. *Pediatrics, 127*, 1034–1042. doi:10.1542/peds.2010-2989

Braddock, M. E., Leutgeb, V., Zhang, L., & Koop, S. E. (2015). Factors influencing recurrent admissions among children with disabilities in a specialty children's hospital. *Journal of Pediatric Rehabilitation Medicine, 8*, 131–139. doi:10.3233/PRM-150326

Brashers, D. E. (2001). Communication and uncertainty management. *Journal of Communication, 51*, 477–497. doi:10.1111/j.1460-2466.2001.tb02892.x

Brewer, K., Pollock, N., & Wright, F. V. (2014). Addressing the challenges of collaborative goal setting with children and their families. *Physical & Occupational Therapy in Pediatrics, 34*, 138–152. doi: 10.3109/01942638.2013.794187

Bruns, D. A. (2000). Leaving home at an early age: Parents' decisions about out-of-home placement for young children with complex medical needs. *Mental Retardation, 38*, 50–60. doi:10.1352/0047-6765(2000)038<0050:LHAAEA>2.0.CO;2

Burke, R. T., & Alverson, B. (2010). Impact of children with medically complex conditions. *Pediatrics, 126*, 789–790. doi:10.1542/peds.2010-1885

Burkhard, A. (2013). A different life: Caring for an adolescent or young adult with severe cerebral palsy. *Journal of Pediatric Nursing, 28*, 357–363. doi:10.1016/j.pedn.2013.01.001

Burns, K. H., Casey, P. H., Lyle, R. E., Bird, M., Fussell, J. J., & Robbins, J. M. (2010). Increasing prevalence of medically complex children in U.S. hospitals. *Pediatrics, 126*, 638–646. doi:10.1542/peds.2009-1658

Butler, A. M., Elkins, S., Kowalkowski, M., & Raphael, J. L. (2015). Shared decision making among parents of children with mental health conditions compared to children with chronic physical conditions. *Maternal and Child Health Journal, 19*, 410–418. doi:10.1007/s10995-014-1523-y

Carnevale, F. A., Alexander, E., Davis, M., Rennick, J., & Troini, R. (2006). Daily living with distress and enrichment: The moral experience of families with ventilator-assisted children at home. *Pediatrics, 117*, e48–e60. doi:10.1542/peds.2005-0789

Carnevale, F. A., Rehm, R. S., Kirk, S., & McKeever, P. (2008). What we know (and do not know) about raising children with complex continuing care needs. *Journal of Child Health Care, 12*, 4–6. doi:10.1177/1367493508088552

Chaney, J. M., Gamwell, K. L., Baraldi, A. N., Ramsey, R. R., Cushing, C. C., Mullins, A. J., . . . Mullins, L. J. (2016). Parent perceptions of illness uncertainty and child depressive symptoms in juvenile rheumatic diseases: Examining caregiver demand and parent distress as mediators. *Journal of Pediatric Psychology, 41*, 941–951. doi:10.1093/jpepsy/jsw004

Chase, C. A. (2012). Beyond the basics in home modification for the pediatric client. *Rehab Management, 25*, 32–35.

Cheak-Zamora, N. C., & Thullen, M. (2017). Disparities in quality and access to care for children with developmental disabilities and multiple health conditions. *Maternal and Child Health Journal, 21*, 36–44. doi:10.1007/s10995-016-2091-0

Chu, J., & Richdale, A. L. (2009). Sleep quality and psychological wellbeing in mothers of children with developmental disabilities. *Research in Developmental Disabilities, 30*, 1512–1522. doi:10.1016/j.ridd.2009.07.007

Cohen, E., Berry, J. G., Camacho, X., Anderson, G., Wodchis, W., & Guttmann, A. (2012). Patterns and costs of health care use of children with medical complexity. *Pediatrics, 130*, e1463-e1470. doi:10.1542/peds.2012-0175

Cohen, E., Kuo, D. Z., Agrawal, R., Berry, J. G., Bhagat, S. K., Simon, T. D., & Srivastava, R. (2011). Children with medical complexity: An emerging population for clinical and research initiatives. *Pediatrics, 127*, 529–538. doi:10.1542/peds.2010-0910

Davey, H., Imms, C., & Fossey, E. (2015). "Our child's significant disability shapes our lives": Experiences of family social participation. *Disability and Rehabilitation, 37*, 2264–2271. doi:10.3109/09638288.2015

Dodds, C., & Rempel, G. (2016). A quality of life model promotes enablement for children with medical complexity. *Journal of Pediatric Rehabilitation Medicine, 9*, 253–255. doi:10.3233/PRM-160402

Drainoni, M.-L., Lee-Hood, E., Tobias, C., Bachman, S. S., Andrew, J., & Maisels, L. (2006). Cross-disability experiences of barriers to health-care access. *Journal of Disability Policy Studies, 17*, 101–115.

Elias, E. R., Murphy, N. A., & Council on Children with Disabilities. (2012). Home care of children and youth with complex health care needs and technology dependencies. *Pediatrics, 129*, 996–1005. doi:10.1542/peds.2012-0606

Fiks, A. G., Mayne, S., Localio, A. R., Alessandrini, E. A., & Guevara, J. P. (2012). Shared decision making and health care expenditures among children with special health care needs. *Pediatrics, 129*, 99–107. doi:10.1542/peds.2011-1352

Forsingdal, S., St. John, W., Miller, V., Harvey, A., & Wearne, P. (2013). Goal setting with mothers in child development services. *Child: Care, Health and Development, 40*, 587–596. doi:10.1111/cch.12075

Friedman, S. L., Norwood, K. W., & Council on Children with Disabilities. (2016). Out-of-home placement for children and adolescents with disabilities—Addendum: Care options for children and adolescents with disabilities and medical complexity. *Pediatrics, 138*, e20163216. doi:10.1542/peds.2016.3216

Golden, S. L., & Nageswaran, S. (2012). Caregiver voices: Coordinating care for children with complex chronic conditions. *Clinical Pediatrics, 51*, 723–729. doi:10.1177/0009922812445920

Goudie, A., Narcisse, M.-R., Hall, D. E., & Kuo, D. Z. (2014). Financial and psychological stressors associated with caring for children with disability. *Families, Systems, & Health, 32*, 280–290. doi:10.1037/fsh0000027

Halfon, N., Houtrow, A., Larson, K., & Newacheck, P. W. (2012). The changing landscape of disability in childhood. *The Future of Children, 22*, 13–42.

Hayles, E., Harvey, D., Plummer, D., & Jones, A. (2015). Parents' experiences of health care for their children with cerebral palsy. *Qualitative Health Research, 25*, 1139–1154. doi:10.1177/1049732315570122

Hellander, I., & Bhargavan, R. (2012). Report from the United States: The U.S. health crisis deepens amid rising inequality—A review of data, fall 2011. *International Journal of Health Services, 42*, 161–175. doi:10.2190/HS.42.2.a

Houtrow, A. J., Okumura, M. J., Hilton, J. F., & Rehm, R. S. (2011). Profiling health and health related services for children with special health care needs with and without disabilities. *Academic Pediatrics, 11*, 508–516. doi:10.1016/j.acap.2011.08.004

Hubner, L. M., Feldman, H. M., & Huffman, L. C. (2016). Parent-reported shared decision making: Autism spectrum disorder and other neurodevelopmental disorders. *Journal of Developmental & Behavioral Pediatrics, 37*, 20–32. doi:10.1097/DBP.0000000000000242

Kerr, A. M., & Haas, S. M. (2014). Parental uncertainty in illness: Managing uncertainty surrounding an "orphan" illness. *Journal of Pediatric Nursing, 29*, 393–400. doi:10.1016/j.pedn.2014.01.008

Kuo, D. Z., Cohen, E., Agrawal, R., Berry, J. G., & Casey, P. H. (2011). A national profile of caregiver challenges among more medically complex children with special health care needs. *Archives of Pediatric & Adolescent Medicine, 165*, 1020–1026. doi:10.1001/archpediatrics.2011.172

Kuo, D., Goudie, A., Cohen, E., Houtrow, A., Agrawal, R., Carle, A. C., & Wells, N. (2014). Inequities in health care needs for children with medical complexity. *Health Affairs, 33*, 2190–2198. doi:10.1377/hlthaff.2014.0273

Kuo, D. Z., & Houtrow, A. J. (2016). Recognition and management of medical complexity. *Pediatrics, 138*, e1–e13. doi:10.1542/peds.2016-3021

Kuo, D. Z., Melguizo-Castro, M., Goudie, A., Nick, T. G., Robbins, J. M., & Casey, P. H. (2015). Variation in child health care utilization by medical complexity. *Maternal Child Health Journal, 19,* 40–48. doi:10.1007/s1095-014-1493-0

Kuo, D. Z., Robbins, J. M., Lyle, R. E., Barrett, K. W., Burns, K. H., & Casey, P. H. (2013). Parent-reported outcomes of comprehensive care for children with medical complexity. *Families, Systems, & Health, 31,* 132–141. doi:10.1037/a0032341

Liberman, D. B., Song, E., Radbill, L. M., Pham, P. K., & Derrington, S. F. (2016). Early introduction of palliative care and advanced care planning for children with complex chronic medical conditions: A pilot study. *Child: Care, Health and Development, 42,* 439–449. doi:10.1111/cch.12332

Lindblad, B. M., Rasmussen, B. H., & Sandman, P. O. (2005). Being invigorating in parenthood: Parents' experiences of being supported by professionals when having a disabled child. *Journal of Pediatric Nursing, 20,* 288–297. doi:10.1016/j.pedn.2005.04.015

Llewellyn, G., Dunn, P., Fante, M., Turnbull, L., & Grace, R. (1999). Family factors of influencing out-of-home placement decisions. *Journal of Intellectual Disabilities Research, 43*(pt 3), 219–233. doi:10.1046/j.1365-2788.1999.00189.x

MacLeod, K., Causton, J. N., Radel, M., & Radel, P. (2017). Rethinking the individualized education plan process: Voices from the other side of the table. *Disability & Society, 32,* 381–400. doi:10.1080/09687599.2017.1294048

Manhas, K. P., & Mitchell, I. (2012). Extremes, uncertainty, and responsibility across boundaries: Facets and challenges of the experience of transition to complex, pediatric home care. *Journal of Child Health Care, 16,* 224–236. doi:10.1177/1367493511430677

Mayes, R., Cant, R., & Clemson, L. (2011). The home and caregiving: Rethinking space and its meaning. *OTJR: Occupation, Participation and Health, 31,* 15–22. doi:10.3928/15394492-20100122-01

McBean, A. L., & Schlosnagle, L. (2016). Sleep, health and memory: Comparing parents of typically developing children and parents of children with special health-care needs. *Journal of Sleep Research, 25,* 78–87. doi:10.1111/jsr.12329

McCann, D., Bull, R., & Winzenberg, T. (2012). The daily patterns of time use for parents of children with complex needs: A systematic review. *Journal of Child Health Care, 16,* 26–52. doi:10.1177/1367493511420186

McCann, D., Bull, R., & Winzenberg, T. (2015). Sleep deprivation in parents caring for children with complex needs at home: A mixed methods systematic review. *Journal of Family Nursing, 21,* 86–118. doi:10.1177/1074840714562026

McDonald, J., McKinlay, E., Keeling, S., & Levack, W. (2015). How family carers engage with technical health procedures in the home: A grounded theory study. *BMJ Open, 5,* e007761. doi:10.1136/bmjopen-2015-007761

McDonald, J., McKinlay, E., Keeling, S., & Levack, W. (2016). Becoming an expert carer: The process of family carers learning to manage technical health procedures at home. *Journal of Advanced Nursing, 72,* 2173–2184. doi:10.1111/jan.12984

Meltzer, L. J., Sanchez-Ortuno, M. J., Edinger, J. D., & Avis, K. T. (2015). Sleep patterns, sleep instability, and health related quality of life in parents of ventilator-assisted children. *Journal of Clinical Sleep Medicine, 15,* 251–258. doi:10.5664/jcsm.4538

Mesman, G. R., Kuo, D. Z., Carroll, J. L., & Ward, W. L. (2013). The impact of technology dependence on children and their families. *Journal of Pediatric Health Care, 27,* 451–459. doi:10.1016.j.pedhc.2012.05.003

Miller, A. R., Condin, C. J., McKellin, W. H., Shaw, N., Klassen, A. F., & Sheps, S. (2009). Continuity of care for children with complex chronic health conditions: Parents' perspectives. *BMC Health Services Research, 9,* 242. doi:10.1186/1472-6963-9-242

Mindell, J. A., Meltzer, L. J., Carskadon, M. A., & Chervin, R. D. (2009). Developmental aspects of sleep hygiene: Findings from the 2004 National Sleep Foundation Sleep in America Poll. *Sleep Medicine, 10,* 771–779. doi:10.1016/j.sleep.2008.07.016

Morgan, D. J., Boniface, G. E., & Reagon, C. (2016). The effects of adapting their home on the meaning of home for families with a disabled child. *Disability & Society, 31,* 481–496.

Øien, I., Fallang, B., & Østensjo, S. (2009). Goal-setting in paediatric rehabilitation: Perceptions of parents and professional. *Child: Care, Health and Development, 36,* 558–565. doi:10.1080/09687599.2016.1183475

Pierce, D. (2013). Designing a child-centered and accessible home. *Exceptional Parent, 43,* 28–32.

Robinson-Shelton, A., & Malow, B. A. (2016). Sleep disturbances in neurodevelopmental disorders. *Current Psychiatry Reports, 18,* 6. doi:10.1007/s11920-015-0638-1

Romley, J. A., Shah, A. K., Chung, P. J., Elliot, M. N., Vestal, K. D., & Schuster, M. A. (2017). Family-provided health care for children with special health care needs. *Pediatrics, 139*, e20161287. doi:10.1542/peds.2016-1287

Rosen-Reynoso, M., Porche, M. V., Kwan, N., Bethell, C., Thomas, V., Robertson, J., . . . Palfrey, J. (2016). Disparities in access to easy-to-use services for children with special health care needs. *Maternal and Child Health Journal, 20*, 1041–1053. doi:10.1007/s10995-015-1890-z

Roy, L., Rousseau, J., Allard, H., Feldman, D., & Majnemer, A. (2008). Parental experience of home adaptation for children with motor disabilities. *Physical & Occupational Therapy in Pediatrics, 28*, 353–368. doi:10.1080/01942630802307101

Sandella, D. E., O'Brien, L. M., Shank, L. K., & Warschausky, S. A. (2011). Sleep and quality of life in children with cerebral palsy. *Sleep Medicine, 12*, 252–256. doi:10.1016/j.sleep.2010.07.019

Schwichtenberg, A. J., & Malow, B. A. (2015). Melatonin treatment in children with developmental disabilities. *Sleep Medicine Clinics, 10*, 181–187. doi:10.1016/j.jsmc.2015.02.008

Simon, T. D., Berry, J., Feudtner, C., Stone, B. L., Sheng, X., Bratton, S. L., . . . Srivastava, R. (2010). Children with complex chronic conditions in inpatient hospital settings in the United States. *Pediatrics, 126*, 647–655. doi:10.1542/peds/2009-3266

Singer, B. (2012). Perceptions of school nurses in the care of students with disabilities. *Journal of School Nursing, 29*, 329–336. doi:10.1177/1059840512462402

Szulczewski, L., Mullins, L. L., Bidwell, S. L., Eddington, A. R., & Pai, A. L. H. (2017). Meta-analysis: Caregiver and youth uncertainty in pediatric chronic illness. *Journal of Pediatric Psychology, 42*, 395–421. doi:10.1093/jpepsy/jsw097

Terwiel, M., Alsem, M. W., Siebes, R. C., Bieleman, K., Verhoef, M., & Ketelaar, M. (2017). Family-centred service: Differences in what parents of children with cerebral palsy rate important. *Child: Care, Health and Development*. Advance online publication. doi:10.1111/cch.12460

Tétreault, S., Blais-Michaud, S., Deschênes, P. M., Beaupré, P., Gascon, H., Boucher, N., & Carrière, M. (2014). How to support families of children with disabilities? An exploratory study of social support services. *Child & Family Social Work, 19*, 272–281. doi:10.1111/j.1365-2206.2012.00898.x

U.S. Department of Education. (2017). Individuals with Disabilities Education Act. Retrieved from https://www2.ed.gov/about/offices/list/osers/osep/osep-idea.html

U.S. Department of Health and Human Services (USDHHS), Health Resources and Services Administration, Maternal and Child Health Bureau. (2013). *The National Survey of Children with Special Health Care Needs Chartbook 2009–2010*. Rockville, MD: U.S. Department of Health and Human Services. Retrieved from https://mchb.hrsa.gov/cshcn0910/more/pdf/nscshcn0910.pdf

Walter, J. K., DeCamp, L. R., Warrier, K. S., Murphy, T. P., & Keefer, P. M. (2013). Care of the complex chronically ill child by generalist pediatricians: Lessons learned from pediatric palliative care. *Hospital Pediatrics, 3*, 129–138.

Wayte, S., McCaughey, E., Holley, S., Annaz, D., & Hill, C. M. (2012). Sleep problems in children with cerebral palsy and their relationship with maternal sleep and depression. *Acta Paediatrica, 101*, 618–623. doi:10.1111/j.1651-2227.2012.02603.x

Whiting, M. (2014a). Support requirements of parents caring for a child with disability and complex health needs. *Nursing Children & Young People, 26*(4), 24–27. doi:10.7748/ncyp2014.05.26.4.24.e389

Whiting, M. (2014b). Children with disability and complex health needs: The impact on family life. *Nursing Children & Young People, 26*(3), 26–30. doi:10.7748/ncyp2014.04.26.3.26.e388

Wiart, L., Ray, L., Darrah, J., & Magill-Evans, J. (2010). Parents' perspectives on occupational therapy and physical therapy goals for children with cerebral palsy. *Disability and Rehabilitation, 32*, 248–258. doi:10.3109/09638280903095890

Woodgate, R. L., Edwards, M., Ripat, J. D., Borton, B., & Rempel, G. (2015). Intense parenting: A qualitative study detailing the experiences of parenting children with complex care needs. *BMC Pediatrics, 15*, 197. doi:10.1186/s12887-015-0514-5

Zan, H., & Scharff, R. L. (2015). The heterogeneity in financial and time burden of caregiving to children with chronic conditions. *Maternal-Child Health Journal, 19*, 615–625. doi:10.1007/s10995-014-1547-3

9

Structuring a Child's Nutritional Care

Janine M. Bamberger

Nature is amazing. Plants require air, water, sunlight, and nutrients to grow. People do as well (if you consider sunlight as our source of vitamin D), but getting the proper nutrient mix tends to be more challenging for people than for plants. Plants mostly sit around in a garden, field, or forest as the seasons change, the precipitation falls, and the sundial teeters between day and night. Infants and children thrive on the same nutrients, but in different amounts based on age, growth velocity, and need to recover from, or prevent, illness or injury. Confounding the situation, nutrients to support all of these needs may come, or not come, from a wide variety of sources and in quite diverse amounts, and even types.

Thinking a little more about how nutrition ties into the life of a child, let us ponder the fact that supporting growth and development throughout the life cycle happens at the intersection of ever-changing nutrient needs and a dynamic activity level. The activity level at any given time is a combination of automatic bodily functions and activities that the individual chooses to pursue or avoid. It is the job of the individual to be sure that nutrient intake (what the individual eats and drinks) supports energy needed for day-to-day activities. Since the body is pretty smart, it normally listens to itself and makes good decisions. The body inherently knows to eat more or less to support growth and activity. It knows to consume more calories when it is setting off on a growth spurt. In the case of infants, children, and even adolescents, the parents and caregivers have a significant role in this nutrient-searching activity. They are the providers, the ones responsible for *what* is offered, as Ellyn Satter (2016) reminds us. Infants and young children can only do so much on their own. Infants can cry, or anxiously open their mouths, to indicate hunger and readiness to eat, and they can lock their lips and turn their head away to signal "Done!" Older children are able to verbalize their desire to eat, or to quit eating. With words, a child or adolescent can state that they like a taste or texture. An infant can, though, express the same with their eyes and lips, the position of their head, or the tongue that pushes or spits the food out. It is really an ingenious game, for both the young and the old, whereby the body speaks, the body reacts, and if all goes well, the "environment" provides. For infants and children, the environment is represented by the adult who physically gathers, prepares, and dishes up the food, even conveying the food all the way to the lips of the child, based on the child's level of physical, mental, and emotional development. As children move into adolescence, they become more and more responsible for gathering their own food from the environment in which they live. The choices become their responsibility. By adolescence, children have hopefully learned how to make, and actually have the ability to access, healthy choices.

For a moment, compare the common car, a machine with which we are all familiar, to the human body. To steer a vehicle effectively, one needs a fit and functioning machine. That is the purpose of routine maintenance. When an automobile is kept fit and functioning as per its original design, it continues to work satisfactorily. For people, a state of health sets the scene for ongoing and appropriate development. That is, health allows the body to be fit and functioning according to its original design. Injury, illness, stunted growth or wasting, or abnormal physical development change the trajectory. This can happen in an instant, as with a fall and the resulting traumatic brain injury, or it can happen over time, as with failure to thrive caused by behavioral issues or food insecurity. For some infants, the change from original design occurs at, or even long before, birth.

The World Health Organization (WHO) presented this definition of health in 1946 in the Preamble to the organization's Constitution: "*Health* is a state of complete physical, mental and social well-being and not merely the absence of disease or infirmity" (World Health Organization, 2018b). The purpose of regular intake of required nutrients is to proactively maintain health. The fact is, though, that life's health is a bumpy ride. The lucky ones are born perfectly healthy, but even they will experience ups and downs. Figure 9.1 offers a simple visual idea of how health changes, sometimes slightly and sometimes dramatically, and how it may or may not return to the base level.

Each period of illness or health change, whether adaptation or recovery is at home or in a healthcare facility, involves an initial stage of instability, a stable but vulnerable time of transition, and then, arrival at the new normal. Ideally, the new normal is at the same level, or possibly at a better level, than the state of health prior to illness or health change. There may be other stages in the mix as well. As an example, consider the

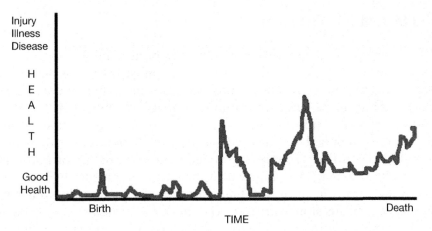

FIGURE 9.1 Lifetime health variability. The line represents the changing nature of health versus injury, illness, and disease over a lifetime.

newborn preterm infant with unstable vitals, immature lungs and gastro-intestinal (GI) tract, and inability to coordinate sucking and swallowing. This period is potentially followed by more complications of prematurity (e.g., infection, osteopenia of prematurity, gastroesophageal [GE] reflux), a calmer time during which the infant can simply eat and grow, and finally move home. Each blip in Figure 9.1, many of which relate to eating and nutrition, has its own ups and downs, as well as new, unexpected complications. Resiliency is the key to coping with lifetime health variability. In short, the American Psychological Association (2016) says that *resilience* "means 'bouncing back' from difficult experiences." The purpose of this chapter is to describe how guided participation teaching and learning, utilized by nurses in particular, can facilitate parental development of an efficacious caregiving practice. Such a practice sets the scene for effective growth and development, for health, from the moment an infant greets the world, or before, to the time he or she sets off to explore life on his or her own, and beyond. Development of resilience to lifetime health trials can be part of this work. Details related to the provision of specific types and amounts of nutrients to meet growth requirements will be left to dietitian and physician consultants, as well as to a variety of specialists who deal with the many diseases and health conditions that plague the age groups from preterm infancy through adolescence. Additionally, to simplify the text, the terms mother and father and parents will be used, but they should always be interpreted broadly to fit the context, and without assumption of who comprises the family unit. Thus, the key caregiver, protector, and teacher may be the mother, father, grandfather, grandmother, a parent, neighbor, aunt, uncle, sister, brother, guardian, daycare worker, babysitter, teacher, or even the family dog (sometimes the best soulmate), and the key caregiver(s) may change hour to hour, day to day, or year to year.

OPTIMUM NUTRITION

Poor growth can negatively affect brain, bones, lungs, and muscles. *Optimal growth*, which can be viewed as the most favorable physical and mental growth for a particular child's genetic, environmental, social, and clinical situation, depends on optimum nutrition. The provision of *optimum nutrition* for infants and children, in turn, requires that all nutrients are both supplied and utilized for (a) normal organ development and function, (b) normal growth and maintenance, (c) repair of body tissue that has been damaged or injured, (d) peak, developmentally appropriate activity, and (e) resistance to inflammation and infection. In your role as a healthcare professional utilizing the guided participation approach to support families, join your attention with the family to scan continuously for roadblocks to optimum nutrition. What is new in the life of the child? What is expected in the near future? Has a physical issue that could affect nutrient intake developed recently? Is a tooth erupting or falling out? Is it time for effective and potentially painful braces to improve teeth or jaw alignment? Is the child uncomfortable due to an ear infection, or the GI effects of the prescribed antibiotic? Is there new peer pressure because the child's friends are now eating hot CHEETOS Crunchy FLAMIN' HOT Cheese Flavored Snacks for breakfast? Are classmates pushing an adolescent toward unhealthy dieting choices? Does anyone in the house actually cook? Is the family meal a thing of the past? Share your observations, not in a condescending, condemning, or prescriptive manner, but in a thoughtful, supportive, and potentially inquisitive manner. Remember that it is the child and the family who ultimately need to climb over the hurdles that present themselves. Invite discussion, problem solving, and a spirit of resilience around new and ongoing nutrition issues.

Assuring that recommendations related to nutrition are met can be a complex task. There are no less than 34 nutrients (macronutrients, minerals, electrolytes, and vitamins) in the list of dietary reference intakes (DRI; Food and Nutrition Board, Institute of Medicine, National Academies, 2016). There are actually many more known nutrients, plus additional ones that are yet to be discovered as scientific methods improve. As if that is not enough, nutrient requirements change with age and health condition. For this chapter, basic nutrient recommendations are listed in Tables 9.1 and 9.2. A review of this information can help you and the families with whom you are working understand that nutrient needs change over time, across gender, and according to a subject's weight. The nutrients addressed in Tables 9.1 and 9.2 are the ones that we tend to focus on first, due to their significance in growth and development and/ or risk for deficiency, when addressing nutrient needs for children and adolescents.

TABLE 9.1 Recommended Daily Energy Requirement

Age	Energy kcal/d (enteral)		Energy kcal/kg/d (parenteral)[c]
Preterm infant	55–525[a]		110–120
	Female[b]	Male[b]	
Infant 0–6 mo	520	570	90–100 (0–1 yr)
Infant 7–12 mo	676	743	90–100 (0–1 yr)
Toddler 1–2 yr	992	1046	75–90 (1–7 yr)
Child 3–8 yr	1642	1742	75–90 (1–7 yr)
Child 9–13 yr	2071	2279	60–75 (7–12 yr)
Teen 14–18 yr	2368	3152	30–60 (12–18 yr)
Adult >18 yr	2403	3067	25–40[d] (adult)

Sources: [a]Preterm infant daily energy needs (enteral intake) based on consensus recommendations of 110 to 150 kcal/kg from the American Academy of Pediatrics, Committee on Nutrition. (2014). Nutritional needs of preterm infants. In R. E. Kleinman & F. R. Greer (Eds.), *Pediatric nutrition handbook* (7th ed.). Elk Grove, IL: Author. Calculated for infants weighing 0.5 to 3.5 kg.

[b]From Dietary Reference Intakes (DRI) for energy from the Food and Nutrition Board, Institute of Medicine of the National Academies. (2005). *Dietary reference intakes for energy, carbohydrate, fiber, fat, fatty acids, cholesterol, protein, and amino acids*. Washington, DC: National Academies Press. Retrieved from https://www.nap.edu/read/10490/chapter/1

[c]From Koletzko, B., Agostoni, C., Ball, P., Carnielli, V., Chaloner, C., Clayton, J., . . . Yaron, A. (2005). ESPEN/ESPGHAN Guidelines on paediatric parenteral nutrition. 2. Energy. *Journal of Pediatric Gastroenterology and Nutrition, 41*, S5–S11. Retrieved from http://www.rch.org.au/uploadedFiles/Main/Content/rchcpg/hospital_clinical_guideline_index/ESPGHAN%20Guidelines_Paediatric_Parenteral_Nutrition_2005.pdf

[d]From Queensland Health. (2015). Estimating energy, protein & fluid requirements for adult clinical conditions. Retrieved from https://www.health.qld.gov.au/nutrition/nemo_nutrsup.asp and https://www.health.qld.gov.au/__data/assets/pdf_file/0022/144175/est_rqts.pdf

TABLE 9.2 DRI: Recommended Dietary Allowances and Adequate Intakes, Vitamins[a]

Age	Total Water (mL/d)		Protein (g/kg)	Sodium (mg/d)	Calcium (mg/d)	Zinc (mg/d)		Fiber (g/d)		Vitamin D (IU/d)
Preterm infant[b]	140–180 mL/kg		3.4–4.4 g//kg	69–115 mg/kg	100–220 mg/kg	1–3 mg/kg		n/a		150–400
Infant 0–6 mo	700		1.5	120	200	2		n/a		400
Infant 6–12 mo	800		1.5	370	260	3		n/a		400
Toddler 1–3 yr	1,300		1.1	1,000	700	3		19		600
Child 4–8 yr	1,700		0.95	1,200	1,000	5		25		600
	Female	Male						Female	Male	
Child 9–13 yr	2,100	2,400	0.95	1,500	1,300	8		26	31	600
						Female	Male			
Teen 14–18 yr	3,300		0.85	1,500	1,300	9	11	26	38	600
Adult 19–30 yr	2,700		0.8	1,500	1,000	8	11	25	38	600

DRI, dietary reference intakes.

Sources: [a]DRI for energy from the Food and Nutrition Board, Institute of Medicine of the National Academies. (2005). *Dietary reference intakes for water, potassium, sodium, chloride, and sulfate.* Washington, DC: National Academies Press. Retrieved from https://www.nap.edu/read/10925/chapter/1; *Dietary reference intakes for calcium, phosphorus, magnesium, and fluoride* (1997). Washington, DC: National Academies Press. Retrieved from https://www.nap.edu/read/5776/chapter/1; *Dietary reference intakes for vitamin A, vitamin K, arsenic, boron, chromium, copper, iodine, iron, manganese, molybdenum, nickel, silicon, vanadium, and zinc* (2001). Washington, DC: National Academies Press. Retrieved from https://www.nap.edu/read/10026/chapter/1; *Dietary reference intakes for energy, carbohydrate, fiber, fat, fatty acids, cholesterol, protein, and amino acids.* Washington, DC: National Academies Press. Retrieved from https://www.nap.edu/read/10490/chapter/1

[b]From the American Academy of Pediatrics, Committee on Nutrition. (2014). Nutritional needs of preterm infants. In R. E. Kleinman & F. R. Greer. (Eds.), *Pediatric nutrition* (7th ed.). Elk Grove, IL: Author.

NORMAL GROWTH EXPECTATIONS: INFANCY THROUGH ADOLESCENCE

Growth during infancy, toddlerhood, childhood, and adolescence follows an expected pattern. Thus, standards can be used to compare a particular child's growth to that of many. Of course, expectations may be exceeded, or not met, usually because of issues such as injury, illness, disease, genetics, environmental factors, social patterns, dietary choices, or food access.

Growth Curves

Infants start off at a variety of sizes. Full-term infants are defined as those born between 39 and 41 weeks of gestation, according to the American Congress of Obstetricians and Gynecologists (ACOG; 2013). Parents may see their child's growth plotted on one curve or another, depending on their doctor's office practices, or their own access to growth charts. The 50th percentile weight for females at birth is 3.399 kg (7 pounds 7.8 ounces) whereas the 50th percentile weight for males at birth is 3.530 kg (7 pounds 12.4 ounces) according to the Centers for Disease Control and Prevention's (CDC) National Center for Health Statistics (NCHS) data (Centers for Disease Control and Prevention, National Center for Health Statistics, 2001). The 50th percentile birth weights in the WHO data tables are slightly lighter (3.232 kg [7 pounds 2 ounces] for girls and 3.346 kg [7 pounds 6 ounces] for boys; WHO Multicentre Growth Reference Study Group, 2009). Parents and other family members are always excited to hear how much the family's newest addition weighs. Health professionals, though, use the birth weight to classify the infant as small- or large-for-gestational age (i.e., birth weight below the 10th percentile [SGA] or above the 90th percentile for gestational age [LGA], respectively), extremely low birth weight (ELBW; birth weight <1,000 g), very low birth weight (VLBW; birth weight <1,500 g), low birth weight (LBW; birth weight <2,500 g), or micropremie (birth weight <750 g; Merck, 2016; Nafday, 2008; World Health Organization, 2011). Additionally, the term intrauterine growth restriction (IUGR), like SGA, is commonly used to describe birth weight less than the 10th percentile on intrauterine growth curves, regardless of whether the infant is born preterm or full term. Unlike SGA, though, IUGR actually implies a pathological process or an in utero insult that inhibited the newborn from reaching its genetic potential (Nafday, 2008). All of these classifications, assigned on the day of birth, foreshadow future growth and development expectations. Many of these infants will travel through trying times with regard to growth and feeding.

The CDC growth charts, released in 2000, describe the size and growth of children in the United States. The data for these growth charts came from nationally representative growth surveys that were conducted 1963 to 1965 (National Health Examination Survey [NHES] II), 1966 to 1970 (NHES III), 1971 to 1974 (National Health and Nutrition Examination Survey [NHANES]), 1976 to 1980 (NHANES II), and 1988 to 1994 (NHANES III), as well as well as from birth certificates and hospital and clinic records from 1968 to 1995. Over 82 million children under the age of 20 years, and over birth weight 1,500 g, were included in the creation of the standards (Grummer-Strawn, 2002). Details of the development of the 16 growth charts, a combination of cross-sectional and some longitudinal data that describe weight, length/height, head circumference, and body mass index (BMI), are available from the CDC (Kuczmarski et al., 2002). Released in 2006, the WHO growth charts, based on cross-sectional and longitudinal data gathered from 8,440 individuals in six countries across the world (Brazil, Ghana, India, Norway, Oman, and the United States), describe the growth of healthy infants and young children from diverse cultural settings and ethnic backgrounds (WHO Multicentre Growth Reference Study Group, 2009). Currently, the CDC recommends that growth from birth to 2 years of age be plotted on the WHO growth charts, available from the CDC's NCHS website. The CDC recommends use of the WHO growth standards to monitor growth for infants and children 0 to 2 years of age in the United States, and the CDC growth charts for children 2 to 20 years of age in the United States (Centers for Disease Control and Prevention, National Center for Health Statistics, 2010a, 2010b). Examples of commonly used growth curves (for boys and girls from birth to 5 years and from 2 to 20 years [percentiles and z-scores]) are included in Figures 9.2 through 9.6.

Choice of growth chart can be challenging because the academic literature contains many different growth charts. Unique conditions may warrant use of one growth chart rather than another. Growth patterns differ between the newest WHO growth standards, earlier reference standards, and the CDC NCHS standards. For children younger than 2 years, the WHO charts better reflect growth of breastfed children, growth during optimal conditions, and growth using longitudinal length and weight data measured at frequent intervals (Centers for Disease Control and Prevention, National Center for Health Statistics, 2010b). Some individuals with abnormal health conditions deserve their own "normal" growth curves. Down syndrome patients fit into that category. In 2015, the CDC published new Growth Charts for Children with Down syndrome from birth to 3 years and age 2 to 20 years (Zemel et al., 2015). It makes sense to assess growth of infants and children with Down syndrome as its own normal, rather than graphing their progress on standard curves that do not reflect the Down syndrome population. Z-score tables can also be used to assign magnitude to extreme values, either high or low, on a growth chart.

Just as standard WHO and CDC growth curves do not include growth data for individuals with specific conditions, such as those with Down syndrome, they also do not reflect growth of infants who are born prematurely. Lubchenco's curves, as well as Babson's, and others reviewed by Fenton, were

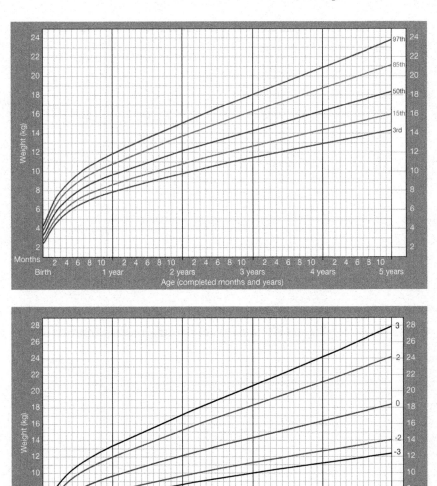

FIGURE 9.2 Weight-for-age BOYS birth to 5 years (percentiles and z-scores).

Source: Reprinted from WHO Child Growth Standards. (2018). http://www.who.int/childgrowth/standards/cht_wfa_boys_p_0_5.pdf?ua=1

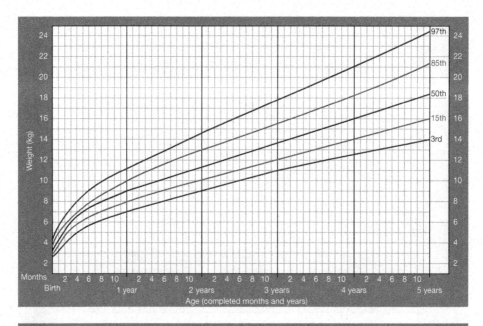

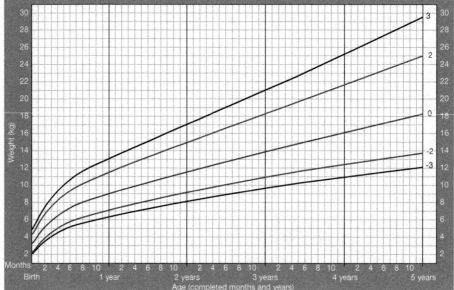

FIGURE 9.3 Weight-for-age GIRLS birth to 5 years (percentiles and z-scores).

Source: Reprinted from WHO Child Growth Standards. (2018). http://www.who.int/childgrowth/en

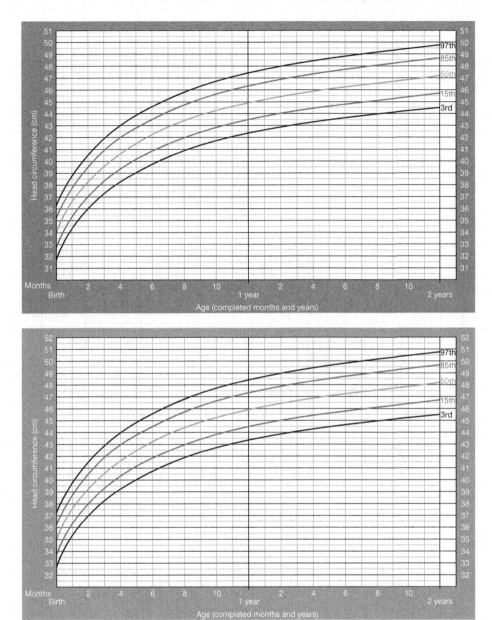

FIGURE 9.4 Head circumference BOYS and GIRLS birth to 2 years (percentiles).

Source: Reprinted from WHO Child Growth Standards. (2018). http://www.who.int/childgrowth/en

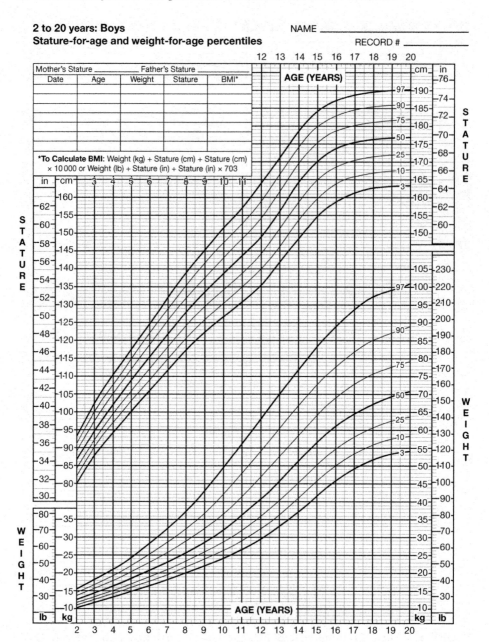

FIGURE 9.5 BOYS stature-for-age and weight-for-age 2 to 20 years (percentiles).

Source: Developed by the National Center for Health Statistics in collaboration with the National Center for Chronic Disease Prevention and Health Promotion (2000). Retrieved from http://www.cdc.gov/growthcharts

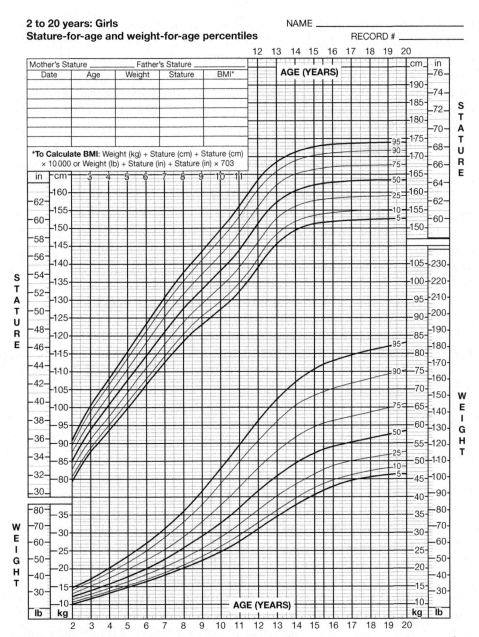

FIGURE 9.6 GIRLS stature-for-age and weight-for-age 2 to 20 years (percentiles).

Source: Developed by the National Center for Health Statistics in collaboration with the National Center for Chronic Disease Prevention and Health Promotion. (2000). Retrieved from http://www.cdc.gov/growthcharts

used to graph growth of premature infants for many years, starting with a grid by Dancis in 1948 (Babson & Benda, 1976; Dancis, O'Connell, & Holt, 1948; Fenton, 2003; Lubchenco, Hansman, & Boyd, 1966; Lubchenco, Hansman, Dressler, & Boyd, 1963). Fenton and Olsen have both developed more recent growth charts for the important and unique premature infant population. Data used to create Olsen's intrauterine growth curves include a racially diverse population of 257,855 singleton infants whose growth was assessed in United States. NICUs across 33 states from 1998 to 2006 (Olsen, Groveman, Lawson, Clark, & Zemel, 2010). Olsen has also created BMI curves, based on U.S. infants born at 22 to 42 weeks gestation (Olsen et al., 2015). The Fenton preterm growth chart, originally published in 2003, but updated in 2013, includes data collected between 1991 and 2007 from six developed countries (Germany, Italy, United States, Australia, Scotland, and Canada). The chart allows for plotting of growth by exact age, not completed week of gestation, from 22 to 50 weeks postmenstrual age, that is, through 10 weeks postterm (Fenton, 2003; Fenton & Kim, 2013), and are considered references, not standards. Though there is a weight shift upwards from 40 to 50 weeks for both girls and boys from the WHO growth standards to the CDC growth references, the WHO growth standards are representative of global fetal and infant growth. The INTERGROWTH-21st project (described on the International Fetal and Newborn Growth Consortium website) is striving to define ideal growth patterns for preterm infant growth through the development of simple, international standards that reflect the diversity of multiple populations (International Fetal and Newborn Growth Consortium, 2009; Villar et al., 2014).

Anthropometry

The NHANES III Anthropometric Procedure Videos describe standardized body measurement procedures for measuring weight, height, limb length, circumferences, skinfolds, and body breadth measurements (Centers for Disease Control and Prevention, National Center for Health Statistics, 2014). Additionally, the website for the INTERBIO-21st Study, which is an extension of the International Fetal and Newborn Growth Consortium for the 21st Century (INTERGROWTH-21st) project, houses an *Anthropometry Manual* that aims to assure that anthropometric measurements are reliable, accurate, and precise. It describes measurement techniques for infant weight, length, and head circumference; adult height, weight, and BMI; and equipment calibration (INTERGROWTH-21st Anthropometry Group, 2012; International Fetal and Newborn Growth Consortium, 2009). Some of the directions are equipment specific, but much of the information is generic to the process of gathering anthropometric data. Training on use of the WHO growth charts (CDC Growth Chart Training) is available for providers who measure and assess child growth, especially RNs, nutritionists, and pediatricians (Centers for Disease Control and Prevention, Division of Nutrition, Physical Activity, and Obesity, National Center for Chronic Disease Prevention and Health Promotion, 2015).

PRACTICAL NUTRITION AND GROWTH CONSIDERATIONS

Neonatal

Parents typically anticipate delivery of healthy newborn infants. It does not always turn out that way, though. Worldwide, the incidence of preterm deliveries is 9% in higher income countries and 12% in lower income countries (World Health Organization, 2018c). In the United States, 9.85% of infants are born prematurely (Centers for Disease Control and Prevention, National Center for Health Statistics, 2018a). For these infants born before completing 37 weeks of gestation, life begins with many trials for both the baby and the parents.

Basic Nutrient Requirements

Premature infants have very limited nutrient stores in the body compared to full-term infants. Therefore, they must be offered food soon after birth. The more immature the infant, the greater the needs, per kilogram of body weight, for calories, fluids, minerals, trace elements, and electrolytes. Table 9.1 provides a look into the complexity of nutrient variation across age groups. Requirements are not based on age itself, but rather on the metabolic and growth needs of the body, the fitness of metabolic pathways and cell function to do their intended jobs, and the ability of the body to acquire and use nutrients. Growth and need for repair (as in trauma, disease, and recovery from illness) up the ante for nutrients. Preterm neonates are not only intensive care patients but are also on this earth ahead of their time. Their nutrient needs, based on body weight, are at the highest of any time throughout their life cycle. When recommending nutrients for young infants, dietitians and physicians, and others who specialize in neonatal care, apply evidence-based principles outlined by groups such as the American Congress of Obstetricians and Gynecologists (acog.org), the American Academy of Pediatrics (AAP; aap.org), the American Society for Enteral and Parenteral Nutrition (ASPEN; nutritioncare.org), and Pediatric Nutrition, a dietetic practice group of the Academy of Nutrition and Dietetics (pnpg.org).

Preterm infants are at risk for inadequate intake of a variety of nutrients due to their very high needs for growth and recovery from neonatal-related illness or injury, if present, and their struggles to consume feedings of adequate volume and nutrient density. Nutrition assessment of these patients focuses on energy, sodium, calcium, phosphorus, zinc, iron, vitamins D and E, and folate. See Tables 9.1 and 9.2 for key nutrient recommendations in comparison to other age groups. Additional details are available in the National Academy of Science's Dietary Reference Intakes publication and the book *Pediatric Nutrition* (7th edition) from the AAP (Kleinman & Greer, 2014, pp. 609–642; Otten, Hellwig, & Meyers, 2006).

Developmental Expectations Related to Nutrient Intake

Preterm infants are born with organs and systems that are developmentally and functionally immature. The types and amounts of nutrients provided to these infants are tied to this fact. The lungs are the last of the major organs to develop during gestation. Immature lungs create a need for respiratory support and the potential for acute and chronic lung disease. A key strategy to avoid such complications is to supply nutrients required for normal, or catch-up growth, from the time the baby is born. The goal is to allow the small infant to grow in a manner that mimics healthy, in utero growth so that the lungs can develop, and thus function, as intended. Infants who develop bronchopulmonary dysplasia require more calories per kilogram, typically in less fluids (restricted to combat pulmonary edema), than infants without chronic lung disease in order to breath successfully and grow due to the work of breathing (Lai, Rajadurai, & Tan, 2006).

Bones of premature infants present another nutritional challenge. Biochemical and radiological monitoring is required during, and sometimes after, neonatal hospitalization until acceptable mineralization is apparent (Rehman & Narchi, 2015). The brain deserves mention, as well, since it is the master of the house, so to speak. The brain and spinal cord begin to develop in the fetus in week 3. The brain continues to grow rapidly throughout early childhood, actually quadrupling in size during the preschool years and reaching 90% of adult volume by age 6. Development is orderly and follows a regular pattern (Stiles & Jernigan, 2010). Fetal and neonatal iron adequacy is important for normal development of the brain (accrued mostly in the last trimester of pregnancy) and central nervous system, as is fat. Iron deficiency can negatively affect brain development. The result can be diminished functioning and development of the central nervous system with adverse effects on attention, intelligence test performance, and, ultimately, school achievement (Larkin & Rai, 1990). Essential fatty acids, linoleic acid (LA [18:2ω-6]) and alpha-linolenic acid (ALA [18:3ω-3]), as well as their long-chain polyunsaturated fat derivatives, arachidonic acid (ARA [20:4ω-6]), eicosapentaenoic acid (EPA [20:5ω-3]), and docosahexaenoic acid (DHA [22:6ω-3]), critical to the functioning of all bodily tissues, contribute greatly to normal nervous system development (Kleinman & Greer, 2014, pp. 407–434). Sepsis, bronchopulmonary dysplasia (BPD), necrotizing enterocolitis (NEC), cerebral pathology (cerebral palsy, seizures, and others), genetic abnormalities, and neuromuscular conditions are disorders that plague infants born prematurely, and negatively affect growth and feeding.

Feeding and swallowing issues, abnormal GI tract anatomy and function, and excessively high or low energy needs make caring for infants born prematurely a challenge for families and the medical community. Nutrition problems, if left unchecked, may result in less than desirable growth and development during infancy, childhood, and adolescence. In the hospital, nurses utilizing the Infant-Driven Feeding (IDF) model of practice, designed to optimize long-term growth and development for preterm and convalescing infants, support parents as they learn about infant communication and care related to their child (Ludwig & Waitzman, 2016). The IDF method helps

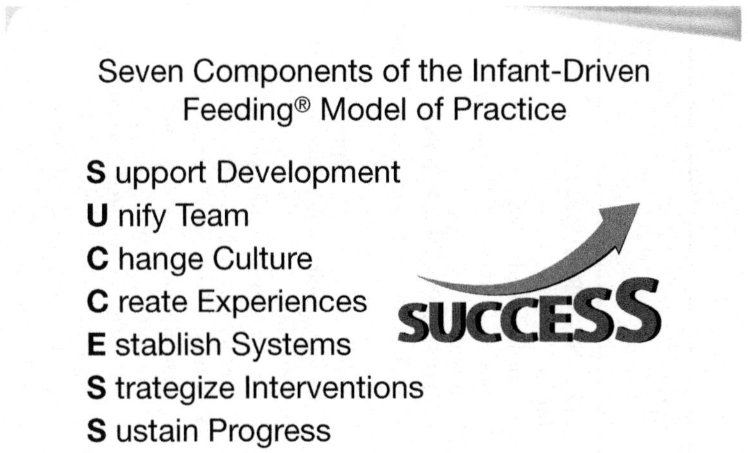

Seven Components of the Infant-Driven
Feeding® Model of Practice

S upport Development
U nify Team
C hange Culture
C reate Experiences
E stablish Systems
S trategize Interventions
S ustain Progress

SUCCESS

FIGURE 9.7 Infant-driven feeding® is a model of practice developed to support infants' transition to oral feeding in the NICU.

Reprinted with permission from Infant-Driven Feeding, LLC

boost parental confidence and competence surrounding feeding. Figure 9.7 contains a list of the seven components of the IDF model. According to Sue Ludwig, an experienced NICU occupational therapist, "It [feeding] is a complex neurodevelopment task for the infant that has to be supported by the family and the staff." The concept of teaching and learning together, baby, mother, and professionals, is foundational in the IDF model (S. Ludwig, personal communication, September 19, 2016).

Table 9.3 describes a recommended progression of foods from birth through 18 months of age, with an option to enter corrected, or adjusted, age for premature infants. For example, an infant born 2 months prematurely would follow the first set of guidelines from 0 to 6 months chronological age, rather than from 0 to 4 months. Additional tools that may also be helpful when working with families of preterm infants, or in developing site-appropriate tools for working with families, include the Neonatal Nutritional Discharge Plan (Figure 9.8) and the Community Provider Support of Growth in Premature Infants (Appendix 9.1).

KEY NUTRITION RECOMMENDATIONS TO SHARE WITH THE FAMILY

1. Breastfeed and/or provide human milk for as much of the first year as possible.
2. Feed preterm infants in the same manner as infants born full term, just start later to adjust for how early the baby was born. Work with medical team, as needed, to individualize.
3. With human milk and supplement(s), or appropriate infant formula, be sure to provide adequate protein, fat, calories, iron, calcium, phosphorus, vitamins D and E, and folic acid for rapid growth, tissue repair, brain development, and building bones and red blood cells.

TABLE 9.3 Guide to Infant Feeding

1 month 2 months 3 months 4 months 5 months 6 months. . . Guide to Infant Feeding

When (months)	Total Daily Food Intake	How	Suggested Foods	Why
— Usually 0–4	HUMAN MILK or FORMULA 14–42 fl oz (__cal/ fl oz) Typically eight to 12 feedings per day if breastfed; five to seven feedings per day if formula fed	If human milk fed, feed exclusively by breast for the first 3–4 weeks, if possible, in order to establish milk supply and prevent nipple confusion. Alternatively, use a: ■ Bottle ■ Small cup ■ Small/medicine spoon If all, or mostly, formula fed, feed by bottle.	Human milk or infant formula (iron fortified) NO cow's milk (or goat, soy, rice, or almond milk) NO juice NO solid foods needed NO water needed unless weather is very hot	**FEEDING/ORAL SKILLS** Infant: ■ can suck and swallow ■ pushes food out of mouth with tongue **OTHER CONSIDERATIONS** ■ Human milk or infant formula has the right nutrients. ■ Solids, fed too early, replace nutrient-rich human milk or infant formula. ■ Overfeeding is easier with solids and may induce obesity. ■ Young infants are affected, more than adults, by additives such as salt, sugar, nitrates. Limit intake. ■ Babies naturally sleep through the night between 1 and 3 months; cereal will not make it happen sooner. ■ Some solids increase renal solute load (which causes more stress on the kidneys).

—
Usually
5–6

HUMAN MILK or FORMULA
26–39 fl oz (____ cal/fl oz)

four to six feedings per day

6 months
Start:
1–2 tbsp dry cereal

Advance to:
2–6 tbsp dry cereal
4 tbsp vegetables
4–8 tbsp fruit

By spoon, not bottle, add:
CEREAL (iron fortified)
Start with dry rice cereal mixed with an equal amount of human milk or formula; give once a day for several days.
Increase to twice a day as infant learns to enjoy the experience.
Advance to ½ cup cereal before adding vegetables or fruit.
VEGETABLES/FRUITS
Start with 1–2 tbsp/feeding; increase to 4 tbsp/feeding.
Add one new vegetable or fruit every 3–4 days.

Human milk may be the exclusive nutrient source for full-term infants during the first 6 months after birth.

■ Begin infant cereal. Start with rice; add wheat and mixed varieties (only after 6 months).

■ Add strained vegetables.
■ Add strained fruit.
■ Add **finger foods** such as graham crackers, teething biscuits, and cheese sticks. **Supervise closely** due to choking risk.

NO cow's milk (or goat, soy, rice or almond milk)
NO juice

FEEDING/ORAL SKILLS:

■ Drooling appears and pancreatic amylase (an enzyme) increases to allow better starch digestion.
■ Acceptance of solids slowly begins.
■ Infant expects food, opens mouth for the spoon, and pushes food out less.

4 months: Normal solid food swallowing pattern appears
5 months: Able to grasp objects voluntarily and beginning to reach mouth with hands
6 months: Sits with balance while using hands; transfers food from front of tongue to back

OTHER CONSIDERATIONS
The purpose of introducing complementary foods (solid or semisolid foods or liquids), added to human milk or formula, is to add nutrients, textures, and flavors that help the infant meet changing needs and move closer to the family's table foods/food routine.

(continued)

TABLE 9.3 Guide to Infant Feeding (*continued*)

		Guide to Infant Feeding		
When (months)	Total Daily Food Intake	How	Suggested Foods	Why
	NOTE: The American Academy of Pediatrics and the World Health Organization recommend exclusive breastfeeding during the first 6 months of life.	ABOUT ALLERGIES Until ____ months (usually 6 months), AVOID foods commonly associated with allergies, including eggs, cow's milk, wheat, soy, peanuts, tree nuts, fish, shellfish. Delaying introduction longer, though, may increase risk of allergy. (doi:10.1016/j.jaip.2012.09.003)	NOTE: Home-prepared beets, spinach, carrots, turnips, and collard greens are potentially high in nitrate. Use commercially prepared, or postpone home-prepared, until infant is at least 6 months old due to risk of methemoglobinemia, "blue baby syndrome."	Introduce new foods one at a time, with 3–5 days between each; observe for possible allergic reaction/intolerance. Dark green and deep yellow vegetables and fruits are good Vitamin A sources.

OPTIONAL: Infant name _____ Birthdate _____ Gestational age _____ weeks Nutrition provider _____ Date _____

. . . 7 months 8 months 9 months 10 months 11 months 12 months . . . 18 months

Usually 7–9

HUMAN MILK or FORMULA
24–32 fl oz (____ cal/fl oz)

four to five feedings per day

GRAINS, two servings
¼–½ cup prepared cereal, ½ slice bread or crackers, or other grain products
VEGETABLES, one to two servings
¼–½ cup vegetables
FRUIT, one to two servings
¼–¾ cup fruit
PROTEIN FOOD (MEAT/MEAT ALTERNATIVES), one to two servings
1–2 tbsp, then ¼–½ cup

- Thicken cereal to lumpier mixture.
- Move to mashed or finely chopped table foods, mashing soft food with a fork or infant food mill.
- Encourage child to eat new textures.
- Introduce **cup** at 6–9 months.
- May feed infant in high chair, with feet supported, once able to sit on own. Do not leave unattended.
- If juice is offered, give 100% fruit/vegetable juice, 2–4 fl oz, from a cup.

- Bite-sized pieces of soft fruits and vegetables
- Ground, and then finely cut, meat/meat alternative, moistened with water or strained vegetables if too dry
- Egg
- Continue finger foods; add Cheerios® or similar.
- Continue human milk or infant formula.

FEEDING/ORAL SKILLS
- Can get spoon in mouth but usually turns it over
- Improved pincer grasp; lateral jaw movements; learns side-to-side "rotary" chewing

OTHER CONSIDERATIONS
- Changing texture helps transition to table foods.
- Feeding self encourages eating only to hunger satiation (i.e., until the child is no longer hungry). Ask child "Is your tummy full?" Watch for cues: slowed rate of eating, decreased attention to eating, utensil dropping. Food acceptance improves if infant is allowed to self-feed.
- Can handle balanced amounts of reasonably soft, moderately seasoned family foods.
- Continue to provide well-cooked mashed or chopped table foods, as needed, until chewing is effective and firmer textures are well tolerated.

(continued)

TABLE 9.3 Guide to Infant Feeding (*continued*)

When (months)	Total Daily Food Intake	How	Suggested Foods	Why
___ – ___ Usually 10–11	**HUMAN MILK** or **FORMULA** 20–24 fl oz (___ cal/fl oz) four to five feedings per day **GRAINS**, four servings ½–1 slice bread or crackers, ¼–½ cup prepared cereal **VEGETABLES/FRUIT**, four servings 3–4 tbsp **PROTEIN FOODS**, two servings 2 tbsp or 1 oz, or equivalent	▪ Transition to all table foods (ground or finely chopped). ▪ Provide meals in a pattern similar to rest of family.	▪ Move to all table foods by 12 months. ▪ Encourage child to try new textures. ▪ Continue baby cereal until ___ months (usually 18 months). ▪ AVOID soda, Kool-Aid, chips and other overly salty or overly sweet foods. ▪ AVOID excess consumption of juice. May include 3–4 fl oz of 100% juice in **a cup**.	▪ Encourage independence and self-feeding (order of foods, amount to feel full, combinations of foods, cup). ▪ Follow growth in relation to intake. ▪ Provide spoon, and fork when safe handling is understood, but allow hands. ▪ PROTEIN FOODS include beef, pork, lamb, fish, poultry, eggs, dried beans, dried peas, lentils, tofu, tempeh, nuts, nut butters (smooth), seeds, seed butters (smooth), cheese, cottage cheese, yogurt. ▪ No need for added sugar and salt.

| —
Usually
12–18 | **DAIRY/MILK/MILK PRODUCTS,** four to five servings (16–24 fl oz HUMAN MILK, WHOLE COW'S MILK, or equivalent yogurt or cheese)

PROTEIN FOODS, two servings
FRUIT, two to three servings
VEGETABLES, two to three servings
GRAINS, six servings (bread, cereal, rice, pasta, other grain; mostly whole grain)
FATS/OILS, three servings (oil, margarine, butter, mayonnaise, salad dressing)
OTHER FOODS, such as jams, jellies, syrup, and sweet desserts in limited amounts. | ■ Provide three meals a day plus a nourishing mid-morning and mid-afternoon snack, as needed in relation to growth and energy demands.

■ Cut/chop food based on child's chewing ability.
■ Offer new foods repeatedly in order to improve child's chance of acceptance.
■ Eliminate use of bottle; move to **cup** for beverages. | ■ NO skim or 1% milk (until 24 months of age)
■ **AVOID** foods that tend to cause choking, such as candy, nuts, whole grapes, raw carrots, popcorn, hot dogs cut in coin shapes, gum.

■ Provide **adequate protein, iron, and zinc** for growth, especially during times when toddlers are typically poor/picky eaters. For iron, consider continued use of infant cereals, or look for adult cereals (for breakfast or snacks) that contain higher amounts of iron as well as low amounts of sugar (ideally <6 g/serving). | **OTHER CONSIDERATIONS**
Daily, include a vitamin C source such as citrus fruits, berries, melons, tomatoes, peppers, cabbage, potatoes, broccoli, cauliflower.

Three to four times a week, include a vitamin A source such as melons, peaches, apricots, carrots, spinach, broccoli, squash, pumpkin, sweet potatoes, tomatoes, brussels sprouts. |

NOTES

fl oz, fluid ounce =15 mL (liquid); tbsp, tablespoon (volume).
EQUIVALENTS: 4 tbsp = ¼ cup; 8 tbsp = ½ cup; 12 tbsp = ¾ cup; 16 tbsp = 1 cup.

Sources: American Academy of Pediatrics. (2015). *Pediatric nutrition* (7th ed. ISBN-13: 978-1-58110-819-4; Academy of Nutrition and Dietetics (2015). *Pediatric nutrition care manual.* ©2017 JM Bamberger. ColtivatoLLC.com.

Neonatal Nutritional Discharge Plan
This Plan was developed to assist in the transition
from the hospital to the community for infants in the
neonatal intensive care unit with special nutritional
needs, It is meant to be completed by the discharge
coordinating nurse, dietitian, or other appropriate
health care professional.

If using printed copy of form,
attach patient label here.

Patient Name _____ Date of Birth _____
Mother's Name _____
Address _____ Phone _____

Diagnosis/Nutrition Problem List   Reset Section

Growth   Reset Section
Birth Weight _____g   Birth Length _____ cm   Birth OFC _____cm Gestational Age at Birth _____
Discharge Date _____ Corrected Age at Discharge _____
Weight at Discharge _____g   Length at Discharge_____ cm
Occipitofrontal Circumference (OFC) (Head Circumference) at Discharge _____ cm
◉ Growth Chart(s) Attached
Concern Exists Regarding
◉ Slow weight gain   ◉ Ability to catch-up   ◉ Rapid weight gain
Weight gain goal: _____

Current Feeding Plan at Discharge   Reset Section
Method of Feeding (select all that apply):
◉ Gavage: **Please select one** ◐   ◉ Cup fed   ◉ Finger fed   ◉ G-tube
◉ Supplemental nursing system   ◉ Bottle   ◉ Breast   ◉ _____
Discharge Feeding-select all that apply and choose appropriate unit:
◉ Breastmilk   ◉ Donor Milk   ◉ Fortified Breastmilk   ◉ Formula
_____ **OZ** ◐ per day   Formula Type:
_____ calories per day
_____ feedings per day
Recipe:

Supplements/Vitamins: _____

Intake Ability Concerns:

◉ Volume   ◉ Calories   ◉ Skill (nippling)   ◉ Gastroesophageal Reflux
Comments: _____

FIGURE 9.8 Neonatal nutritional discharge plan. (*continued*)

Current Feeding Plan at Discharge (continued)   <kbd>Reset Section</kbd>

Comments/Goals/Recommendations:

◯ Need for special formula feeding until _____ (age)
  due to: ◯ Tolerance   ◯ Adequacy/Rate Advancement   ◯ _____
◯ Recommended daily volume to support growth: _____ (Goal: At least ____ mL/kg/day)
◯ Recommended progression from current feeding/feeding therapies:

Breastfeeding Status at Discharge   <kbd>Reset Section</kbd>

Mother:
Production **Please select one**   ⊙
Nipple condition **Please select one**   ⊙ _____
Breastpump type available past infant's discharge: _____

Baby:
Infant's latch **Please select one**   ⊙ _____
Suckling behavior **Please select one**   ⊙ _____
Signs of disorganized or dysfunctional suckling or swallowing **Please select one**   ⊙
Interventions planned:

Comments: <kbd>Reset Section</kbd>

Contact person:
Name (print): _____   Organization: _____
Address: _____
Phone: _____   Fax: _____
Email: _____

Signature: _____   Date: _____

Send to: <kbd>Reset Section</kbd>

◯ Primary provider   ◯ Home care   ◯ Public health   ◯ WIC   ◯ Parent(s)
◯ _____

Funded in part the MCH Title V services Block Grant, Maternal and Child Health Bureau, Health Resources and Services Administration, U.S. Department of Health and Human Services and the Perinatal Foundation

FIGURE 9.8 Neonatal nutritional discharge plan.

Reprinted with permission. Wisconsin Association for Perinatal Care, www.perinatalweb.org.

Infancy

A newborn infant is a mystery that unfolds in the arms of his or her parents. The infant displays clues and the parents need to decode the clues. In the ideal situation, the child exhibits expected behaviors in expected ways at expected times. For instance, if the newborn baby is hungry, she cries and turns her head in a way that she hopes will easily allow her to find the nipple she so desires, and the perfect food that comes from it—breast milk. If she is tired, her eyelids grow heavy, and soon close. Possibly she sucks on her fist or thumb or pacifier to self-soothe. If the baby wets her diaper, or poops, she squirms as if doing so will free her of the mess which soon becomes cooler than body temperature and not nearly as comfortable as a soft, fluffy diaper, or no diaper. These three activities—eating, sleeping, and eliminating unused nutrients—take up much of every 24 hours in the life of a newborn. The child does what comes naturally. It is the parent who is often confused by the child's actions. The healthcare professional, nurse or other medical caregiver, is a step removed from the baby–parent duo. In the midst of the chaos of the day or night, the professional can remind the mother to listen, observe, and feel the messages the infant is working to convey.

Fortunate parents attend childbirth education classes prior to delivery. In the class, they learn about the birth process, normal infant development, how to feed a baby, how to diaper and dress the infant, and how to put their child "back to sleep," as parents are reminded in order to prevent sudden infant death syndrome (SIDS; NIH, 2016). A 2003 U.S. study on childbirth education classes noted that two-thirds (66%) of mothers of children from 4 to 35 months of age had attended childbirth education classes before giving birth (Lu et al., 2003). White mothers were twice as likely as African American or Hispanic mothers to attend, though, plus attendance rates varied by household income, education, and marital status. A 2006 study showed that childbirth education class attendance of surveyed mothers fell from 70% in 2000, for first-time mothers, to 56% in 2005 (Declercq, Sakala, Corry, & Applebaum, 2006). Families may not be aware of the help they need, or the education they could have, to make the journey with their infant easier. They may not be aware that the child is actually teaching the parent on a regular basis. The **guided participation** approach of teaching and learning, together, may be particularly useful to parents who have not attended childbirth education classes.

Whether a child is the first for a parent, or the tenth, everything is new when a baby enters the world. The look in each newborn's eyes is new. One infant may settle when held over mom's shoulder while another may cry until his little face is nestled close to her heart. The way one young infant responds to hunger pangs, a full belly, sleepiness, or a desire to be awake and explore the world, may be very different from sibling to sibling. Thus, the fact that parents have mastered the newborn language of one child does not mean that they are skilled in the dialect of the next. Experience is a good thing, but parents must be willing to start afresh with each child. A reminder of this fact at just the right time by a nurse confidante, for example, may be particularly encouraging to a parent.

Basic Nutrient Requirements

During infancy, rapid growth of the whole body, especially the brain, requires a significant nutrient load per kilogram of body weight. Energy needs must be met despite the limited stomach capacity of an infant, about 1 tablespoon (10–20 mL) at birth and about 1 cup (240 mL) at a year. Therefore, eight to 12 feedings per day for breastfed infants (six to eight for formula-fed infants since formula is less easily and more slowly digested than breast milk) are commonly required in the early months of infancy. Feedings of only human milk or infant formula are recommended for the first 6 months of life. From 6 to 12 months, infants typically make the transition from an all liquid diet to the mixed diet of the family. During this time, solid foods become a main source of key nutrients such as iron, zinc, calcium, vitamin B_{12} in vegan families, and, of course, protein. Fluoride, to prevent dental caries, may be recommended after 6 months of age, but dosage is based on a review of potential sources and the challenging goal of preventing both dental caries (from too little fluoride) and fluorosis (from too much fluoride). Vitamin D is also a nutrient of concern for infants. If exposure to adequate sunlight is not feasible due to the angle of the sun in a particular geographic location (far northern or far southern latitude); presence of tall, sun-blocking buildings, clouds or smog; or inability to take the infant outside regularly, for example, vitamin D supplementation may be needed. See Table 9.3 for a recommended progression of foods from birth through 18 months of age.

Developmental Expectations Related to Nutrient Intake

By the time a full-term infant is born, organ systems generally work rather well. Kidneys are not totally up to speed, so dehydration and electrolyte losses during illness may be a concern, but the heart and lungs work efficiently, for example, in contrast to those of a preterm infant. For infants who have passed 40 weeks gestation, the focus is on strengthening muscles and fine-tuning the way muscles work. Infants convey need for food, based on changes in appetite, through episodic crying spells. Attentive parents, especially breastfeeding mothers, come to understand this routine over time (Lampl, 2002).

Developmental issues related to nutrient intake during infancy, that is, during the first 12 months of life, are often addressed month-by-month, or according to a list of developmental landmarks. For the purpose of guided participation teaching and learning, skills development can be considered from the perspective of parents dealing with a new member of the family, and what they must watch for, and assist with, in order to support their child during this yearlong transition.

Infant feeding development, or the changes required to move an infant from all breastfeeding to eating at the table with the family, primarily revolves around the (a) ability to sit up; (b) variety (acceptance of new tastes and textures); (c) grasp, grip, and eye–hand coordination; (d) ability to bite and chew; and (e) ability to control liquid coming from a cup. Until an infant is able to sit up independently in an infant seat, somewhere around 4 to 7 months, feeding solid foods is risky since choking is a greater possibility for a person, including a little one, who is lying down. Infant cereal is typically the first "solid" introduced by spoon. It is a good source of iron and it is something that can be prepared at an appropriate consistency, fairly thin at first and then thicker as the infant improves in ability to successfully move food from the front of the mouth to the back. The AAP currently recommends that the introduction to solid foods begin at 6 months, both as a developmentally and a nutritionally appropriate activity (Kleinman & Greer, 2014, pp. 123–139).

Once an infant can sit independently and start solids, what is next with regard to food and nutrition? Variety is next. First there is variety of consistency. Companies that produce packaged baby foods, for example, classify foods by stages (Heinz Stage 1, Stage 2, Stage 3, Stage 4; Gerber 1st Foods®, 2nd Foods, 3rd Foods; Sprout Stage 1, Stage 2, Stage 3; Beech-Nut Stage 1, Stage 2, Stage 3, Stage 4; and others). The main reason parents may wish to purchase prepared baby food is ease. It is usually more expensive than home-prepared food, but for some families, the ease of having something ready to go, and the comfort of knowing that the texture is right for the infant, is valuable. The websites for infant food companies are quite robust. They provide lots of information about the developmental readiness and nutritional appropriateness for a certain set of products. They often review general infant/child feeding concepts as well, so such websites can be helpful to parents who are looking for answers or just wanting to learn more about feeding. Along with progression of consistency, infants also get to progress to new flavors. It is a great idea for parents to introduce their youngsters to the many flavors and textures typically consumed by the family, but it does not have to stop there. Nonstandard home-prepared foods can be offered. Foods not usually served, possibly broccoli or apricots, can be purchased from the infant product shelves, if desired. One tip to discuss with parents is that texture progression should be based on the infant's ability, not the age on the jar's label, whether using commercial or home-prepared foods. Mashed banana may work well at the start, but it might not be long until the infant is able to gum small pieces. On the other hand, it may be a very long time until teeth come in and small chunks of chicken are a safe possibility! Eruption of teeth, and the baby's ability to chew, at first, and then eventually take bites of food, plays a big part in the progression to new foods for a particular infant. Remind parents that the goal is for the infant to be eating all, or nearly all, family foods by 1 year of age. Foods may need to be cut finer, or cooked more, depending on the number of teeth and the infant's chewing competency, but the actual foods offered can be the same for the whole family.

During the latter half of an infant's first year, more developmental changes come into play. The palmar grasp develops at about 5 to 7 months, allowing the infant to begin to hold simple biscuits and move them to the mouth. Little ones can be challenged, and rewarded, with the fun of picking up small food items such as Cheerios or small pieces of carrot or pear, as the pincer grip develops around 9 to 11 months, and eye–hand coordination improves, or a spoon with oatmeal or mashed potatoes. Finally, by

12 months, most infants are able to drink from a cup. Thus, between 6 and 12 months, significant developmental changes occur. The result is that the infant becomes a junior member of the family who is able to eat the same foods as the rest of the family, in most cases, though size and texture of some items may need to be modified.

KEY NUTRITION RECOMMENDATIONS TO SHARE WITH THE FAMILY

1. Breastfeed and/or provide human milk for as much of the first year as possible.
2. Introduce solid food, including iron-fortified infant cereal, at age 6 months.
3. By 12 months of age, provide all food as table food, modified in texture and bite size as needed, and provide all, or nearly all, beverages by cup.

Childhood

"Eat your vegetables" can be a fun and a positive mantra for parents to use as children are growing up, though it is only positive if spoken in an upbeat and enjoyable manner, not in a punitive fashion, or as a threat. A common theme for good health throughout life is to include a variety of food, especially vegetables, and to eat in moderation. The DASH Eating Plan, the Mediterranean Diet, Choose My Plate, and the Dietary Guidelines for Americans, for example, all recommend inclusion of a variety of brightly colored, tasty vegetables (see 'Useful Websites [and Books] for Nutrition and Growth' at the end of this chapter for websites). For children, the "eat your vegetables" lesson begins at home as soon as they are learners, that is, as soon as they are watching and taking cues from parents and siblings. Additional information is available online through the Springer Publishing website at **www.springerpub.com/pridham**, Chapter 9. These documents include "First Meals" and "Nutrition Education."

Basic Nutrient Requirements

Energy needs for children from 1 through 13 years of age vary rather dramatically, as noted in Table 9.1. Typical intake requirements generally double from age 1 to 2 years (approximately 1,000 kcal/d) to the end of childhood (about 2,000–2,300 kcal/d for the 9- to 13-year-olds). In between, the average 3- to 8-year-old requires about 1,600 to 1,700 kcal per day. After infancy and early childhood, protein needs, relative to the size of the child, decrease. At 1 to 3 years of age, young children require about 1.1 g/kg/d, but from 4 to 13 years of age, they only need 0.95 g/kg/d (see Table 9.2). The absolute protein requirement nearly triples, though, from 13 to 34 g/d, in the stretch from 1 to 13 years of age (Food and Nutrition Board, Institute of Medicine, National Academies, 2016). Other nutrients of particular significance in childhood include calcium (for rapid bone growth), vitamin D (to facilitate adequate calcium absorption), iron (to prevent iron deficiency in light of rapid cell growth), zinc (essential for growth), and fluoride (to inhibit tooth decay). Fat (about 30%–35% of total calories), fiber (14 g/1,000 kcal), and fluid (from 1,300 mL for toddlers to approximately 2,300 mL [girls]/3,300 mL [boys] per day) round out significant nutrient concerns. The website ChooseMyPlate.gov is useful for exploring actual food options and ideas, recommended numbers of servings, and portion size in relation to age and gender (United States Department of Agriculture, 2016).

Developmental Expectations Related to Nutrient Intake

In the years between infancy and adolescence, hunger and satiety cues continue to be important tools to guide intake of food and beverages. During toddlerhood, parents (or those taking the role of parent anywhere along the way) are responsible for purchasing, preparing, and offering food that is need-appropriate. The food and beverages offered must meet the nutrient and developmental needs of the child. Though providing food for an infant was the same in many ways, the game changes in toddlerhood as the child begins to exert more and more independence. It should be of no surprise that a 1- to 2-year-old toddler begins to do more than just open or close his mouth at meal time, or turn her head away when her tummy is full. Hunger and satiety counts, but so does the toddler's attraction to explore, and even set limits, of their own. Thus, food jags (the desire by toddlers or young children to eat the same food, or foods, meal after meal) becomes the center of attention with regard to food purchase and preparation.

Cognitive and emotional development plays a role in how a child addresses food. Physical changes, such as the adolescent growth spurt, connect to internal cues to search for more energy (calories) per kg. The height spurt occurs between 9.5 and 14.5 years of age for girls, and 10.5 and 16 years of age for boys (Marshall & Tanner, 1970). According to Lampl (2002), "Growth saltations are accompanied by changes in behavior: agitation, sleep and appetite increase, and illness episodes co-occur with growth saltations more than can be explained by chance alone." In fact, Lampl (2002) says, "children grow by leaps and bounds, intermittently." Children experience appetite changes (increases) in relation to growth which can be described as "distinct, stepwise (**salutatory**) increases or jumps separated by intervals of no change," according to Lampl (Lampl, 1996; Lampl, Velhuis & Johnson, 1992). Parents are faced with the need to morph their own approach to purchasing and preparing food, and feeding and offering food, as the child grows physically ("by leaps and bounds, intermittently") and matures cognitively and emotionally. The time frame from age 1 through 13 years requires continuous learning and teaching on the part of both the child and the parents. It is also important, during these years, to teach and model the importance of breakfast.

Breakfast skipping is common for school-age children. Twenty percent of 9- to 13-year-olds skip the first meal of the day (Deshmuhk-Takar, Radcliffe, Lu, & Nicklaus, 2010), resulting in the potential for nutrient deficiencies, decreased energy intake, decreased ability to concentrate, and increased risk of becoming overweight or obese. During childhood, overweight is a serious concern. Frequent and/or excessive snacking may be to blame. Seven percent of U.S. 6- to 11-year-olds were overweight in 1980; by 2012, the number rose to 18% (Centers for Disease Control and Prevention, 2017). In contrast, underweight and failure to thrive can occur during childhood; either or both may be connected to food insecurity. Additionally, autism spectrum disorder (Privett, 2013) and attention deficit hyperactivity disorder (ADHD; McCann et al., 2007), two conditions linked to food hypersensitivities, may develop in childhood, along with food allergies and food intolerances. Nutrient needs during childhood vary based on age, sex, and activity level, as well as stage of physical development and health condition. Cognitive and emotional development play a significant role in how a child accepts or rejects food, makes decisions about food, and accepts guidance related to food. Nurturing a positive feeding relationship is just as important for toddlers and school-age children as it is for infants. It is positive and productive to allow children to explore food and make food decisions appropriate to stage of development (Satter, 2008).

KEY NUTRITION RECOMMENDATIONS TO SHARE WITH THE FAMILY

1. Propose food choices (such as "either/or" options), rather than restrictions, and always offer food in a form the child can manage.
2. Go with the food jags (unless unsafe). They are part of normal development, and they will not last forever.
3. Make mealtimes enjoyable with positive discussion at a level in which the child can participate.

Adolescence

Adolescence, the exciting and awkward time between childhood and adulthood, is a period of physical, psychological, and cognitive change. Adolescence is variously defined as the period between 12 and 18 years of age, or 12 and 21 years of age, or, for example, 10 to 19 years of age (World Health Organization, 2018a). Despite the actual age in years, this time known as adolescence is marked by preoccupation with body size and shape; by cognitive, emotional, and psychosocial development; by social, emotional, and financial independence; and by a significant amount of growth. Approximately half of adult body weight is gained during adolescence along with 20% of adult height. Food, therefore, plays a key role in adolescence.

Basic Nutrient Requirements

Energy needs during adolescence vary considerably since they are based on height, weight, gender, age, physical activity, and an additional caloric allotment for growth. Protein needs per kilogram of body weight are lower for

9- to 13-year-olds (0.95 g/kg/d) than for younger children, but higher than needs of 14- to 18-year-olds (0.85 g/kg/d; Table 9.2). The Dietary Reference Intake for protein increases, though, from 34 g/d for 9- to 13-year-olds to 46 g/d for females and 52 g/d for males age 14 to 18 years. Other nutrients of particular concern during adolescence include calcium (due to rapid bone, endocrine, and muscle development), iron (for increased muscle mass and blood volume [as well as blood loss for girls, once menstruation begins]), folic acid (to support accretion of lean body mass, and neurological development for the fetus should an adolescent get pregnant), vitamin D (for calcium and phosphorus absorption), as well as micronutrients and vitamins required for growth.

Developmental Expectations Related to Nutrient Intake

As with younger children, appetite is a factor in the development that takes place during adolescence. Appetite surges as the body calls for an increase in food to support rapid growth. Adolescents are far more capable than they were as children to meet the nutrient needs of their own body. That is, unlike their younger self, they are cognitively able to determine that they need food to assuage their hunger, and they are physically able to search for food (e.g., at home or school, at a friend's house, or out in the big world via a bus or car). They are tall enough to reach food, possibly skilled enough to prepare food, and potentially independent enough to purchase food. Not all adolescent behaviors support the needs of the growing adolescent body, though. Image becomes a driver. The media and peers get the better of a certain number of adolescents. For them, the need to diet takes over. Some adolescents, unfortunately, head down the path to anorexia, bulimia, or some other disordered eating behavior. For others, the choices are not quite so debilitating. Rather, activities such as snacking, meal skipping, eating away from home, and eating at irregular times become the norm. These patterns have the potential to keep adolescents from obtaining all of the nutrients their bodies crave, or of setting the scene for obesity. Some adolescents try out new eating styles or diets, such as vegetarianism. Making the choice to become a vegetarian, or the more extreme vegan, may be done for health reasons, animal rights, or rebellion. No matter what the motivation, B vitamins, calcium, iron, and zinc requirements may need to be addressed. Unfortunately, though the adolescent period can very well be a time of positive, healthy development, in recent years it has also become a time for the birth of hyperlipidemia, hypertension, weight gain, and diabetes. It is imperative to prevent or limit the development of such conditions since not doing so will set the individual up for early and difficult health trials.

Young children are given a significant amount of attention. They thrive over time, though, if they are allowed to make healthy decisions on their own. This is true, also, for the adolescent. When it comes to food and food choices, empowering adolescents to make healthy choices is a great plan. Invite them to remain a part of the family, to share meals together, to prepare food at home (to eat either at home or on the run), to choose wisely when selecting restaurants, and to be physically active. Weight-bearing activities and a nutrient-rich diet help to build strong bones at a time (puberty) when bone growth is rapid. According to Berge et al. (2015), adolescents who eat meals with their families on a regular basis, even a minimal number of meals, are less likely to become overweight or obese compared to teens who never eat with their families. This is an important concept for all members of the family to support. The family table can be a place to model healthy eating behaviors and make positive emotional connections.

KEY NUTRITION RECOMMENDATIONS TO SHARE WITH THE FAMILY

1. Always provide access to healthy food at a manageable cost and in a reasonable location.
2. Make family meals a family value.
3. Encourage independence through participation in meal preparation and choice in meal offerings.

AN EXEMPLAR: A PRETERM INFANT

Baby L. D. weighed 570 g when she was born 12 weeks early at 28 weeks gestation. Her birth length was 30.5 cm and birth head circumference was 22 cm. Based on the revised Fenton growth chart for girls (Fenton & Kim, 2013), L. D.'s weight at birth was less than the 10th percentile; so she was classified as small-for-gestational age (Merck, 2016) (see Figure 9.9). Growth restriction probably began early in pregnancy since weight, length, and head circumference were all affected in a nearly symmetric manner. Her parents are average height, so the small size is most likely not merely genetic in origin. Unfortunately, weight (and length) continued to drift further below the 3rd percentile. That is, the z-score fell below –2.0, or greater than 2 standard deviations below the mean, throughout her time in the NICU and she did not maintain weight or length parallel to the growth curves, as recommended (Kleinman & Greer, 2014, pp. 609–642).

L. D.'s mother was planning to breastfeed, even though L. D. was her first baby and, as a new mother, she knew very little about the process. She had heard it was the right thing to do for her baby, but she was not sure why. During the first weeks in the hospital, L. D.'s mother and father came to the hospital daily. Mom brought pumped breast milk for L. D. at each visit, and she also pumped during the visit. As she handed it to the nurse, she and her husband always asked, "How much does L. D. weigh today?" Most days, L. D.'s weight was higher than the day before, but occasionally, her weight went down. On those days, L. D.'s mother quickly became quiet as she anticipated her next hurdle—pumping breast milk as she considers why L. D. lost weight, and whether it was her fault as the provider of life-giving nutrients.

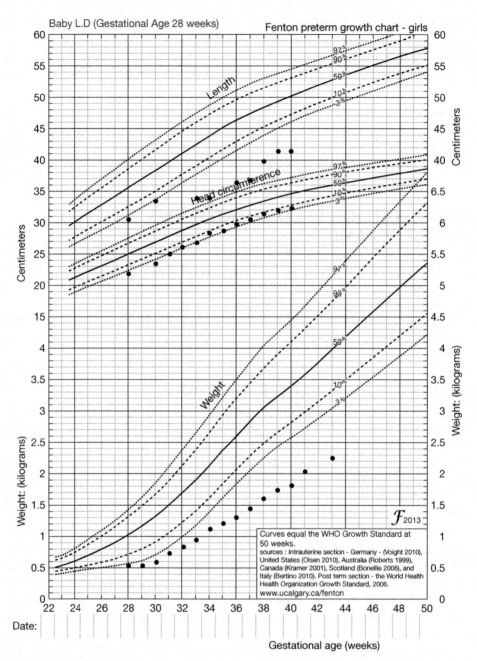

FIGURE 9.9 Weight, length, and head circumference of baby L. D. from birth (28 weeks gestation) to 43 weeks postconceptional age.

Reprinted with permission, tfenton@ucalgary.ca

Throughout the hospitalization, L. D. encountered breathing problems (due to her immature lungs), bouts of constipation (especially when she was fed infant formula due to limited supply of human milk), infection (as a result of a line infection during her first weeks), and then esophageal reflux. In the hospital, L. D. was started on parenteral nutrition and intravenous lipids within her first days. Small amounts of human milk were added by the end of L. D.'s first week of life. As time went on, L. D.'s mother struggled with pumping breast milk in hopes of avoiding the need for L. D. to be fed infant formula. L. D. met a number of bumps on the growth road. To cope with the stress of L. D.'s medical issues, on top of her need for more rapid growth, L. D. was fed 24, 27, and even 30 cal/ounce (fortified) human milk and preterm infant formula, sometimes with the addition of protein powder and/ or medium-chain triglyceride (MCT) oil. L. D. struggled to gain weight effectively when she transitioned from parenteral nutrition to all enteral feedings, when she made the leap from tube feeding to all breast/bottle-feeding, and then again when she went home and moved to mostly breastfeeding. Though the day-to-day weight dips, spread throughout the weeks of slow weight increases, were not obvious on the growth chart that depicted weekly measurements, L. D.'s mother noticed each one. Fortunately, L. D.'s head growth continued at rates parallel to the growth chart, and even improved a bit, though just up to the 3rd percentile. Length increased, but not nearly as much as the medical team was hoping for. L. D.'s weight progress was affected the most. At the time of discharge from the hospital, her weight was farther below the reference standards than at any previous time, due to gaining at rates much slower than the growth curves. Not unlike parents of most sick or preterm infants, L. D.'s mother and father had so many concerns on their minds: poor intake, frequent feedings, irregular feedings, proper nutrition, GI problems, difficulties weaning to new food flavors and textures, anemia, underweight, overweight, poor weight gain, rapid weight gain, short stature, and more (Cho, Lee, Youn, Kim, & Sung, 2012). With the help of L. D.'s supportive medical team, L. D.'s parents left the hospital anticipating that their still-tiny bundle would, over time and with close attention, grow to the size that was healthy for her.

How might I begin to use guided participation with L. D.'s parents as they develop their own practice of caregiving, day to day, in relation to their child's changing (advancing or delayed) feeding skills and nutritional needs?

- Explore the concept of breastfeeding. What is on the mom's/dad's mind? Consider time to pump, comfort/discomfort of the procedure, volume of human milk available, privacy, time required, desire to provide some or all of L. D.'s feeding, its nutritional (and emotional) value, alternatives (risks/benefits) to breastfeeding/pumping, and dad's role in breastfeeding.
- Ask what the parents think about the most in relation to their hospitalized infant—during the day, and during the night. What makes them smile? What makes them sad or anxious?
- Discuss feeding options, benefits, and concerns. If L. D.s' mother decides to continue breastfeeding throughout the newborn hospitalization, what does that mean to her life, her free-time, her body, the infant's health?
- Invite a discussion about what they want the future to look like for their child, and how they, as parents, may be able to facilitate that outcome. How will L. D. be fed? How will the process and the food change over the next weeks, months, or years?

- Consider, with the parents, what they feel they need to care for L. D. effectively (during the hospitalization and at home)—knowledge, skills, physical tools, emotional support, an extra pair of hands, more sleep? Walk L. D.'s parents through a plan to acquire what is needed, but let the parents lead the discussion. Encourage them to review the plan with you regularly and to adjust the plan as needed to accommodate the needs of both infant and parents.
- Reflect on how L. D.'s growth, weight gain in particular, affects her mom and dad, and how to decide what is concerning and what is not.

What could we (parents, child, and clinician) do together to make connections and build trust around feeding decisions?

- Share the burden. Each day, when L. D.'s mother and father visit their daughter, ask them to share (verbally and in writing) the best part of the visit. Did L. D. gain weight, have less apneic spells, remain alert a minute longer during a feeding, nurse at the breast?
- Assist the family with thinking about the tools they will need for feeding L. D. immediately after discharge from the hospital, and in the coming months, as well as where the tools, formula, and food will come from, and how costs will be covered.
- Together, anticipate next steps. Schedule times for in-person visits, phone calls, and virtual meetings (via secure web conferencing). Arrange for Health Insurance Portability and Accountability Act (HIPAA)-compliant messaging (text or email). Decide on communication routes that meet the needs, skill levels, and time constraints of L. D.'s parents.

CONCLUSION

- **Continuous growth, though at varying rates, is expected from birth (premature or term) throughout adolescence.** The need to support growth differentiates nutritional care of infants and children from that of adults. Nutrient needs in the pediatric population vary with normal growth rate, diminishing at times and increasing at others. Additionally, requirements vary at unexpected times for individuals who need to achieve catch-up growth after a period of deficient intake, and for those who need to recover after illness or injury. Wound healing and pregnancy always increase nutrients requirements above baseline needs for age.
- **Growth patterns that diverge significantly from normal have a cause.** Learning together, as with the guided participation approach, can help families find the cause of a divergent growth pattern which may be clinical- or knowledge-related, behavioral, or social in nature, for example, and then discover a feasible means of improvement. For some individuals, divergence from a standard is acceptable and genetically appropriate. When either suboptimal growth or excessive weight gain is noted, though, a child (infant through adolescent) will benefit the most

if professional caregivers and the family work together to reflect on reasons for inadequate or excessive nutrient intake in relation to decreased or excessive energy expenditure. Consider activity, healing, illness, or disease.

■ **Food habits form at an early age.** Parents have an obligation to offer foods and beverages that are nutrient- and texture-appropriate for age, for developmental stage, and for health condition. By learning and teaching together, the process of guided participation can help parents support their children in the investigation of new flavors, colors, forms, and types of food. Exploration of foods can be a fun, healthy lifelong adventure.

REFERENCES

American Academy of Pediatrics, Committee on Nutrition. (2014). Nutritional needs of preterm infants. In R. E. Kleinman & F. R. Greer (Eds.), *Pediatric nutrition handbook* (7th ed.). Elk Grove, IL: Author.

American College of Obstetricians and Gynecologists. (2016). *Ob-Gyns redefine the meaning of "Term Pregnancy."* Retrieved from http://www.acog.org/About-ACOG/News-Room/News-Releases/2013/Ob-Gyns-Redefine-Meaning-of-Term-Pregnancy

American Psychological Association. (2016). *The road to resilience: What is resilience?* Retrieved from www.apa.org/helpcenter/road-resilience.aspx

Babson, S. G., & Benda, G. I. (1976). Growth graphs for the clinical assessment of infants of varying gestational age. *Journal of Pediatrics*, 89(5), 814–820.

Berge, J. M., Wall, M., Hsueh, T.-F., Fulkerson, J. A., Laron, N., & Neumark-Sztainer, D. (2015). The protective role of family meals for youth obesity: 10-year longitudinal associations. *The Journal of Pediatrics*, 166(2), 296–301.

Centers for Disease Control and Prevention. (2017). *Growth charts for children with down syndrome.* Retrieved from http://www.cdc.gov/ncbddd/birthdefects/downsyndrome/growth-charts.html

Centers for Disease Control and Prevention, Division of Nutrition, Physical Activity, and Obesity, National Center for Chronic Disease Prevention and Health Promotion. (2015). *Growth chart training.* Retrieved from http://www.cdc.gov/nccdphp/dnpao/growthcharts/index.htm

Centers for Disease Control and Prevention, Healthy Schools. (2017). *Childhood obesity facts.* Retrieved from http://www.cdc.gov/healthyschools/obesity/facts.htm

Centers for Disease Control and Prevention, National Center for Health Statistics. (2001). *Data table of infant weight-for-age chart.* Retrieved from http://www.cdc.gov/growthcharts/html_charts/wtageinf.htm

Centers for Disease Control and Prevention, National Center for Health Statistics. (2010a). *Growth charts.* Retrieved from http://www.cdc.gov/growthcharts

Centers for Disease Control and Prevention, National Center for Health Statistics. (2010b). *WHO Growth standards are recommended for use in the U.S. for infants and children 0 to 2 years of age.* Retrieved from http://www.cdc.gov/growthcharts/who_charts.htm#The%20WHO%20Growth%20Charts

Centers for Disease Control and Prevention, National Center for Health Statistics. (2014). *The NHANES story.* Retrieved from https://wwwn.cdc.gov/nchs/nhanes/nhanes3/anthropometricvideos.aspx

Centers for Disease Control and Prevention, National Center for Health Statistics. (2018). *Births: Final data for 2016.* Retrieved from https://www.cdc.gov/nchs/data/nvsr/nvsr67/nvsr67_01.pdf

Cho, J-Y., Lee, J., Youn, Y. A., Kim, S. Y., & Sung, I. K. (2012). Parenteral concerns about their premature infants' health after discharge from the neonatal intensive care unit: A questionnaire survey for anticipated guidance in a neonatal follow-up clinic. *Korean Journal of Pediatrics*, 55(8), 272–279. doi:10.3345/kjp.2012.55.8.272

Dancis, J., O'Connell, F. R., & Holt, L. E., Jr. (1948). A grid for recording the weight of premature infants. *Journal of Pediatrics*, 33(11), 570–572.

Declercq, E. R., Sakala, C., Corry, M. P., & Applebaum, S. (2006). *Listening to mothers II: Report of the second national U.S. survey of women's childbearing experiences.* New York, NY: Childbirth Connection.

Deshmuhk-Takar, P. R., Radcliffe, J. D., Lu, Y., & Nicklaus, T. A. (2010). The relationship of breakfast skipping and type of breakfast consumption with nutrient intake and weight status in children and adolescents: The national health and nutrition examination survey 1999–2006. *Journal of the Academy of Nutrition and Dietetics, 110,* 869–878. doi:10.1016/j.jada.2010.03.023

Fenton, T. R. (2003). A new growth chart for preterm babies: Babson and Benda's chart updated with recent data and a new format. *BMC Pediatrics, 3*(13). doi:10.1186/1471-2431-3-13

Fenton, T. R., & Kim, J. H. (2013). A systematic review and meta-analysis to revise the Fenton growth chart for premature infants. *BMC Pediatrics, 13*(59). doi:10.1186/1471-2431-13-59

Food and Nutrition Board, Institute of Medicine of the National Academies. (2005). *Dietary reference intakes for energy, carbohydrate, fiber, fat, fatty acids, cholesterol, protein and amino acids.* Washington, DC: National Academies Press. Retrieved from https://www.nap.edu/read/10490/chapter/1

Food and Nutrition Board, Institute of Medicine, National Academies. (2016). *Dietary reference intakes: Estimated average requirements, recommended intakes, acceptable macronutrient distribution ranges, and tolerable upper intake levels.* Retrieved from https://fnic.nal.usda.gov/dietary-guidance/dietary-reference-intakes/dri-tables-and-application-reports

Grummer-Strawn, L. M. (2002). *The use of NCHS and CDC growth charts in nutritional assessment of infants* (White paper, 3903B1–04). Retrieved from http://www.fda.gov/ohrms/dockets/ac/02/briefing/3903b1-04.pdf

INTERGROWTH-21st Anthropometry Group. (2012). *Anthropometry manual.* Retrieved from http://www.medscinet.net/Interbio/Uploads/ProtocolDocs/Anthropometry%20Handbook.pdf

International Fetal and Newborn Growth Consortium. (2009). *The international fetal and newborn growth standards for the 21st century (INTERGROWTH-21st) study protocol.* Retrieved from http://www.medscinet.net/Intergrowth/patientinfodocs/Intergrowth%20Protocol%20Sept%202009.pdf

Kleinman, R. E., & Greer, F. R. (Eds.) (2014). *Pediatric nutrition* (7th ed.). Elk Village, IL: American Academy of Pediatrics.

Koletzko, B., Agostoni, C., Ball, P., Carnielli, V., Chaloner, C., Clayton, J., . . . Yaron, A. (2005). ESPEN/ESPGHAN guidelines on paediatric parenteral nutrition. 2. Energy. *Journal of Pediatric Gastroenterology and Nutrition, 41,* S5–S11. Retrieved from http://www.rch.org.au/uploadedFiles/Main/Content/rchcpg/hospital_clinical_guideline_index/ESPGHAN%20Guidelines_Paediatric_Parenteral_Nutrition_2005.pdf

Kuczmarski, R. J., Ogden, C. L., Guo, S. S., Grummer-Strawn, L. M., Flegal, K. M., Mei, Z., . . . Johnson, C. L. (2002). *2000 CDC growth charts for the United States: Methods and development.* DHHS Publication no. (PHS) 2002–1696. Hyattsville, MD: National Center for Health Statistics. Retrieved from http://www.cdc.gov/nchs/data/series/sr_11/sr11_246.pdf

Lai, N. M., Rajadurai S. V., & Tan K. (2006). Increased energy intake for preterm infants with (or developing) bronchopulmonary dysplasia/chronic lung disease. *Chochrane Database of Systematic Reviews, 3,* CD005093. doi:10.1002/14651858.CD005093.pub2

Lampl, M. (1996). Saltatory growth and illness patterns. *American Journal of Physical Anthropology, 22*(Suppl.), 45.

Lampl, M. (2002). Saltation and stasis. In N. Cameron & N. Cameron (Eds.), *Human growth and development* (pp. 253–270). San Diego, CA: Academic Press.

Lampl, M., Velhuis, J. D., & Johnson, M. L. (1992). Saltation and stasis: A model of human growth. *Science, 258,* 801–803.

Larkin, E. C., & Rai, A. (1990). Importance of fetal and neonatal iron: Adequacy for normal development of central nervous system. In J. Dobbing (Ed.), *Brain, behaviour, and iron in the infant diet* (pp. 43–62). New York, NY: Springer-Verlag.

Lu, M. C., Prentice, J., Yu, S. M., Inkelas, M., Lange, L., & Halfon, N. (2003). Childbirth education classes: Sociodemographic disparities in attendance and the association of attendance with breastfeeding initiation. *Maternal and Child Health Journal, 7*(2), 87–93.

Lubchenco, L., Hansman, C., & Boyd, E. (1966). Intrauterine growth in length and head circumferences estimated from live births at gestational ages from 26 to 42 weeks. *Pediatrics, 37,* 403–408.

Lubchenco, L., Hansman, C., Dressler, M., & Boyd, E. (1963). Intrauterine growth as estimated from liveborn weight data at 24 to 42 weeks of gestation. *Pediatrics, 32,* 793–800.

Ludwig, S., & Waitzman, K. A. (2016). Infant-driven feeding®: A practice model to optimize long-term growth and development [Video]. Retrieved from www.anhi.org

Marshall, W. A., & Tanner, J. M. (1970). Variations in the pattern of pubertal changes in boys. *Archives of Disease in Childhood, 45*(13), 13–23.

McCann, D., Barrett, A., Crumpler, D., Dalen, L., Grimshaw, K., Kitchin, E., . . . Stevenson, J. (2007). Food additives and hyperactive behaviour in 3-year-old and 8/9-year-old children in the community: A randomised, double-blinded, placebo-controlled trial. *Lancet, 370* (9598), 1560–1567.

Merck Sharp & Dohme Corp., a subsidiary of Merck & Co., Inc. (2016). *Merck manual professional edition*. Retrieved from http://www.merckmanuals.com/professional

Nafday, S. M. (2008). Neonatal medical conditions. In T. K. McInerny, H. M. Adam, D. E. Campbell, D. M. Kamat, & K. J. Kelleher (Eds.), *Textbook of pediatric care* (pp. 883–892). Elk Grove Village, IL: American Academy of Pediatrics.

NIH Eunice Kennedy Shriver National Institute of Child Health and Human Development. (2016). *Safe to sleep® public education campaign*. Retrieved from https://www.nichd.nih.gov/sts/Pages/default.aspx

Olsen, I. E., Groveman, S. A., Lawson, M. L., Clark, R. H., & Zemel, B. S. (2010). New Intrauterine growth curves based on United States data. *Pediatrics, 125*, e214–e224. doi:10.1542/peds.2009-0913

Olsen, I. E., Lawson, M. L., Ferguson, A. N., Cantrell, R., Grabich, S. C., Zemel, B. S., & Clark, R. H. (2015). BMI curves for preterm infants. *Pediatrics, 135*, e572–e581. doi:10.1542/peds.2014-2777

Otten, J. Hellwig, J. P., & Meyers, L. D. (Eds). (2006). *Dietary reference intakes: The essential guide to nutrient requirements*. Washington, DC: National Academies Press.

Privett, D. (2013). Autism spectrum disorder—Research suggests good nutrition may manage symptoms. *Today's Dietitian, 15*(1), 43–46.

Queensland Health. (2015). Estimating energy, protein & fluid requirements for adult clinical conditions. Retrieved from https://www.health.qld.gov.au/nutrition/nemo_nutrsup.asp

Rehman, M. U., & Narchi, S. (2015). Metabolic bone disease in the preterm infant: Current state and future directions. *World Journal of Methodology, 5*(3), 115–121. doi:10.5662/wjm.v5.i3.115

Satter, E. (2008). *Secrets of feeding a healthy family* (2nd ed.). Madison, WI: Kelcy Press.

Satter, E. (2016). *Ellen Satter's division of responsibility in eating*. Retrieved from http://ellynsatterinstitute.org/dor/divisionofresponsibilityinfeeding.php

Stiles, J., & Jernigan, T. L. (2010). The basics of brain development. *Neuropsychological Rehabilitation, 20*, 327–438. doi:10.1007/s11065-010-9148-4

United States Department of Agriculture. (2016). *ChooseMyPlate.gov*. Retrieved from https://www.choosemyplate.gov

Villar, J., Papageorghiou, A. T., Pang, R., Ohuma, E. O., Ismail, L.C., Barros, F.C., . . . Kennedy, S. (2014). The likeness of fetal growth and newborn size across non-isolated populations in the INTERGROWTH-21st Project: The fetal growth longitudinal study and newborn cross-sectional study. *The Lancet, 2*(10), 781–792.

World Health Organization. (2011). *Guidelines on optimal feeding of low birthweight infants in low-and middle-income countries*. Retrieved from http://www.who.int/maternal_child_adolescent/documents/infant_feeding_low_bw/en

World Health Organization. (2018a). *Adolescent development*. Retrieved from http://www.who.int/maternal_child_adolescent/topics/adolescence/dev/en/

World Health Organization. (2018b). *Constitution of WHO: Principles*. Retrieved from http://www.who.int/about/mission/en

World Health Organization. (2018c). *Preterm birth*. Retrieved from www.who.int/mediacentre/factsheets/f2e6e/en

World Health Organization Multicentre Growth Reference Study Group. (2009). *WHO child growth standards: Length/height-for-age, weight-for-age, weight-for-length, weight-for-height and body mass index-for-age: Methods and development*. Geneva, Switzerland: World Health Organization. Retrieved from http://www.who.int/childgrowth/publications/technical_report_velocity/en

Zemel, B. S., Pipan, M., Stallings, V. A., Hall, W., Schadt, K., Freedman, D. S., & Thorpe, P. (2015). Growth charts for children with Down syndrome in the United States. *Pediatrics, 136*(5), e1204–e1211. doi:10.1542/peds.2015-1652

APPENDIX 9.1 COMMUNITY PROVIDER SUPPORT OF GROWTH IN PREMATURE INFANTS

Community care providers are critical in supporting premature infants and their families in attaining healthy outcomes. These providers include primary physicians (family physicians and pediatricians), public health nurses, nurse practitioners, birth to 3 months providers, registered dietitians, and WIC nutritionists. Growth is a reflection of a young child's well-being. Compared to good growth, inappropriate growth is more often associated with frequent illnesses and hospitalizations (Hack et al.,1993), lower bone density (Fewtrell, Prentice, Cole & Lucas, 2000), and adiposity (Euser et al., 2005). Quality of care affects growth (Steward & Pridham, 2002). Evidence-based care to support growth begins with adjusting a premature infant's chronological age for prematurity. Quality care includes close monitoring of growth parameters to allow for early recognition of an abnormal trajectory, immediate efforts to encourage appropriate growth (e.g., nutritional supplementation), and early detection and treatment of illness.

THE PURPOSES OF THIS STATEMENT ARE THE FOLLOWING

- To describe the method for adjusting an infant's age for prematurity
- To define appropriate parameters for monitoring an infant's growth
- To provide resources and intervention strategies for community care providers in their efforts to support optimal growth in premature infants

ADJUSTING AGE FOR PREMATURITY

Adjusting age for prematurity (birth prior to 37 weeks gestation) helps healthcare providers set realistic expectations for the infant's growth and development. The provider can then communicate these expectations to parents and other individuals caring for the infant. For as long as the first 2 to 3 years of life, premature infants are likely to exhibit lower than average weight and length unless allowance is made for gestational age. Therefore, what is normal may not seem normal unless one adjusts for prematurity.

TIPS FOR ADJUSTING AN INFANT'S AGE FOR PREMATURITY

- Use infant's due date for calculating adjusted age. For example, an infant born on March 30 and due on June 30 would be approximately 1 month old (or 4 weeks) on July 30.
- Round off the adjusted age to the nearest week.
- Continue to adjust at least through 24 months (2 years).

Plotting Anthropometric Measurements

It is important to plot an infant's measurements routinely on a consistent growth chart. Incremental weight charts (measuring velocity) provide more graphic illustration than standard growth charts regarding the changes in weight over time (Desch, 1993), but these charts may not be readily available or applicable to current age (e.g., when an infant has not reached term). Current growth charts (weight for age, length for age, head circumference for age, weight for length), available in English, Spanish, and French, can be downloaded from www.cdc.gov/growthcharts/.

TIPS FOR OBTAINING ACCURATE AND RELIABLE MEASUREMENTS

- Measuring length requires two people and a length board with a head and foot piece. One person holds the head in position. The second person straightens the knees and brings the ankles to a right angle with the foot piece. Lengths done on exam tables using a tape measure are approximations at best, and often useless in accurately tracking growth.
- Weigh on a digital scale.

Measuring and Plotting BMI

Experts recommend following the BMI because of its accessibility and correlation with total body fat and risk factors for obesity-related morbidity in adults (Krebs, et al., 2007). BMI is defined as the individual's body weight (kg) divided by the square of his or her length/height (m). Calculating BMI of an infant requires accurate measures of weight and recumbent length/ height. BMI tables, nomograms, and calculator programs are available from a number of sources. Current BMI standards are based on term infants; data for prematurely born infants are not available.

Online Resources for BMI Tables and Nomograms

- www.who.int/childgrowth/standards/bmi_for_age/en/index.html
- www.cdc.gov/nccdphp/dnpa/bmi/calc-bmi.htm
- https://www.nhlbi.nih.gov/health/educational/lose_wt/bmitools.htm

GROWTH FALTERING

Growth faltering means that attained growth is inadequate or growth veloc- ity is reduced compared to expected growth velocity. Alternatively, growth faltering describes the situation when one or more parameters drop two or more channels on the growth chart (e.g., from the 50th to 75th percentiles to the 5th to 10th). Generally, growth faltering happens first in weight, then length, then head circumference. Poor head growth is a late, and more ominous, sign of nutritional deficits.

Early identification and close monitoring of growth faltering, combined with appropriate nutritional intervention, may reverse the downward growth trajectory before it affects the infant's brain and overall development.

Sometimes clinicians are deceived about growth by how a baby looks, or the clinician might think, "Well, the parents are small." Remember, to judge adequate growth, you need accurate anthropometric measurements.

CATCH-UP GROWTH

Inadequate

A premature infant's weight, length, and head circumference frequently fall below the 50th percentile when plotted on a growth grid, even when the infant's age is adjusted for prematurity. The distance between where the infant's growth actually falls and the 50th percentile is considered to be his or her growth potential, or the gap that needs to be closed in order to say that the infant has "caught up" with peers. Catch-up growth is dependent on growth velocity (the rate of change in growth over time) that exceeds expected velocity. The velocity excess during catchup equals the deficit during growth faltering (Forbes, 1974). Factors that influence catch-up growth include gestational age at birth, size for gestational age at birth, genetic potential, neurological injury, illness, and nutritional intake. Generally, catchup occurs first in head circumference, then length, then weight.

Excessive

While earlier studies indicated a beneficial effect of catch-up growth on head circumference and infant development (Ehrenkranz et al., 2006; Georgieff, Hoffman, Pereira, Bernbaum, & Hoffman-Williamson, 1985) recent research has suggested an association between rapid postnatal weight gain and the metabolic syndrome. Increased global and central adiposity have been associated with rapid postnatal weight gain in both premature and full-term infants, changes which increase concerns about the development of insulin resistance and the metabolic syndrome (Cooke & Griffin, 2009; Demerath et al., 2009).

However, adult behaviors and lifestyle are stronger predictors of metabolic syndrome than rapid postnatal growth (Greer, 2007; Yeung, 2010). Thus, there is insufficient evidence at this time to recommend submaximal nutrition support for premature infants, but further study is necessary.

CONSIDERATIONS

- Infant head circumference growth and development are positively associated with catch-up growth.
- Excessive catch-up growth has been associated with global and central adiposity and has been associated with metabolic syndrome in adults.

PROVIDING OPTIMUM NUTRITION TO PREMATURE INFANTS

Breast milk is the nutrient of choice for premature infants (Vohr et al., 2006). Breast milk protects against infection, is easily digested and well tolerated, contains species-specific nutrients, enhances cognitive development, and reduces cost of both healthcare and infant feeding.

- Premature infants who are breastfed, as well as those fed either breast milk or formula, may need additional calories and nutrients through supplementary feedings (Meier, 2003). To determine appropriate supplementary feedings, consultation with someone with expertise in premature infant nutrition and growth may be necessary.
- All premature infants (including late preterm infants) need closer monitoring than full-term infants (Santos et al., 2009).
- Nutritional management of premature infants should consider such factors as degree of prematurity and presence of other medical conditions which could affect metabolic demands.

Premature infants are often discharged to home on nutrient-enriched formula to facilitate "catch-up" growth. A meta-analysis of seven trials, enrolling a total of 631 infants, provided no strong evidence that feeding with nutrient-enriched formula following hospital discharge affects growth and development (Henderson, Fahey, & McGuire, 2007a). Similarly, randomized controlled trials have provided insufficient evidence to determine whether multicomponent-fortified breast milk is superior to unfortified breast milk for premature infants following discharge (Henderson, Fahey, & McGuire, 2007b).

ADDITIONAL RESOURCES

- "Gaining and Growing: Assuring Nutritional Care of Premature Infants" (www.depts.washington.edu/growing) is a source of good information on nutrition and growth of premature infants.

SUMMARY

The goal of monitoring the growth of premature infants is twofold: to prevent or arrest growth faltering and to improve the odds of achieving appropriate catch-up growth in a timely manner. For the newborn premature infant, care should focus on support of the infant's return to his or her in utero growth trajectory prior to hospital discharge (Radmacher, Looney, Rafail, & Adamkin, 2003). For the premature infant who is already living in the community at large, family and healthcare services should focus on provision of nutrients to support appropriate catch-up growth. While not every premature infant will achieve the 50th percentile, or even the 10th percentile weight, length, and/or head circumference for adjusted age, with few exceptions, the goal should continue to be achievement of, or return to, the growth pattern the infant would have followed if he or she had been born at term.

Authors: Janine Bamberger, MS, RD, CD, Aurora Sinai Medical Center, Milwaukee; Rana Limbo, PhD, RN, PMHCNS-BC, Gundersen Lutheran Medical Foundation, Inc.

Reviewers: Jill Paradowski, RN, MSN, Karen Pridham, PhD, RN, FAAN; Anne Weinfurter, RN; Judy Zunk, MS, RD, CSP, CD; Eva Fassbinder Brummel, MPH, WAPC Staff, and Ann Conway, RN, MS, MPA, WAPC staff

Authors of 1st edition (formerly titled "Catch-up Growth in Premature Infants"): Sherie Sondel, MEd, RD, CD, DHFS, Division of Public Health, Madison; Janine Bamberger, MS, RD, CD, Aurora Sinai Medical Center, Milwaukee; and Rana Limbo, PhD, RN, CS, WAPC staff

Reviewers: Lorna Cisler-Cahill, RN, MS; Kyle Mounts, MD; Jill Paradowski, RN, MSN, City of Milwaukee Health Department; Karen Pridham, PhD, RN, FAAN; Judy Zunk, MS, RD, CSP, CD; and Ann Conway, RN, MS, MPA, WAPC staff

REFERENCES TO APPENDIX 9.1

Cooke, R. J. & Griffin, I. (2009). Altered body composition in preterm infants at hospital discharge. *Acta Paediatrica, 98,* 1269–1273.

Demerath, E. W., Reed, D., Choh, A. C., Soloway, L., Lee, M., Czerwinski, S. A., . . . Towne, B. (2009). Rapid postnatal weight gain and visceral adiposity in adulthood: The Fels longitudinal study. *Obesity, 17*(11), 2060–2066.

Desch, L. W. (1993). Use of incremental weight charts with follow-up of high-risk infants. *Journal of Perinatology, 13*(5), 361–367.

Ehrenkranz, R. A., Dusick, A. M., Vohr, B. R., Wright, L. L., Wrage, L. A., & Poole, W. K. (2006). Growth in the neonatal intensive care unit influences neurodevelopmental and growth outcomes of extremely low birth weight infants. *Pediatrics, 117,* 1253–1261.

Euser, A. M., Finken, M. J., Keijzer-Veen, M. G., Hille, E. T., Wit, J. M., Dekker, F. W., & Dutch POPS-19 Collaborative Study Group. (2005). Associations between prenatal and infancy weight gain and BMI, fat mass, and fat distribution in young adulthood: A prospective cohort study in males and females born very preterm. *American Journal of Clinical Nutrition, 81*(2), 480–487.

Fewtrell, M., Prentice, A., Cole, T. J., & Lucas, A. (2000). Effects of growth during infancy and childhood on bone mineralization and turnover in preterm children aged 8-12 years. *Acta Paediatrica, 89*(2), 148–153.

Forbes, G. B. (1974). A note on the mathematics of "catch-up" growth. *Pediatric Research*, *8*, 931–934.

Georgieff, M. K., Hoffman, J. S., Pereira, G. R., Bernbaum, J., & Hoffman-Williamson, M. (1985). Effect of neonatal caloric deprivation on head growth and 1-year developmental status in preterm infants. *Journal of Pediatrics*, *107*(4), 581–587.

Greer, F. R. (2007). Long-term adverse outcomes of low birth weight, increased somatic growth rates, and alterations of body composition in the premature infant: Review of the evidence. *Journal of Pediatric Gastroenterology and Nutrition*, *45*, S147–S151.

Hack, M., Weissman, B., Breslau, N., Klein, N., Borawski-Clark, E., & Fanaroff, A. A. (1993). Health of very low birth weight children during their first eight years. *Journal of Pediatrics*, *122*(6), 887–892.

Henderson, G., Fahey, T., & McGuire, W. (2007a). Nutrient-enriched formula versus standard term formula for preterm infants following hospital discharge. *Cochrane Database Systemic Reviews*, *4*, CD004696.

Henderson, G., Fahey, T., & McGuire, W. (2007b). Multicomponent fortification of human breast milk for preterm infants following hospital discharge. *Cochrane Database of Systematic Reviews*, *4*, CD004866.

Krebs, N. F., Himes, J. H., Jacobson, D., Nicklas, T. A., Guilday, P., & Styne, D. (2007). Assessment of child and adolescent overweight and obesity. *Pediatrics*, *120*, S193–S228.

Meier, P. P. (2003). Supporting lactation in mothers with very low birth weight infants. *Pediatric Annals*, *32*(5), 317–325.

Radmacher, P. G., Looney, S. W., Rafail, S. T., & Adamkin, D. H. (2003). Prediction of extrauterine growth retardation (EUGR) in VLBW infants. *Journal of Perinatology*, *23*, 392–395.

Santos, I. S., Matijasevich, A., Domingues, M. R., Barros, A. J., Victora, C. G., & Barros, F. C. (2009). Late preterm birth is a risk factor for growth faltering in early childhood: A cohort study. *BMC Pediatrics*, *9*, 71.

Steward, D. K., & Pridham, K. F. (2002). Growth patterns of extremely low-birth-weight hospitalized premature infants. *Journal of Obstetric, Gynecologic, and Neonatal Nursing*, *31*, 57–65.

Vohr, B. R., Poindexter, B. B., Dusick, A. M., McKinley, L. T., Wright, L. L., Langer, J. C., & Poole, W. K. (2006). Beneficial effects of breast milk in the neonatal intensive care unit on the developmental outcome of extremely low birth weight infants at 18 months of age. *Pediatrics*, *118*(1), 115–123.

Yeung, E. H., Hu, F. B., Solomon, C. G., Chen, L., Louis, G. M., Schisterman, E., . . . Zhang, C. (2010). Life-course weight characteristics and the risk of gestational diabetes. *Diabetologia*, *53*(4), 668–678.

Reprinted with permission. Wisconsin Association for Perinatal Care, www .perinatalweb.org.

APPENDIX 9.2 USEFUL WEBSITES [AND BOOKS] FOR NUTRITION AND GROWTH

For Parents (and Professionals)

Academy of Nutrition and Dietetics

www.eatright.org

Academy of Nutrition and Dietetics (Kids Eat Right)

www.eatright.org/resources/for-kids

American Academy of Pediatrics

healthychildren.org

DASH Eating Plan

www.nhlbi.nih.gov/health/health-topics/topics/dash

Dietary Guidelines for Americans

health.gov/dietaryguidelines/2015/

Choose My Plate

www.choosemyplate.gov/healthy-eating-style (Healthy Eating Style)
www.choosemyplate.gov/meals-and-snacks (Meals and Snacks)
www.choosemyplate.gov/MyPlate-Daily-Checklist (Daily Checklist by age)
www.choosemyplate.gov/MyPlate-Daily-Checklist-input (MyPlate Checklist Calculator)

Ellyn Satter Institute (see "How to Eat")

ellynsatterinstitute.org/hte/howtoeat.php
Satter, E. (2008). *Secrets of feeding a healthy family.* Madison, WI: Kelcy Press.

Fruits and Veggies More Matters

www.fruitsandveggiesmorematters.org/

Mediterranean Diet (OLDWAYS version)

oldwayspt.org/traditional-diets/mediterranean-diet

Nutrition for Kids

nutritionforkids.com

Wisconsin Association for Perinatal Care (see "For Parents & Consumers")

www.perinatalweb.org

For Professionals

Abbott Nutrition Health Institute

anhi.org

Academy of Nutrition and Dietetics

www.eatright.org or www.eatrightpro.org
ncpt.webauthor.com/ (see "eNCPT" [subscription required for Nutrition Care Process and
  Terminology site access])

American Academy of Pediatrics

www.aap.org
Kleinman, R. E., & Greer, F. R. (Eds.). (2014). *Pediatric nutrition* (7th ed.). Elk Village, IL:
  American Academy of Pediatrics

BMI calculator

http://www.nhlbi.nih.gov/health/educational/lose_wt/BMI/bmicalc.htm

CDC Growth Chart Training

www.cdc.gov/nccdphp/dnpao/growthcharts/
www.cdc.gov/nccdphp/dnpao/growthcharts/training/overview/page1.html

Ellyn Satter Institute

www.ellynsatterinstitute.org/

Feeding Guidelines for Infants and Young Toddlers: A Responsive Parenting Approach

healthyeatingresearch.org/wp-content/uploads/2017/02/her_feeding_guidelines_
  report_021416-1.pdf

Guide to Infant Feeding
docs.wixstatic.com/ugd/71c36f_c82f7b3bb6b6467bbaed5bae0bb4bbe7.pdf

Growth of Children with Special Healthcare Needs
depts.washington.edu/growth/cshcn/text/page1a.htm

Healthy Eating Research
healthyeatingresearch.org/who-we-are/about-us/

Infant-Driven Feeding
www.infantdrivenfeeding.com

Nestlé Nutrition Institute
www.nestlenutrition-institute.org

Nutrition Detectives
www.davidkatzmd.com/nutritiondetectives.aspx

PediTools Clinical Tools for Pediatric Providers
peditools.org

Wisconsin Association for Perinatal Care (see "For Healthcare Professionals" and "For Parents & Consumers")
www.perinatalweb.org

Growth Charts

NHANESIII Anthropometric Videos (VIDEO)
wwwn.cdc.gov/nchs/nhanes/nhanes3/anthropometricvideos.aspx

TERM—CDC Growth Curves
www.cdc.gov/growthcharts/cdc_charts.htm

TERM—CDC Growth Curves—Children With Down Syndrome
www.cdc.gov/ncbddd/birthdefects/downsyndrome/growth-charts.html

TERM—WHO Growth Curves
www.cdc.gov/growthcharts/who_charts.htm

PRETERM—Fenton Growth Chart
ucalgary.ca/fenton

Infant Formula and Food (A Sample of Commercial Vendors)

Beech-Nut
www.beechnut.com/foods/

Gerber
www.gerber.com/products/baby-food

Enfamil Products (Baby Formula, Toddler Milk Drinks and Nutritional Products)
www.enfamil.com/products

Heinz
www.heinzbaby.com/en-ca/products

Similac Products (For Baby, For Toddler)
similac.com/baby-formula

Sprout Foods, Inc.
www.sproutorganicfoods.com

Teaching and Learning Nutrition Education at Mealtime

By Janine M. Bamberger, MS, RDN, CD

These educational tools are most effective when used as the base of a discussion with moms and dads, and/or other caregivers, of young children.

- Have you had any experiences like this with your child? Talk about them.
- What skills have you taught your child, and how?
- What are some things you have learned while teaching your child?
- If you have more than one child, how have your food-related experiences with your children been the same? How have they differed?
- What food skills do you think are important to teach your child, and at what ages?

MEALTIME WITH A TODDLER: TEACHING AND PRACTICING SELF-FEEDING (VIDEO [0:44 MIN])

YOUTU.BE/4QRV_YOTGDO

> In this video clip of a 28-month-old boy eating chicken with a fork, the parents are teaching and learning with their son. They are calm and supportive as they guide him to hold the fork right-side up. They learn that he enjoys the activity, and while they guide him to focus on self-feeding as he practices fork use, they downplay the tapping on the plate and reward him with respectful, encouraging words. The grandparent, who is also present, complements the parental support by also reassuring the boy that the new skill is well accepted by the family.

MEALTIME WITH A TODDLER: TEACHING AND PRACTICING KNIFE SKILLS (VIDEO [0:52 MIN])

YOUTU.BE/YBE9GK0WSXE

> In this video clip, a 28-month-old boy is practicing early knife skills with his family. It is clear that they have previously taught him about the safety concerns of knives, probably during the many times they cut food in front of him, since he knows that the blade is "owie!" While it would be inappropriate to give a 2-year old a serrated metal knife with which to practice cutting, a plastic utensil is a reasonable way to allow him to transition from play (with plastic knives in

his play kitchen) to real life experiences. Of course, an adult continues to watch the boy during this lesson to be sure he does not hurt himself. In this case, the toddler is learning part of the process of preparing his own food, with guidance, and he is enjoying the activity and the result—that he has chiseled his very own bite away from the apple. The session helps the parents understand their son's current skill level, and it helps the little one prepare for increasingly more complicated food preparation skills.

MEAL PREPARATION THROUGH THE EYES OF A 6-YEAR-OLD: TEACHING AND PRACTICING SETTING THE TABLE (VIDEO [2:46 MIN])

YOUTU.BE/HNZ0_JUS7V0

In this video, a 6-year-old first-grader sets the table. Based on her upbeat attitude, she appears to enjoy this duty, and is interested in doing the job well. Napkins are situated around the table next to the plates, and forks are placed atop the napkins. She thinks twice when setting the spoons down, placing the first one on the left, then moving it to the right. Finally, when it is time to add the knives, she demonstrates her version of understanding how to handle knives safely. Though some gentle adult guidance factors into this activity, the young girl is allowed to also make decisions on her own, such as choosing the order for laying out the place settings, while completing the chore.

MEAL PREPARATION THROUGH THE EYES OF A 6-YEAR-OLD: TEACHING AND PRACTICING HOME-MADE SPRING ROLLS (VIDEO [2:39 MIN])

YOUTU.BE/4NJ0P4OKPAS

The 6-year-old first-grader in this video demonstrates the fact that food preparation can be both productive and fun. After washing her hands, to remove unwanted germs, she starts the process of assembling a spring roll using two of her favorite vegetables (celery and carrots). This experience provides mom the opportunity to offer support while overseeing the development of a new skill. The young girl enjoys the activity that allows her to be creative and independent, but she does get a little annoyed with her mom for helping with the process. Quickly, though, she refocuses on the job at hand. She is proud of her end product, and clear that it does not have to be perfect to be a success.

MEAL PREPARATION THROUGH THE EYES OF A 6-YEAR-OLD: TEACHING AND PRACTICING PREPARING LUNCH (VIDEO [1:38 MIN])

YOUTU.BE/XTC1HFZCJKU

In this video, a 6-year-old happily jumps into the activity of preparing her lunch. She knows how to seal the bag containing her pita, but explains why—according to what is on her mind (taste, not dryness). The task of peeling a hard-boiled egg demands concentration, but is clearly enjoyable. She has a brief conversation with the onlooker about the risk, from her perspective, of eating egg shells (that it could "cut your lungs!"). Correcting that notion is not particularly important. What is important is that the egg gets peeled and the child looks forward to eating it at mealtime!

MEAL PREPARATION THROUGH THE EYES OF A 6-YEAR-OLD: TEACHING AND PRACTICING PACKING LUNCH (VIDEO [4:49 MIN])

YOUTU.BE/UTWEKY1PTLM

In this video, a 6-year-old first grader peels two hard-boiled eggs as she begins to pack her lunch. She puts the eggs, vegetable spring rolls, and sliced apples in containers of varying sizes. She speaks fondly of her mom and dad, acknowledging the fact that they both work with her in the kitchen, happily describing skills she has learned from them, such as how to peel eggs and make monkey bread! In her mind, they are great teachers. As she packs her lunch box, she is allowed to use her spatial skills to arrange, and rearrange, the containers she plans to take to school. Preparation ends as she adds an ice pack to the lunch box, slings the strap over her shoulder, and then turns to the next item that catches her attention, asking "What are these for?"

FIRST MEALS: HEALTHY FROM THE START

TINYURL.COM/YAKMTPF6 [PDF]

Through pictures and simple descriptions, this presentation demonstrates the value of capturing teachable moments. Parents and others can learn what is on the mind of youngsters and offer opportunities for children to understand and participate in food activities from a very early age. The focus is birth through age 6.

Online Supplemental Resources (For Parents and Professionals)

2015–2020 Dietary Guidelines for Americans
Office of Disease Prevention and Health Promotion, U.S. Department of Health and Human Services
health.gov/dietaryguidelines/2015/

ChooseMyPlate.gov

Daily Checklist by Age

U.S. Department of Agriculture (USDA), ChooseMyPlate.gov
www.choosemyplate.gov/MyPlate-Daily-Checklist

Healthy Eating Style

U.S. Department of Agriculture (USDA), ChooseMyPlate.gov
www.choosemyplate.gov/healthy-eating-style

Meals and Snacks

U.S. Department of Agriculture (USDA), ChooseMyPlate.gov
www.choosemyplate.gov/meals-and-snacks

MyPlate Checklist Calculator

U.S. Department of Agriculture (USDA), ChooseMyPlate.gov
www.choosemyplate.gov/MyPlate-Daily-Checklist-input

Description of the DASH Eating Plan

*U.S. Department of Health & Human Services, National Heart, Lung and Blood
    Institute (NIH)*
www.nhlbi.nih.gov/health/health-topics/topics/dash

Eat Right
Academy of Nutrition and Dietetics (AND)
www.eatright.org

Fruits and Veggies More Matters
Produce for Better Health Foundation
www.fruitsandveggiesmorematters.org/

healthychildren.org
American Academy of Pediatrics (AAP)
healthychildren.org

How to Eat
Ellyn Satter Institute
ellynsatterinstitute.org/hte/howtoeat.php

Kids Eat Right
Academy of Nutrition and Dietetics (AND)
www.eatright.org/resources/for-kids

Mediterranean Diet
OLDWAYS
oldwayspt.org/traditional-diets/mediterranean-diet

Nutrition for Kids
Connie Evers, MS, RD, CSSD, LD
nutritionforkids.com

Wisconsin Association for Perinatal Care (WAPC)
Wisconsin Association for Perinatal Care
www.perinatalweb.org

Online Supplemental Resources (for Professionals)

Abbott Nutrition Health Institute
Abbott Laboratories
anhi.org

Abridged Nutrition Care Process Terminology (NCPT)
Academy of Nutrition and Dietetics' Nutrition Care Process and Terminology (NCPT)
ncpt.webauthor.com/

American Academy of Pediatrics

American Academy of Pediatrics (AAP)

www.aap.org

Calculate Your Body Mass Index (BMI calculator)

U.S. Department of Health & Human Services, National Heart, Lung and Blood Institute

www.nhlbi.nih.gov/health/educational/lose_wt/BMI/bmicalc.htm

Eat Right PRO

Academy of Nutrition and Dietetics (AND)

www.eatrightpro.org

Ellyn Satter Institute

www.ellynsatterinstitute.org

Feeding Guidelines for Infants and Young Toddlers: A Responsive Parenting Approach

Healthy Eating Research, a national program of the Robert Wood Johnson Foundation

healthyeatingresearch.org/wp-content/uploads/2017/02/her_feeding_guidelines_report_021416-1.pdf

First Meals: Healthy From the Start

Janine M. Bamberger

tinyurl.com/yakmtpf6

Growth Charts

CDC Growth Charts

Centers for Disease Control and Prevention, National Center for Health Statistics

www.cdc.gov/growthcharts/cdc_charts.htm

Growth Charts for Children With Down Syndrome

Division of Birth Defects and Developmental Disabilities, National Center on Birth Defects and Developmental Disabilities (NCBDDD), Centers for Disease Control and Prevention

www.cdc.gov/ncbddd/birthdefects/downsyndrome/growth-charts.html

Growth of Children With Special Healthcare Needs

U.S. Department of Health & Human Services, Health Resources and Services Administration, Maternal and Child Health Bureau

depts.washington.edu/growth/cshcn/text/page1a.htm

The NHANES Story (videos contain the standardized anthropometric procedures)

Centers for Disease Control and Prevention, National Center for Health Statistics

wwwn.cdc.gov/nchs/nhanes/nhanes3/anthropometricvideos.aspx

Welcome to the Fenton Preterm Growth Chart Webpage

University of Calgary

ucalgary.ca/fenton

*WHO Growth Charts (WHO Growth Standards Are Recommended for Use in the
    United States for Infants and Children 0 to 2 Years of Age)*

Centers for Disease Control and Prevention, National Center for Health Statistics
www.cdc.gov/growthcharts/who_charts.htm

Growth Chart Training

Growth Chart Training: Introduction

U.S. Department of Health & Human Services, Centers for Disease Control and Prevention
www.cdc.gov/nccdphp/dnpao/growthcharts

Growth Chart Training: What Growth Charts Are Recommended for Use?

U.S. Department of Health & Human Services, Centers for Disease Control and Prevention
www.cdc.gov/nccdphp/dnpao/growthcharts/training/overview/page1.html

Guide to Infant Feeding

J. M. Bamberger
tinyurl.com/ya6wlgfb

Healthy Eating Research

A Robert Wood Johnson Program
healthyeatingresearch.org/who-we-are/about-us

Infant Formula & Food (A Sample of Commercial Vendors)

Beech-Nut Real Food for Babies

Beech-Nut
www.beechnut.com/foods/

Enfamil Family Beginnings

Mead Johnson & Company
www.enfamil.com/

Gerber Tools, Guidance, Savings, and More

Nestlé
www.gerber.com/products/baby-food

Heinz Baby Products

Heinz
www.heinzbaby.com/en-ca/products

Similac Products

Abbott Laboratories
similac.com/baby-formula

Sprout

Sprout Foods, Inc.
www.sproutorganicfoods.com

Infant-Driven Feeding® (IDF)
Sue Ludwig and Kara Ann Waitzman
www.infantdrivenfeeding.com

Mealtime With a Toddler

Mealtime With a Toddler: Teaching and Practicing Knife Skills
Janine M. Bamberger
youtu.be/YBe9Gk0wSxE

Mealtime With a Toddler: Teaching and Practicing Self-feeding
Janine M. Bamberger
youtu.be/4qrv_yoTGdo

Meal Preparation Through the Eyes of a 6-Year-Old

Meal Preparation Through the Eyes of a 6-Year-Old: Teaching and Practicing Home-Made Spring Rolls
Janine M. Bamberger
youtu.be/4NJ0P4okpas

Meal Preparation Through the Eyes of a 6-Year-Old: Teaching and Practicing Packing Lunch
Janine M. Bamberger
youtu.be/UtwEKy1PTlM

Meal Preparation Through the Eyes of a 6-Year-Old: Teaching and Practicing Preparing Lunch
Janine M. Bamberger
youtu.be/XtC1hfzCJKU

Meal Preparation Through the Eyes of a 6-Year-Old: Teaching and Practicing Setting the Table
Janine M. Bamberger
youtu.be/HNz0_Jus7v0

Nestlé Nutrition Institute (NNI)
www.nestlenutrition-institute.org

NUTRITION DETECTIVES™ "Teaching Kids to Make Healthy Choices"
David L. Katz
www.davidkatzmd.com/nutritiondetectives.aspx

PediTools: Clinical Tools for Pediatric Providers
Joseph Chou
peditools.org

Wisconsin Association for Perinatal Nutrition (WAPC)
www.perinatalweb.org

10

Caring for an Adolescent With a Concussion

Traci R. Snedden

The developmental stage of adolescence is a period of substantial physical, cognitive, social, and emotional growth. Guided participation (GP) is central to theory for supporting adolescents and their families during this transitional phase. Through the application of partnered teaching and learning, this clinical model aids in developing competencies that are personally and socially meaningful to adolescent everyday life (Pridham, Limbo, Schroeder, Thoyre, & Van Riper, 1998; Rogoff, 1990). During adolescence, a child transitions to a young adult, reaching for independence and self-identity through a variety of activities that contribute to their personal definition of self. For many adolescents, engagement in school- and club-based sports activities plays a large role in their identity as an athlete, in addition to that of a student. Coaches, athletic trainers, school nurses, healthcare providers, and teammates join parents in providing a source of knowledge and encouragement, serving as guides for sport competency, injury prevention and recognition, and overall safety.

Despite the numerous benefits of sports participation, it is not without risk. Recent scientific and media attention has brought the issue of sport-related concussion to an unprecedented international forefront of science, sports, and politics. There is not a day that goes by without attention to the all too common incidence of concussion, its complex presentation and the potential risk for life-changing, long-term effects. Concussion is known to disturb an adolescent's life in broad and complicated ways, through the presence of individualized responses to this injury across a number of domains (Kontos et al., 2012; Lovell & Collins, 1998; Pardini et al., 2004; Snedden, 2013). Amid this complexity, concussed adolescents and their families are challenged to sift through fact versus fiction to determine next steps and evidence-based direction that will support a safe and timely return to what adolescents frame as their self-identify, in the classroom, in their sport, and amid their social interactions.

Nurses play an important role in competency development that supports an adolescent's concussion recovery. For example, the emergency department (ED) nurse serves as the frontline clinician/first contact with concussed adolescents and their caregivers, providing initial assessment and guidance. In addition, the ED nurse is the source of discharge instruction clarification and important teaching. The nurse practitioner (NP), as a healthcare provider across the care continuum, and the school nurse, as a member of a school-based multidisciplinary team, also contribute to concussion competency development through their role in adolescent healthcare, teaching, and advocacy. Nurses act as vital guides, for both caregivers and adolescents during the concussion recovery process.

Just as in other activities of adolescent life, GP offers the opportunity to support adolescents and their caregivers to competently engage in sports participation and, if injured, subsequent healing processes. As guides, ED nurses, NPs, and school nurses are perfectly positioned to use this clinical practice model to grow caregiver competencies that mitigate the effects of injury. Furthermore, guides using the five processes of GP—(a) getting and staying connected, (b) joining and maintaining attention, (c) bridging, (d) structuring the task/learning, and (e) transferring responsibility—can support caregiver and adolescent competency development for concussion symptom support and overall recovery, and for adolescent development of identity as an effective agent. A supportive and dynamic process of teaching and learning within the context of a relationship in the sport and school setting is vital to a timely and positive concussion outcome.

The purpose of this chapter is to apply GP to the clinical context of adolescent concussion. It reviews concussion and its effect on everyday adolescent and family life, describes the role of the ED nurse, NP, and school nurse in developing caregiver and adolescent concussion competencies, and then discusses GP as a sensitive and responsive clinical practice that is able to support the unique needs of adolescents who sustain this type of injury. A clinical vignette follows to illustrate the complexities of adolescent concussion and subsequent recovery. A series of reflective questions encourages the reader to incorporate GP processes into their response to the clinical vignette, using the partnered relationship of the adolescent, caregiver, and nurse to navigate a safe and timely postconcussion return to sport, classroom, and all aspects of adolescent life. This chapter closes with key GP concepts important to working with concussed adolescents and their caregivers.

BACKGROUND

Scope and Significance of Adolescent Concussion

The collision between science, sports, and politics has shifted the pendulum of concussion recognition and management from that of "part of the game" to a significant public health concern. Historically, most concussions were not considered serious, and athletes who sustained them were said to have been "dinged" or had their "bell rung." The injured player would "shake it off" and return to play, usually under the coach's direction or with parents' encouragement and no further action occurred (Institute of Medicine [IOM] & National Research Council [NRC], 2013).

However, recent years have noted an expansion of knowledge that has led to an increased awareness and understanding that all concussions include some level of injury to the brain, and that an athlete suspected of having a concussion should be immediately removed from play for further evaluation and management (Centers for Disease Control and Prevention [CDC], 2017; Halstead, Walter, & Council on Sports Medicine and Fitness, 2010; Harmon et al., 2013; McCrory et al., 2005, 2009, 2013, 2017). Concussion has been estimated to occur in 1.6 to 3.8 million athletes in the United States on an annual basis, with a majority of these injuries occurring in pediatric populations (CDC, 2017; Gilchrist, 2011; Langlois, Rutland-Brown, & Wald, 2006). Of this number, although assumedly underreported, it is estimated that the etiology of 300,000 concussions annually are sports related (Halstead et al., 2010; Marar, McIlvain, Fields, & Comstock, 2012). Among individuals 15 to 24 years of age, sports are second only to motor vehicle accidents as the leading cause of concussions (Marar et al., 2012). Football, ice hockey, and lacrosse post the highest concussion rates for boys, with the sports of soccer, lacrosse, and basketball leading girls' high school rates (Marar et al., 2012).

A sport-related concussion is formally defined as "a traumatic brain injury induced by biochemical forces" (McCrory et al., 2013, p. 251). This commonly utilized definition, along with its associated constructs, was generated in 2016 by the fifth International Concussion in Sport workgroup (McCrory et al., 2017, p. 2). The traumatic forces and subsequent biochemical cascade result in a complex set of symptoms that affect physical, cognitive, emotional, and sleep-related domains as unique presentations in every individual (Kontos et al., 2012; Lovell & Collins, 1998; Pardini et al., 2004; Snedden, 2013). Common postinjury symptoms typically include headache, nausea, vomiting, balance problems, dizziness, fatigue, trouble falling asleep, sleeping more or less than usual, drowsiness, sensitivity to light and/or noise, irritability, sadness, nervousness, feeling more emotional, numbness or tingling, feeling slowed down, feeling mentally "foggy," difficulty concentrating or remembering, and visual problems (CDC, 2017; Lovell & Collins, 1998). Although symptomatic recovery in the adolescent is typically reached within

2 weeks of injury, recent studies suggest that 21% to 73% of children and adolescents who sustain a concussion will still be experiencing symptoms at 1 month after injury (Babcock et al., 2013; Corwin et al., 2014; Eisenberg, Meehan, & Mannix, 2014; Grubenhoff et al., 2014).

Adolescents are also at risk for psychological and emotional disturbance following injury, including depression, anxiety, social isolation and loneliness, frustration, anger, and guilt (Bloom, Horton, McCrory, & Johnston, 2004; Mainwaring, Hutchison, Bisschop, Comper, & Richards, 2010; Mainwaring et al., 2004; Putukian & Echemendia, 2003). Comparable to the complexity and individualization of humans, the outcomes of concussion injury span a varied and somewhat unknown continuum of severity encompassing short- and long-term cognitive and physical deficits, and negative alterations in overall quality of life, in addition to mental health concerns (McCrory et al., 2009; Reeves & Panguluri, 2011). Finally, returning to contact sports or physical activities prior to full recovery may have rare but catastrophic consequences, including second-impact syndrome, a poorly understood phenomenon of severe cerebral edema that risks the loss of life in just moments of onset when an additional head trauma occurs prior to brain healing from the first concussion (Boden, Tachetti, & Cantu, 2007; Cantu, 1998).

Effects of Concussion on the Adolescent and Family

Concussion in the adolescent athlete is a substantial public health concern with potential short- and long-term sequelae in multiple cognitive and functional domains. These sequelae risk interruption in academic, sport, social, and family processes over the time of recovery and beyond. Symptoms alone have the potential to disrupt ability to perform in the classroom, engage in social activities, and maintain what adolescents know as their "normal" life and self-identity. To further complicate the recovery process, every adolescent has a unique injury response, symptom experience, and recovery pattern that is based on their own history of injury, comorbidities and internal working model of concussion effects, and overall recovery. The individualized injury response requires a coordinated application of evidence-based strategies to promote recovery.

Understanding how to best promote concussion recovery may be a significant challenge for caregivers, placing a considerable emotional and financial burden upon them. Factors that contribute to this caregiver burden include challenges related to complex symptom management, the coordination of multiple care providers, and the navigation of return to class and sport, all while attempting to develop and integrate care competencies that are evidence based (Sady, Vaughan, & Gioia, 2011). Additionally, caregivers can become easily overwhelmed with the abundance of concussion information that is available in public domains (e.g., Internet, social networking sites), some fraught with inaccuracies and outdated guidance (Ahmed, Sullivan, Schneiders, & McCrory, 2010; Fahy, Hardikar,

Fox, & Mackay, 2014). Caregivers may also receive conflicting information from friends, colleagues, and even clinicians who are not aware of recent updates in guidelines and recommendations. Resultant information overload makes it difficult for caregivers to discern which approaches are effective and appropriate for their adolescent, resulting in frustration, exhaustion, or even emotional paralysis.

GP is a clinical practice that develops caregiver competencies through a built and respectful relationship around a shared goal. In this clinical context, that goal is the health and safety of a concussed adolescent (recovery from existing head injury and protection from subsequent injury). GP is flexible, adaptive, and responsive to unique adolescent and family needs and provides a fitting clinical practice model for the individualized and complex response to concussion recovery.

The Role of the ED Nurse, NP, and School Nurse in Concussion Recovery

The ED nurse, NP, and school nurse share the ability to holistically assess individual biopsychosocial needs and to plan, deliver, and evaluate the care of patients across the healthcare continuum. They provide care in large academic medical centers, community settings, ambulatory care offices, and schools. In addition, these clinicians are skilled in communication, knowledge assessment, anticipatory guidance, and access to evidence-based resources, all important qualities for the provision of concussion care. The ED nurse, NP, and school nurse are also competent teachers who strive to build relationships with their patients to more fully understand their illness or injury experience and to increase engagement in health behaviors that improve patient outcomes and overall quality of life. Finally, they work in collaborative and complex environments, often coordinating multidisciplinary contributions to meet a unified goal. These skills align well with the complicated process of concussion recovery, a process that requires coordinated and collaborative strategies for best outcomes (McCarty et al., 2016). The ED nurse, NP, and school nurse hold a vital role in GP in the clinical context of adolescent concussion.

THE APPLICATION OF GP TO THE CARE OF AN ADOLESCENT WITH CONCUSSION

In the application of GP to the care of an adolescent with concussion, both the caregiver and the adolescent are initially "learners." The clinicians (ED nurse, NP, and school nurse) serve as the "teachers" or "guides." However, with growth in competency, the caregiver may transition from learner to teacher, joining the clinicians in providing guidance for their adolescent and family, their adolescent's teachers, and their adolescent's sport staff throughout the recovery process, resulting in the building of the adolescent's own self-agency in addition to the competency of others. Using the five processes of GP, mentioned earlier in this chapter, the guide can support and promote caregiver and adolescent competency development for concussion recovery. GP is an effective clinical practice to jointly achieve the overall shared goal of symptom management and a safe and timely return to classroom, sport, and "normal" life after a concussion injury.

The following section provides context to how each aforementioned GP process can be applied to competency building for adolescent concussion recovery from the perspective of the clinician (ED nurse, NP, and school nurse) in addition to the caregiver. It is important to note that these processes are not sequential or meant to be used in a specific/prescribed order or frequency. Instead they are a fluid set of processes that offer the guide a set of tools to apply throughout the partnered competency development process. The contents of this section, coupled with the GP process conversation prompts and strategies within Table 10.1, will guide the reader's application of GP to the chapter's Case Example.

Getting and Staying Connected

The process of *getting and staying connected* centers on the goal of engaging interest from the caregiver and the adolescent to grow a commitment to competency development. A common issue with sport-related concussion lies in the fact that many caregivers and adolescents have inaccurate beliefs and knowledge about concussion. For example, a large number of caregivers and student athletes still believe that a concussion injury requires a direct hit to the head and/or a loss of consciousness. If symptoms are transient or minimal at the time of injury, they may believe that a concussion did not occur. Additionally, some caregivers have a personal experience of sport injury from their own childhood that encouraged a response of toughness and subsequent risk-taking and may consider the current focus on concussion as too conservative or even "soft" in comparison to their own experience. Other adolescents and their caregivers may hold the fearful assumption that as a result of a concussion, the adolescent is at guaranteed risk for serious long-term cognitive or mental health issues, based on overwhelming media focus and their interpretation of it. These inaccuracies offer the clinician the opportunity to connect and to engage in competency development that dispels caregiver and student athlete myths while supporting adolescent recovery from concussion.

However, a prerequisite to the overall GP goal of competency development is to first build a trusting relationship with the caregiver, and then to become connected and stay connected through the strategic application of conversation that elicits this bond. This relationship centers on the common goal of successfully undertaking activities that promote competency development specific to concussion recovery. Existing caregiver strategies

TABLE 10.1 Adolescent Concussion: Conversation Prompts and Strategies to Support GP Processes

GP Process	Getting and Staying Connected	Joining and Maintaining Attention	Bridging	Structuring the Task/Learning	Transferring Responsibility
Conversation Prompts	"Will you take some time to summarize your past experience with concussion, either your own or your adolescent's?" "How might this concussion affect your adolescent's typical day as a student? As an athlete? How do you feel about that?" "What are your thoughts about the knowledge you gained today and how this could be shared with your family? Your adolescent's teacher(s)? Coach? Friends/teammates?"	"Tell me about what has changed since the last time we met." "What concerns do you have today?" "Were you able to connect with your adolescent's teacher(s) and coach? How did that go?" "What have the doctors said?" (If visits were made since last encounter.)	"Has your adolescent had a previous concussion or other injury? How does this experience compare to that one?" "If you had questions or concerns about your adolescent in the past, what did you do? Who did you contact? What knowledge did you gain from them? Does any of that knowledge apply to this concussion injury?" "How do these struggles compare to last week/last month? Are there any strategies we discussed that could help?"	"We have talked about ways to ensure your adolescent's teacher/coach and teammates can support their recovery. How can we bring them into our conversation?" "What are your biggest concerns at this time? How could we work together to strategize support or solutions for those?"	"What do you plan to share with your adolescent's family, school or athletic staff about this visit?" "What challenges do you anticipate ahead? How could you apply the strategies we talked about today?" "Are there any other successful strategies that you are using that we have not discussed? These are very helpful for my work with other families."

(continued)

TABLE 10.1 Adolescent Concussion: Conversation Prompts and Strategies to Support GP Processes (*continued*)

GP Process	Getting and Staying Connected	Joining and Maintaining Attention	Bridging	Structuring the Task/Learning	Transferring Responsibility
Strategies	Encourage sharing of caregiver personal experience with concussion.	Continue to gather information during all caregiver encounters, allowing the caregiver to share positive and challenging situations related to the adolescent's recovery process.	Jointly make connections to previous experiences, learning situations.	Offer written resources and summaries from your clinical encounters.	Encourage the caregivers and adolescent to share their knowledge with others (family members, peers, school and athletic staff). Ask how they can best accomplish that sharing.
	Seek to understand the daily life of the concussed adolescent through the lens of the caregiver.	Respect the caregivers' expectations and intentions.	Encourage the caregivers and adolescent by telling them that they have skills from previous experiences that will support concussion recovery.	Use role-playing to practice anticipated issues that may arise. Offer guidance and feedback that will support a successful outcome during those potential situations.	Value the knowledge you gain from the caregivers and adolescent, incorporating it into your own working model, as a clinician.

Identify caregiver goal for adolescent's concussion recovery.

Assess for the need for additional ways to connect through in-person appointments, phone conversations, and electronic communication, as appropriate.

Listen with focus and empathy, exhibiting true concern for the caregivers and adolescent as they describe their past experiences and sources of support.

Use storytelling from previous patients (or the clinical vignette within this chapter) to offer a context for structured learning.

Inquire regarding the caregivers and adolescent's input for best ways to manage certain symptoms, scenarios (actual and potential).

Assess knowledge and beliefs about concussion.

Consider simulated situations to grow understanding of current or potential challenges surrounding concussion recovery.

Determine existing sources of caregiver support and knowledge.

Refer to credible peers, clinician experts, or electronic sources of information.

Share written evidence-based resources with caregiver.

GP, guided participation.

to reach this goal may be influenced by past experiences, worries, fears, and concerns specific to concussion. Additionally, strategies may embody caregiver reflections of future adolescent aspirations, such as elite academic institution attendance and/or continued participation in their sport at the collegiate or higher level. Adolescents may possess similar internal strategies that center on toughness, resiliency and risk-taking to achieve their personal goals as an athlete, some which may be deeply woven into their identity. These strategies may be a reflection of the adolescent and/or caregiver's internal working model about concussion and recovery. Listening for components of this internal working model through caring conversations centered on shared goals provides a foundation for connecting and staying connected.

Connecting begins with the first encounter and is an important process in GP. This first encounter may occur in the ED, primary care clinic, or school setting, offering the ED nurse, NP, or school nurse the opportunity to "bring the other into the activity" in this clinical context. It is during this time that an agenda and expectations are set in a partnership between the caregiver and clinician. As an example, the clinician's genuine interest in the adolescent's typical day, through the storytelling lens of the student athlete and/or caregiver, brings the other into the activity and supports a better understanding of the adolescent's personal identity. GP clinical practice begins with *getting connected*. Continued success in GP is grounded in the guide and learner continuing to *stay connected*. These interactions provide the opportunity to assess caregiver and adolescent competency gaps, identify potential challenges, gain a commitment to competency development, and identify resources to support a safe and timely return to classroom and sport after a concussion injury.

Joining and Maintaining Attention

The GP process of *joining and maintaining attention* incorporates actual or potential situations to engage in learning activities. This process is best utilized to gain interest and commitment to problem-solving issues that already exist and to anticipate issues that may arise in the future. Conversations that center on assessing how things are going, what has changed, what new concerns have arisen, and what additional resources they may have learned about are all effective for meeting the goals of this GP process. In the context of concussion recovery, asking the caregiver and/or adolescent about the planned meeting with their teacher, coach, and/or athletic trainer serves as an example of a conversation that will foster a shared attention on progress toward returning to the classroom and/or sport in a safe and timely manner.

Continuing the discussion by asking about strategies (or accommodations) the teacher is offering to support academic success provides the clinician with an opportunity to talk about strategies that are helpful in the classroom, based on the symptoms of the adolescent. In parallel, asking the caregiver and/or adolescent about what "return to sport" stage they are at, offers the opportunity to discuss evidence-based steps and timelines for a safe return that lessens the possibility of another injury and prolonged concussion effects. Following each of these inquires with further questions specific to emotional reactions is also imperative. For example, "How did that make you feel?" and "Was that the outcome you expected?" are helpful for better understanding the expectations of the caregiver and/or adolescent regarding those interactions.

In summary, the GP process of *joining and maintaining attention* is vital to keeping the guide and learner active and engaged. This process maintains the clinician and caregiver/adolescent relationship by focusing energies on shared goals through discussion that incorporates what may be new or different since the last interaction into the central conversation, which is focused on the progress of the adolescent's concussion recovery.

Bridging

The GP process of *bridging* provides an opportunity for the guide and the learner to make connections between previous experiences and new situations. Although situations may seem new, or even overwhelming to the caregiver, the process of bridging can encourage the caregiver to apply competencies from a past situation that are applicable and helpful in the context of concussion recovery. For instance, asking the caregiver if they have experience with a past concussion injury or any previous injury or illness for this adolescent (or another child, or even themselves) is an appropriate initial question of this process. Having conversation about that experience may elicit some existing competencies that can be applied to concussion recovery. Including questions specific to whether that past injury brought challenges to school attendance, learning or sports performance, or social interactions offers a starting point for the assessment of strategies previously utilized and how those may support concussion recovery. These conversations additionally offer the clinician the opportunity to learn more about support systems, resources, healthcare experiences, and stressors that contribute to competency gaps specific to this situation.

In the clinical context of concussion recovery, any past injury or illness that an adolescent has incurred is helpful in the process of *bridging*. During the previous illness or injury, it is likely that the caregiver needed to devote time to focus on the adolescent's medical appointment needs and needed to take time away from work to remain at home while they healed or recovered. They likely experienced some stress due to the adolescent's missed school and potentially due to their own work/life demands. That experience may even have resulted in financial or relationship difficulties resulting from the needs of the adolescent. Gaining insight from any injury or illness experience will aid the clinician in better understanding how the caregiver may react emotionally to this situation. Additionally, the insight will provide the clinician with opportunities for bridging the elements of that experience to that of concussion recovery, offering strategies and sources of support for best outcomes. In summary, *bridging* plays a vital role in GP clinical practice as it supports the application of past experience and related learning to concussion, lessening the complexity of the recovery process.

Structuring the Task/Learning

The GP process of *structuring the task/learning* incorporates education into action. This process guides the learner to apply what has been taught or discussed to actual situations that have occurred or are anticipated to occur. *Structuring the task/learning* is similar to eliciting answers to a "What if . . .?" game or role-play event. In the clinical context of concussion recovery, an example of this process involves anticipating concussion symptoms that may worsen or occur when returning to the classroom environment. Through partnered discussion, the adolescent can present their current classroom experience to the caregiver and clinician, if they have returned to school, or the clinician can prepare the adolescent and caregiver for what to expect as they return to the classroom and academic demands. The clinician can then provide guidance, offering strategies known to be successful in mitigating those effects, including advocating for specific classroom accommodations.

An additional example of this GP process could be the preparation that would be involved in planning for the adolescent and/or caregiver to meet with academic staff and/or athletics staff to discuss next steps for their concussion recovery. Using role-playing strategies and posing "what if" questions or scenarios supports a successful outcome through the structuring of the task before the meeting occurs. This example would also be applicable to the adolescent's discussion with coaches, athletic trainers, friends, and teammates. In summary, the GP process of *structuring the task/learning* supports the shared goal of concussion recovery by integrating structured learning into the recovery process.

Transferring Responsibility

The GP process of *transferring responsibility* supports initial sharing and eventual shifting of accountability between the clinician, caregiver, and adolescent. Through the integrated processes of GP, the caregiver and adolescent grow in competency and become able to manage the components of the shared goal because of their knowledge and their ability to problem solve actual or anticipated issues. The clinician, who once served as the guide, now transitions to the role of consultant to both the caregiver and adolescent. In the clinical context of concussion recovery, GP practice supports the caregiver in growing their competencies about concussion, its effects, evidence-based care, school- and sport-based recommendations, and overall symptom management within a partnered relationship. Through the application of GP clinical practice, the caregiver's competency eventually develops enough to serve as the "teacher" to the adolescent, who then grows their competency and self-agency specific to concussion recovery. In addition, as the adolescent's competency develops, the adolescent begins to serve as the guide for peers, school and academic staff, and even some clinicians, who can deepen their knowledge through the personal shared experience of the adolescent.

Concussion recovery is complex and the science is expanding exponentially at record pace. It is not uncommon for academic and/or sports staff to not be fully aware of recent changes or findings. Many parent and student athlete–led concussion advocacy groups have sprung from their personal awareness of the broad knowledge differences surrounding concussion and its recovery process. Caregivers and adolescents have become guides for many, as a result of their newly gained competency, self-agency, and eventual transferred responsibility. It is these individuals who are making a difference at the "grassroots" level with adolescent peers and their caregivers. The GP process of *transferring responsibility* will continue to play an important role in caregiver and adolescent competency development in addition to knowledge translation that reaches others in the area of adolescent concussion care.

The following case is a real-life example of a concussion injury in a typical self-driven adolescent student athlete. As you read through this scenario, attempt to immerse yourself in the experience through the lens of the clinician (ED nurse, NP, and school nurse), the caregiver/parent, and the adolescent. Although you are given a limited amount of details, challenge yourself to apply GP to this clinical context. Strive to support the student athlete and caregiver in reaching a shared goal of symptom management and a safe and timely return to classroom, sport, and life by applying GP processes that were previously discussed.

Case Example 10.1

RJ, a 17-year-old male basketball point guard, with a history of migraines, attention deficit hyperactivity disorder (ADHD), and one previous concussion (approximately 3 months ago), sustained a concussion in a tournament game during his junior year in a top-ranked, academically rigorous high school. RJ was pinned between two players and was elbowed on the left side of his head. He was fouled on the play and recalled feeling dizzy and light-headed at the time, but managed to make both free throws and complete the rest of the game. Despite a state law requiring the removal from play if a concussion is suspected, neither the licensed athletic trainer (LAT) nor the coaching staff saw any sign of concern at the time of injury, so he was not removed from the game for further evaluation. (Later in his recovery, RJ admitted that he should have removed himself from the game and brought those symptoms to their attention. Instead he decided to hide the symptoms, as he didn't want to let his team down.)

Immediately following the game, he was quiet and noted a headache, nausea, loss of appetite, and fatigue. As the night progressed, he felt increasingly "foggy" and even confused. He began crying for no particular reason. Before bed, he took ibuprofen. Despite previous mandatory concussion education, he did not share these symptoms with his team or his parents and continued to hide them as best as he could. The day after, RJ participated in another tournament game. He performed uncharacteristically poorly during this game as, typically, he was an aggressive player but did not perform in the same manner. He fouled out early in the game, in part because he was called for three charging fouls. (RJ later stated that these came from his lack of depth perception; unable to perceive where the opposing players were in relation to him and he believes he miscalculated the contact with them.)

The following day, a Monday, RJ felt forced to inform the LAT of the signs and symptoms he was experiencing because he had arrived at school with a continued headache, was bothered by the lights and noise, and couldn't find the room for his math class, although it was late in the semester and he had been there many times. He was diagnosed with a concussion and his high school's multidisciplinary concussion plan was implemented. Per Berlin guidelines (McCrory et al., 2017), he was removed from all physical and cognitive activity. Symptoms and signs of recovery were to be reassessed every 24 hours. A team, comprised of the school nurse, LAT, with oversight from a physician, homeroom teacher, guidance counselor, psychologist, and athletic director, collaborated to coordinate a plan to support his recovery and ensure he had adequate classroom-based accommodations and appropriate return to full sport play when ready.

RJ met with the LAT and school nurse regularly to assess his recovery and advance his return to school and sport. As his symptoms continued without improvement, he became significantly stressed about schoolwork and upcoming college application deadlines, and over time, grew increasingly anxious and depressed. Because his friends were primarily sport based, he missed out on the socialization and found himself withdrawn during the recovery process. His parents, who both work full time, do not recall receiving any written or verbal communications/instructions, were not included in the regular meetings with the LAT or school nurse, and were unaware of the school's concussion plan. They relied on their son for updates.

However, when they noted their son's ongoing low morale, lack of energy, continual time in his bed, and his uncharacteristically quiet and irritable personality, they phoned the high school and talked with the psychologist who stated they should ask their son to bring his concerns to the school nurse. From the time of injury, it took 3 weeks for RJ to fully return to the classroom and 4 weeks to fully return to his sport. During that time, his teachers grew frustrated with his continued needs for accommodations in the classroom, as he looked "fine." His grades dropped, he lost interest in school, and he lost his starting position as point guard. He was no longer the same adolescent!

CONCLUSION

This chapter examines the application of GP methods to the situation of managing adolescent concussion recovery in ways that optimize health and well-being. In summary, key concepts of GP and implications in caring for a concussed adolescent and their family include the following:

- The response to and recovery from adolescent concussion is personally and socially meaningful to adolescent life.
- GP is grounded in a trusting relationship between the caregiver and clinician who share a common goal for the adolescent's concussion recovery and return to what the adolescent knows as "normal" life.
- GP replaces the usual asynchronous method of telling/lecturing about concussion care with a clinical practice that encourages partnered competency development and eventual transfer of responsibility.
- GP aids in the development of caregiver competencies for the complex and multifaceted process of concussion recovery by adapting teaching and learning for unique family needs.

Questions for Reflection

- What would GP offer the adolescent and his family in the case example? What makes it an appropriate approach to teaching and learning for concussed adolescents and their parent(s)?
- How could GP benefit the complex process of postconcussion return to classroom and sport?
- How is GP unique compared to traditional teaching/educational paradigms in concussion care?
- What could all (parents, adolescent, clinicians, school, and sports staff) do together to make connections and build trust around reporting of concussion, return to classroom, and return to sport processes postconcussion?
- How could the relationship-based teaching–learning practice of GP support improved health and quality of life outcomes for concussed adolescents?

REFERENCES

Ahmed, O. H., Sullivan, S. J., Schneiders, A. G., & McCrory, P. (2010). iSupport: Do social networking sites have a role to play in concussion awareness? *Disability Rehabilitation*, *32*, 1877–1883. doi:10.3109/09638281003734409

Babcock, L., Byczkowksi, T., Wade, S. L., Ho, M., Mookerjee, S., & Bazarian, J. J. (2013). Predicting postconcussion syndrome after mild traumatic brain injury in children and adolescents who present to the emergency department. *JAMA Pediatrics*, *167*, 156–161.

Bloom, G. A., Horton, A. S., McCrory, P., & Johnston, K. (2004). Sport psychology and concussion: New impacts to explore. *British Journal of Sports Medicine*, *38*, 519–521. doi:10.1136/bjsm.2004.011999

Boden, B. P., Tachetti, R. L., & Cantu, R. C. (2007). Catastrophic head injuries in high school and college football players. *American Journal of Sports Medicine, 35,* 1075–1081. doi:10.1177/0363546507299239

Cantu, R. (1998). Second impact syndrome. *Clinics in Sports Medicine, 17,* 37–44.

Centers for Disease Control and Prevention (CDC). (2017). Concussion in sports. Retrieved from http://www.cdc.gov/concussion/sports/inde.htm

Corwin, D. J., Zonfrillo, M. R., Master, C. L., Arbogast, K. B., Grady, M. F., Robinson, R. L., . . . Wiebe, D. J. (2014). Characteristics of prolonged concussion recovery in a pediatric subspecialty referral population. *Journal of Pediatrics, 165,* 1207–1215.

Eisenberg, M. A., Meehan, W. P., III, & Mannix, R. (2014). Duration and course of post-concussive symptoms. *Pediatrics, 133,* 999–1006.

Fahy, E., Hardikar, R., Fox, A., & Mackay, S. (2014). Quality of patient health information on the Internet: Reviewing a complex and evolving landscape. *Australasian Medical Journal, 4,* 24–28.

Grubenhoff, J. A., Deakyne, S. J., Brou, L., Bajaj, L., Comstock, R. D., & Kirkwood, M. W. (2014). Acute concussion symptom severity and delayed symptom resolution. *Pediatrics, 134,* 54–62.

Halstead, M. E., Walter, K. D., & Council on Sports Medicine and Fitness. (2010). American Academy of Pediatrics. Clinical report—Sport-related concussion in children and adolescents. *Pediatrics, 126,* 597–615. doi:10.1542/peds.2010-2005

Harmon, K. G., Drezner, J. A., Gammons, M., Guskiewicz, K. M., Halstead, M., Herring, S. A., . . . Roberts, W. O. (2013). American Medical Society position statement: Concussion in sport. *British Journal of Sports Medicine, 47,* 15–26. doi:10.1136/bjsports-2012-091941

Institute of Medicine (IOM) & National Research Council (NRC). (2013). *Sports-related concussions in youth: Improving the science, changing the culture.* Washington, DC: National Academies Press.

Kontos, A. P., Elbin, R. J., Schatz, P., Covassin, T., Henry, L., Pardini, J., & Collins, M. W. (2012). A revised factor structure for the post-concussion symptom scale: Baseline and postconcussion factors. *American Journal of Sports Medicine, 40,* 2375–2384. doi:10.1177/0363546512455400

Langlois, J., Rutland-Brown, W., & Wald, M. (2006). The epidemiology and impact of traumatic brain injury. *Journal of Head and Trauma Rehabilitation, 21,* 375–378.

Lovell, M. R., & Collins, M. W. (1998). Relationship between concussion and neuropsychological performance in college football players. *Journal of Head Trauma Rehabilitation, 13,* 964–970.

Mainwaring, L. M., Bisschop, S. M., Green, R. E. A., Antoniazzi, M., Comper, P., Kristman, V., . . . Richards, D. W. (2004). Emotional reaction of varsity athletes to sports-related concussion. *Journal of Sport and Exercise Psychology, 26,* 119–135.

Mainwaring, L. M., Hutchison, M., Bisschop, S. M., Comper, P., & Richards, D. W. (2010). Emotional response to sport concussion compared to ACL injury. *Brain Injury, 24,* 589–597. doi:10.3109/02699051003610508

Marar, M., McIlvain, N. M., Fields, S. K., & Comstock, R. D. (2012). Epidemiology of concussions among United States high school athletes in 20 sports. *American Journal of Sports Medicine, 40,* 747–755. doi:10.1177/0363546511435626

McCarty, C. A., Zatzick, D., Stein, E., Wang, J., Hilt, R., & Rivara, F. P. (2016). Collaborative care for adolescents with persistent postconcussive symptoms: A randomized trial. *Pediatrics, 138*(4), e20160459.

McCrory, P., Johnston, K., Meeuwisse, W., Aubry, M., Cantu, R., Dvorak, J., . . . Schamasch, P. (2005). Summary and agreement statement of the 2nd International Conference on Concussion in Sport, Prague, 2004. *British Journal of Sports Medicine, 39,* 196–204. doi:10.1136/bjsm.2005.018614

McCrory, P., Meeuwisse, W. H., Aubry, M., Cantu, B., Dvorak, J., Echemendia, R. J., . . . Turner, M. (2013). Consensus statement on concussion in sport: The 4th International Conference on Concussion in Sport, Zurich, November 2012. *British Journal of Sports Medicine, 47,* 250–258. doi:10.1136/bjsports-2013-092313

McCrory, P., Meeuwisse, W., Dvorak, J., Aubry, M., Bailes, J., Broglio, S., . . . Vos, P. E. (2017). Consensus statement on concussion in sport: The 5th International Conference on Concussion in Sport, Berlin, October 2016. *British Journal of Sports Medicine, 51,* 838–847. doi:10.1136/bjsports-2017-097699

McCrory, P., Meeuwisse, W., Johnston, K., Dvorak, J., Aubry, M., Malloy, M., & Cantu, R. (2009). Consensus statement on concussion in sport: The 3rd International Conference on Concussion in Sport, Zurich, November 2008. *Journal of Clinical Neuroscience, 16,* 755–763.

Pardini, J., Stump, J., Lovell, M. R., Collins, M. W., Moritz, K., & Fu, F. (2004). The Postconcussion Symptom Scale (PCSS): A factor analysis [abstract]. *British Journal of Sports Medicine, 38,* 661–662.

Pridham, K. F., Limbo, R., Schroeder, M., Thoyre, S., & Van Riper, M. (1998). Guided participation and development of care-giving competencies for families of low birth-weight infants. *Journal of Advanced Nursing, 28*, 948–958.

Putukian, M., & Echemendia, R. J. (2003). Psychological aspects of head injury in the competitive athlete. *Clinical Sports Medicine, 22*, 617–630.

Reeves, R. R., & Panguluri, R. L. (2011). Neuropsychiatric complications of traumatic brain injury. *Journal of Psychosocial Nursing and Mental Health Services, 49*, 42–50. doi:10.3928/02793695-20110201-03

Rogoff, B. (1990). *Apprenticeship in thinking: Cognitive development in social context.* New York, NY: Oxford University Press.

Rogoff, B., & Lave, J. (1984). *Everyday cognition in the social context.* Cambridge, MA: Harvard University Press.

Sady, M. D., Vaughan, C. G., & Gioia, G. (2011). School and the concussed youth: Recommendations for concussion education and management. *Physical Medicine Rehabilitation Clinics North America, 22*, 701–719.

Snedden, T. R. (2013). Concussion: A concept analysis. *Journal of Specialists in Pediatric Nursing, 18*, 211–220. doi:10.1111/jspn.12038

11

Transitioning From Hospital to Home Care for a Child Who Is Technology Dependent

Michele M. Schroeder, Barbara J. Byrne, Laura J. Ahola, and Lori J. Williams

Preparing families with a child who is technology dependent to transition from the hospital healthcare team (subsequently referred to as "team") holding primary responsibility for caregiving to a state of readiness for family-independent caregiving at home is a complex process layered with many physical, mental, and emotional challenges. To help illustrate these challenges and an approach to addressing them through guided participation, we introduce you to Sarah and her parents, Mary and John (family names changed to protect privacy). Their journey from observers of care to expert deliverers of care exemplifies what many families and pediatric hospital team members experience while navigating similar circumstances.

The advancement of life-saving and life-enhancing treatments, technology, and services has dramatically improved survival and developmental outcomes for technology-dependent children (Elias, Murphy, & the Council on Children with Disabilities, 2012). Supporting families in developing competencies needed to manage home care for a child who is technology dependent, often in a community with limited resources, is essential. How that process is supported makes a difference for all involved. The story we share with you illustrates the common concerns and triumphs experienced by families and clinicians alike and highlights learnings discovered through working with Sarah and her family. It is our hope, and the purpose of this chapter, that the telling of this story supports nurses and interdisciplinary team members in better understanding their patients' challenges and care, and in turn helps them be better prepared to partner with families via guided participation to achieve a successful transition to care at home.

Case Example 11.1

Sarah is the first-born child to Mary (mother) and John (father), who have been married for approximately 5 years and live on a farm in a rural community. Sarah was born at 26 weeks and 2 days gestation via a cesarean birth after a pregnancy complicated by oligohydramnios, intrauterine growth retardation, and preeclampsia. Her Apgar scores were 2/7 and she weighed 500 g at birth. She was diagnosed with pulmonary interstitial glycogenosis (Deterding, 2010), alveolar hypoplasia, and subglottic stenosis, which resulted in ventilator dependency and the need for a gastrostomy and tracheostomy. By 5 months of age, she had transitioned from the neonatal intensive care unit (NICU) to the pediatric intensive care unit (PICU), then to the pediatric universal care unit (PUCU), where she resided for the next 7 months or so. Sarah was ultimately discharged to home after a total of 363 days in the hospital, just shy of her first birthday.

The Caregiving Team

Sarah's PUCU caregiving team included a number of people, first and foremost her mother and father. Her team members included a primary nurse, two associate nurses (coprimary nurses), pediatric clinical nurse specialist, respiratory therapists, case manager, physical therapist, occupational therapist, speech therapist, social worker, registered dietician, child life specialist, spiritual care provider, physician teams, pharmacists, and a pulmonary clinical nurse specialist. This large team of clinicians worked together with Sarah's family to develop, coordinate, and implement the transition plan of care to home.

Description of Hospital and Pediatric Universal Care Unit

The UW Health American Family Children's Hospital (AFCH) is an 101 bed pediatric hospital within a larger university hospital setting. In their annual rankings of Best Children's Hospitals, *U.S. News & World Report* listed UW Health AFCH among the top 50 children's hospitals in six medical and surgical specialties. The PUCU is a 12-bed progressive care step-down unit from the NICU and the PICU. It is a transitional unit that specializes in the care of complex and technology-dependent children, which engages with and prepares families for the transition of their children to home, especially those children and families experiencing home-going for the first time since the child's birth. The emphasis is on family education, confidence building, and comprehensive home care planning.

TEAM CARE FOR TRANSITION TO HOME

The largest overall issue or goal was preparing Sarah and her family for the transition from hospital to home care. Figure 11.1 summarizes the different components needed to achieve that transition. This document is one of the first items shared with families. It serves to assist the family and team with the initial work of getting connected, joining and maintaining attention, sharing understanding, bridging from the known to the new, and structuring the tasks/learning ahead. Further, it foreshadows for families and team members the journey before them, reinforcing that each needs the other in order to achieve a smooth, safe, and effective transition to home for Sarah and her family.

In reflecting on the complexities of care for Sarah, her family, and the team, we spoke with Sarah's family (see Table 11.1) and those team members primarily responsible for transition care planning and implementation once Sarah was medically stable (see Table 11.2) in order to capture the richness and depth of their experiences. We used internal working model concepts (see Chapter 1) to develop the questions asked to guide the dialogue. Asking about goals, expectations, intentions, meanings, emotions, and evaluations assists in making the internal working model for the issue at hand explicit and accessible to all caregivers involved. The information gathered can then be used to assess, plan, implement, and evaluate the competencies embedded in individualized caregiving activities in the moment as well as those likely to be in the future (Pridham, 1993).

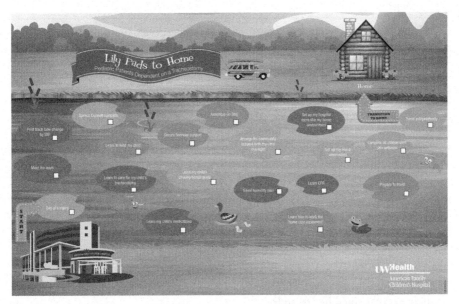

FIGURE 11.1 Lily Pads to Home—transition to home care map for pediatric patients dependent on a tracheostomy.

Source: Shared with permission from UW Health Marketing and Communications.

TABLE 11.1 Dialogue Guide—Family

Dialogue Guide With Family Issue: Getting Ready to Go Home	Internal Working Model Components
Thank you for taking the time to share your insights and experiences with me regarding your experiences in getting ready to take Sarah home. Please let me know if the questions aren't clear or if you need further explanation as we go along.	
1. What did you see as the top three to five most important things in getting ready to take Sarah home? Examples to use if needed: a. Learning about her care b. Learning about the equipment c. Communicating with the healthcare team (nurses, doctors, specialists) d. Developing confidence e. Getting your family ready f. Having the right stuff at home (supplies, equipment, nurses)	Goals
2. What were you hoping would happen as you were getting ready?	Intentions, expectations
3. What told you whether or not it was working?	Evaluations
4. What told you that Sarah and you were ready to go home?	Meanings, evaluations
5. In hindsight, thinking back to before you left the hospital, a. What lessons, if any, were learned in getting ready to go home? b. What do you wish you had known more about before going home? c. What, if anything, do you think would be important to share with healthcare team members about getting ready to go home? d. What, if anything, do you think would be important to share with other families about getting ready to go home?	Goals, meanings, expectations, evaluations
6. Is there anything we haven't talked about yet that you'd like to add?	

(continued)

TABLE 11.1 Dialogue Guide—Family (*continued*)

Dialogue Guide With Family Issue: Getting Ready to Go Home	Internal Working Model Components
Follow-up questions to help draw out more specific thoughts, answers:	
1. Tell me more about [XXX] . . .	Meanings, emotions
2. I wonder what [XXX] might mean to you, why that might be important . . .	Meanings, emotions
3. How was that for you?	Meanings, emotions, evaluations

TABLE 11.2 Dialogue Guide—Healthcare Team Members

Dialogue Guide With Healthcare Team Members Issue: Getting Ready to Go Home	Internal Working Model Components
Thank you for taking the time to share your insights and experiences with me regarding Sarah and her family. Please let me know if the questions aren't clear or if you need further explanation as we go along.	
1. What did you see as the top three to five priorities in preparing Sarah and her family for the transition from our unit to their home? Examples to use if needed: a. Learning about her care b. Learning about the equipment c. Communicating with the healthcare team (nurses, doctors, specialists) d. Developing confidence e. Getting her family ready f. Having the right stuff at home (supplies, equipment, nurses)	Goals
2. As you were developing the plan of care, what were you trying to accomplish?	Intentions
3. What were you hoping would happen?	Expectations
4. What told you whether or not the plan of care was working?	Evaluations

(*continued*)

TABLE 11.2 Dialogue Guide—Healthcare Team Members (*continued*)

Dialogue Guide With Healthcare Team Members Issue: Getting Ready to Go Home	Internal Working Model Components
5. What told you that Sarah and her family were ready to go home?	Meanings, evaluations

6. In hindsight, thinking about Sarah and her family,
  a. What lessons, if any, were learned in working with Sarah and her family?
  b. What, if anything, have you found yourself doing differently with other children/families on the unit since working with Sarah and her family?
  c. What, if anything, do you think would be important to share with other healthcare team members?
	Goals, meanings, expectations, evaluations

7. Is there anything we haven't talked about yet that you'd like to add?	
Follow-up questions to help draw out more specific thoughts, answers:	
1. Tell me more about [XXX] . . .	Meanings, emotions
2. I wonder what [XXX] might mean to you, why that might be important . . .	Meanings, emotions
3. How was that for you?	Meanings, emotions, evaluations

We heard thoughtful, insightful comments, and stories regarding preparation for transitioning from hospital to home care, which we discuss next.

Communicating and Engaging

A variety of services, programs, and clinicians are needed to provide care for children with complex healthcare needs. The role of the parent cannot be underestimated when creating plans of care. Strategies to ensure communication and engagement between the patient, families, clinicians, and services are necessary to support continuous and coordinated care during hospitalization (Swartwout, Drenkard, McGuinn, Grant, & El-Zein, 2016; Taylor et al., 2013). The exchange of information between parents and clinicians, and among clinicians and services, has been found to be essential during hospitalization (Zanello et al., 2015). Explaining clinical information in a way parents can understand significantly influences their understanding of and learning about their child's care (Zanello et al., 2015).

For example, parents may already know how to change a diaper or give a bath for a typically developing infant, but may need assistance from the primary nurse to take what they already know and apply it to the new situation of caring for an infant with a tracheostomy—that is, bridging from the known to the new. At discharge, the transition from hospital to home changes responsibilities and relationships between parents and healthcare clinicians (Brenner et al., 2015). After discharge, many parents feel compelled to ensure continuity of information across healthcare settings and services by physically carrying medical reports or orally communicating information about their child's condition (Zanello et al., 2015).

A framework that guides team members to anticipate and plan for the family's education and support needs is necessary for a successful transition from hospital to home (Bowles, Jnah, Newberry, Hubbard, & Roberston, 2016). Use of a family-focused or family-centered care model is an effective strategy to encourage and sustain communication and parent involvement. Activities imbedded in these models have led to better informed and confident parents (Cooper et al., 2007). Guided participation practice provides a framework to guide communication and engagement activities for the team and family. Planned communication facilitates all participants in developing a shared internal working model of the issue at hand—another way to think about "being on the same page." Structured communication promotes every voice being heard, which contributes to the development of shared understanding and/or agreement about goals or expectations of care. Accompanying emotions can be acknowledged or recognized, allowing problem solving to occur together.

Planned communication can take many forms. Sarah's family and the team used a variety of methods available in the PUCU, as described next.

Rounds

Many different types of rounds are used to assist with communication among the caregiving team. Family participation can be encouraged and achieved successfully, most effectively when team members (a) prepare the family regarding what to expect, (b) assist them with identifying concerns and developing questions, and (c) respectfully support their desire and efforts to participate in the process.

Pulmonary service interdisciplinary rounds provide a weekly opportunity for all disciplines to together formulate, evaluate, and/or revise a plan of care while meeting face to face. The child's discharge criteria are identified, and steps toward achieving those criteria are reviewed from week to week. Tracheostomy rounds is another weekly method employed to keep the discharge process moving forward. The family, case manager, pulmonary clinical nurse specialist, respiratory care discharge planner, and unit clinical nurse specialist review a checklist of items that need to be accomplished prior to discharge. Outstanding items are assigned to the appropriate person for completion by the identified dates. An example would be identifying a primary care provider, which the family would be responsible for finding. Daily medical rounds are another structured opportunity that families may participate in as able (i.e., when able to be present on the unit).

Nurse-led rounds are a structured approach geared to ensuring family questions and concerns are addressed during the rounding process (American Hospital Association, 2013). Incorporating "5 minutes at the bedside" at the beginning of the shift provides an opportunity for the nurse and family to develop a clear and shared understanding of the family's and child's (if old enough to indicate) goals for the day (i.e., plan for the day) and for the hospital stay (i.e., plan for the stay). These goals are then incorporated into the daily medical rounds as the medical plan is determined.

Video Technology

Use of bedside technology such as Vidyo® (Williams, 2016) is another structured approach to support family engagement and participation in rounding processes. Family who cannot be physically present for rounds are included "virtually" when the team is at their child's bedside for rounds. This technology helps families and the team stay connected regardless of physical presence—an important point for families who need to be at work when rounds typically occur.

White Boards

In the PUCU, dry erase boards have been templated to drive aspects of care and discharge planning that we have learned it helps to consistently address. These aspects include spaces for the names of the child and family and for team members such as physicians, primary nurse, the shift nurse, respiratory care, physical therapist, or speech pathologist. There is a large section for the day's tests and treatments, allowing visualization of times for laboratory tests, x-rays, therapies, or other planned activities. Another large section is designated for family or team members to write out the plan of care, or list elements to be completed prior to discharge. For families of children with complex care needs who are learning cares, it is not uncommon to have a list (mirroring the Lily Pads to Home document) that may include completion of classes, equipment training, obtaining home care nurses, and setting up the home environment with equipment.

Care Conferences

Care conferences are another structured approach to communication that can be used to convey information, verify understanding of information, formulate goals, and develop an interdisciplinary approach to achieve a desired outcome. Parental participation is critical to the success of this process (Nelson & Mahant, 2014).

Becoming Competent and Confident in Daily Caregiving Skills, Child Development, and Emergency Care

Competence and confidence seem to go hand in hand. Discussing one almost always involves discussing the other, both for families and the team; that is, confidence grows as one becomes more competent and vice versa. Therefore, in this section, we reflect on the two together.

The transition to home with a technology-dependent child is complex (Callans, Bleiler, Flanagan, & Carroll, 2016). Families not only need to learn basic caregiving for their child but they also need to learn the technology (equipment) and critical-thinking problem-solving skills. Families may often feel they are under scrutiny by team members to perform, a scrutiny that is not always welcome. Likewise, staff may feel they are under scrutiny by family members to give safe and effective care individualized to their child. Guided participation practice offers a way for families and team members to instead cocreate an atmosphere of mutual teaching and learning as partners (see Chapter 1). Development of trust in the partnership is key to success when undertaking guided participation (see Chapter 1). In this partnership, nursing staff daily assess the family's competence and confidence along with the health and well-being of the child in order to fine-tune the ongoing teaching and learning both in the moment (Rogoff, Mejia-Arauz, & Correa-Chavez, 2015) and via structured education programs.

Organized education programs build upon and extend the family's knowledge, thereby increasing competence in needed caregiving skills and building confidence via a systematic process that is individualized to meet the learning needs of each family member for their child (Graf, Montagnino, Hueckel, & McPherson, 2008; Joseph, 2011). The components of an organized education program include the following:

1. Team member identification—initial and with each transition. Therapists may be constant across inpatient settings, but typically providers and nursing staff change as the child transitions from unit to unit, as service rotations occur, as shifts change.
2. Family assessment—assessing the family's understanding of the medical complexities of their child, their goals for their child, home life routines
3. Expectations shared for
   a. The amount of time dedicated to classroom education
   b. The skills that will be learned in the classroom
   c. The skills to be learned/demonstrated at the bedside
   d. The required number of trained home caregivers, inclusive of home health
4. Review of tasks to accomplish, such as suctioning, tracheostomy tube changes, independent care sessions, and independent off-unit trips (e.g., taking their child on walks outside of the hospital)

Program education can start early. For example, the classroom portion of the education can be completed either before or just after the child has surgery to create the tracheostomy. Completing the classroom education prior to surgery can have a positive benefit for the family, as described by Sarah's father: "It was good to do the classroom part before Sarah had her trach; after she had surgery we were able to focus on her. We did not need to leave her for [classroom] education."

Once the family completes the classroom components regarding physiology and anatomy and basic skills, they are ready to begin hands-on learning about how to care for their child's technology. Together, the team and the family assess daily the plan for the day and the plan for the stay, and identify what is still needed for the transition to home. The primary nurse is instrumental in the development of the plan. The nurse works very closely with the family and the entire team to coordinate the daily activities, helping to balance the family's priorities with those of the team. It is important to support families in developing a sense of accomplishment, such as successfully suctioning the tracheostomy tube, as this helps families achieve a level of confidence.

Team members partner with and guide families at the bedside while giving care to the child. For example, when the child's condition changes or when equipment becomes nonfunctional, the nurse guides the family by structuring the task at hand using methods such as role modeling, talking through a situation, and demonstrating the task or skill that the family will need to learn. At the family's pace, the team will begin to transfer responsibility for the care or skill over to the family. This takes place as the healthcare provider asks the family questions such as "What do you see or hear? What do you make of that? What do you think is happening? What, if anything, should we do about it?" in order to understand what the family is making of their child's care and condition. This activity helps families develop the skill to critically think through a situation and take appropriate action. When a family member is able to role model and/or relay this critical thinking to other family members, they build confidence in and for each other. Sarah's father described his experience with the process in this way:

> During my independent session, Sarah was making a noise that I did not recognize. Our nurse asked questions such as "What do you hear, what does Sarah look like, what do you think is going on?" I was not sure, she gave me clues; Sarah's trach was plugged. I told Mary [Sarah's mother] what happened and described it to her.

Sarah's mother then described her subsequent experience with a similar situation: "During my independent session, Sarah starting making that noise, just like he [John] described it, I called the nurse and said, 'I think Sarah has a plug, we should change the trach.' I was right." In this vignette, Sarah's parents describe engaging in bridging for each other, a crucial step toward becoming central to Sarah's care.

The confidence of family members is important. As the child transitions to home, family members need both the confidence and competence to safely problem solve and care for their child. Once the child transitions to home, family members may not have the benefit of healthcare providers in their home or in the community to assist if their child experiences a medical emergency. Even with community healthcare clinicians present, family members will often be the experts in such a situation. Supporting family members in developing competencies needed to manage home care for a child who is technology dependent, often in a community with limited resources, is critical for the long-term outcomes for the child. Nurses have the joy and the responsibility of helping family members develop confidence and competence in caregiving while preparing for the transition to home. Guided participation practice as a model for guiding the development of confidence and competence is efficient and effective.

Assessing and promoting the family's development of both competence and confidence occurs throughout the child's hospital stay. Sarah's primary nurse identified that "Providing a safe environment for Sarah, to teach the cares, the critical thinking, and building confidence, was a top priority for me as her primary nurse. We needed to help Mary gain confidence to be a mom, to see her baby, not the equipment, to look past the medical stuff."

Managing the unexpected is necessary when preparing the family for transition to home. Guiding families through structuring the task of how to care for their child (i.e., recognize what is happening, problem solve and make decisions about what to do, then carry out the necessary skills needed to correct the situation) during emergent situations is essential for the safety of the child. These emergent situations include simulated unplanned decannulations, mucus plugging, power failure, and signs and symptoms of infection. Mary described it this way: "We were going to go home, but she developed a cold. I was upset that we could not go home, but it was good to know what a cold would look and sound like."

The team needs to be mindful of gradually transferring daily care activities to the family, the importance of which Mary identified: "I knew we needed to practice for when the trach fell out; you don't want the first time to be when you are home." The team can engage in activities that simulate the home environment, as Sarah's primary nurse explained: "Helping the family set up the hospital room to match the child's designated room at home, placing emergent equipment where you believe it will be located in the home in proximity to the child helps with developing 'muscle memory' for the family." Transitioning the family from accompanied walks to independent walks with their child helps to solidify the family's growing level of confidence.

Do any of these methods make a difference? Can we assure families are moving along the trajectory we envision for and with them? A review of responses from our dialogues with Sarah's mother, father, and team provides insight. Members from each discipline indicated they knew the process was working when the family stated they felt competent and confident that they could care for their child. Competence was described as confidence with tracheostomy care and changes, and the ability to independently troubleshoot and respond appropriately to equipment challenges, alarms, and concerning changes in Sarah's condition. Confidence was evident when the parents no longer needed prompts for activities like suctioning Sarah or going on walks, were able to independently utilize equipment at the bedside, and were able to think/plan in advance. Being prepared for a safe and smooth transition to home was mentioned several times. This was evidenced by the family's description of feeling well prepared to take their child home and having everything they needed to successfully care for her at home. Sarah's mother and father described the checklists and visual displays such as the dry erase board as helpful. They also described that the ability to perform care for Sarah independently was confidence building.

Becoming a Parent

Parenting a technology-dependent child alters the meaning of being a parent (Kirk, Glendinning, & Callery, 2005). Providing care has been found to have a substantial emotional dimension for parents (Kirk et al., 2005). Parents need opportunities to discuss their feelings about assuming the role of caregiver, what it means for their parenting identity, and their relationship with their child (Kirk et al., 2005). Guided participation processes are ideal for assisting parents with developing the competency of regulating emotions. Parents routinely address a wide range of needs for their children, including physical care, security, love, protection, and developmental encouragement. Parents of technology-dependent children address these needs while grieving the loss of their "normal" child and the parenting experience that was anticipated, hoped for, dreamed for. The parenting role is very different for these parents as they learn "interventions" commonly observed as being done by nurses and now necessary for the care of their child, with the learning occurring in the public arena of the hospital versus the privacy of their home.

Kirk et al.'s (2005) exploration of the parent experience of caring for a technologically dependent child found the parental role to be multifaceted. In addition to the usual parenting activities, these parents could be found organizing home support services, administering oxygen, suctioning airways, changing tracheostomy tubes, replacing gastric tubes, and administering medications. Performing clinical procedures on their own child was found to be the most distressing part of caregiving due to the perceived pain inflicted. Parents in this study desired to see themselves as parents first. They did not want their relationship with their child to be defined by "nursing interventions."

For technology-dependent children, parents need to acquire the usual skills of parenting in addition to learning skilled nursing procedures. These procedures require technical competencies as well as the ability to make complex medical decisions. Learning and giving care in this manner has an emotional dimension that is important to address. Helping parents develop competency at regulating their emotions can be achieved by assisting with identifying and acknowledging the range of emotions experienced, reassuring that they are not alone in feeling them, and discussing ways to manage them.

Parents need opportunities to discuss their feelings about their dual role as "nurse" and parent. Healthcare clinicians can support strategies used by parents to see themselves as parents first. Discussing their expectations and experiences while parenting (i.e., identifying their internal working model of parenting) and implementing problem-solving processes can lead to parenting success. Parents and team members can pool their growing body of individualized knowledge regarding the child, enabling all to pick up and act on subtle changes in the child's condition and/or demeanor. Ideally, parents can be included in the process of making decisions about modifying care routines (like withholding therapies) in response to changes in the child's condition.

Is there evidence that our organized education approach to parent education is working to help parents fully embrace the parent role, while incorporating the technology-dependent child into the family? The primary nurse identified her top priority as "helping the mother gain the confidence to be a mom; to see her baby, not the equipment; and to look past the medical stuff." The primary nurse's plan was to be sure that nursing and respiratory cares became "just the usual care," like a diaper change or teaching the alphabet or reading stories. It was important that the mother could "look past the task of things like suctioning, and to have tasks become something that are routinely done." Turning the task of cares into a caring action was hoped to help Mary "feel like she was the mom, not the nurse." As an advocate for both Sarah and her family, the primary nurse attempted to help Mary and John develop relationship competencies, meaning coming to understand their child, get to know her, learn her likes and dislikes, while learning about typical infant behaviors. Success was defined in part as the parents' ability to read and respond to their daughter's cues.

In addition, the nursing care plan was synchronized with the parents' plan for the day. For example, Mary wanted to have time to read out loud to Sarah, so it was important to carve out time each day for that activity. The primary nurse grew to recognize that what she felt was best and what the family thought was best were not always the same—and that was okay, even desirable.

> I was working on a plan of care that would help Sarah thrive, developmentally as well as physically. At some point, I realized that Mom and Dad's plan of care was becoming aligned with the nursing plan of care, gradually over time. It is important to remember that my plan of care was not always the same or even equal to the parents' plan of care.

Arranging and Confirming Home Care Resources

Making sure home care arrangements are in place and ready to go at the moment of discharge is crucial to a successful transition to home, especially when it is the child and family's inaugural discharge. Much work goes into planning, organizing, and preparing for this momentous occasion. All involved would prefer not to see the child readmitted soon after discharge as a result of inadequate home care resource planning. This includes attention to:

- Adequate in-home 24/7 caregiving help, often via trained caregivers (e.g., agency or independent nurses), family members, neighbors, or (typically) a combination
- Therapies as ordered (e.g., speech, physical, occupational)—either community- or home-based
- Provider follow-up appointments made
- Transportation mode determined
- Home care supplies and equipment delivered, installed, organized, and in good working order
- Home medications on hand, stored, and organized with appropriate administration supplies ready
- Local emergency medical services (EMS) notified with a plan of care on file
- Adequate insurance coverage (private or public) confirmed

When asked "What do you wish you had known more about, if anything, before going home?" Sarah's parents discussed the following related to home care resources and services:

- "We didn't realize how much time it would take to organize the home health supplies and equipment. The home health company is not always organized; orders get screwed up, the company can be stingy with supplies. Use electronic ordering, because then you have an email chain for follow-up."
- "Home nursing is not like the hospital nurses—they are not always reliable; be prepared that you will need to teach them [about your child and their care]."
- "We didn't know we could arrange to have a therapist do all therapies (e.g., speech, physical, occupational) in the home. It is really hard to travel with Sarah, so in-home services are very important."
- "Use mail order for all medications—faster and simpler."

These comments might suggest the need to either find ways to prepare families predischarge for typical problem-solving challenges like these that crop up after the transition to home or extend problem-solving support postdischarge. Questions to consider could include the following:

- How might guided participation processes be brought to bear on situations like this (i.e., how to determine which potential postdischarge challenges to focus education efforts on while trying to accomplish the actual transition home)?
- What resources might be available to assist families with situations like these postdischarge?

Transferring Responsibility for Managing Caregiving

Previous themes have identified the importance of parents being competent and confident in their caregiving abilities with their child—including physical activities and critical thinking and problem-solving skills when confronted with unexpected events or situations. In this section, we reflect further on how parents might move from being on the periphery of caregiving with minimal responsibility in the hospital setting (i.e., observing team members give care to their child) to being central to caregiving with primary responsibility. With guided participation in mind, we attempt to answer the question "How is responsibility for managing caregiving activities and problem solving transferred to parents in preparation for transitioning to care at home?" by exploring what the experience was like with Sarah and her family.

When asked "What were you hoping would happen as you were getting ready to take Sarah home?" her mother replied:

> That the nurses and other people would let us take charge in the hospital. Like when we were still in the PICU and it was time for Sarah to have a bath. Her nurse unhooked her from the cardiac monitor, helped set up the bath supplies, told us to call her if we needed anything and left, shutting the door behind her. We felt nervous, but this forced us to stop looking at the monitors and look instead at Sarah. We had done a lot of her cares before this, but a nurse was always right there. By the time Sarah came to the PUCU, we wanted to be in the loop and present. We felt responsible for her cares. It was better toward the end of Sarah's hospital stay in that we took the lead in caring for her. That's very important to accomplish before you go home.

Even in hindsight, this vignette illustrates several key guided participation practice elements. First, the question asked gives the team members explicit information about the mother's internal working model (goals, expectations, intentions, meanings, emotions, evaluations) regarding the transition to home. That information can be validated with the family and used to tailor the degree of responsibility offered with each caregiving opportunity.

One small change that may have made this transfer of responsibility to the parents less abrupt would have been the use of "structuring the activity." The nurse could have given the parents a clearer notion of caregiving goals (independence), while letting the parents more clearly understand what to expect. For example, the nurse could have said, "This will be your first time bathing Sarah by yourself. I'm wondering what you need from me in order for this to go smoothly. Shall I stay with you for a few minutes and we can decide together if you are ready for me to leave? Would you like me to check back with you in a certain amount of time that we decide on together?" Second, Mary is drawing upon her experiences with independent caregiving in one setting (the PICU) and extending what she learned there to the new caregiving setting in the PUCU—that is, she is independently making connections or bridging lessons learned from the prior unit to the "new" unit.

When asked "What do you wish you had known more about, if anything, before going home?" Sarah's father replied:

> How to focus on Sarah's symptoms. For example, instead of the nurse or respiratory therapist saying "She needs to be suctioned," use words like, "Okay, she sounds funny, what do you think might be going on?" Use words to help parents develop skill at how to think through it. Talk out loud about the smells and sounds, what you see as a nurse. And remind us—this entire process is a marathon, not a sprint.

John's description clearly and succinctly outlines for team members and families how to make use of an in-the-moment occurrence (the need for Sarah to be suctioned) that triggers joining and maintaining attention to engage in developing competencies of doing the task (e.g., assessment skills, suctioning skills), which ultimately supports the process of transferring responsibility for caregiving from the nurse to the parent.

Team members will witness families move from watching cares to independently completing cares without prompt. The primary nurse described this as "I knew we—the team and the parents—had succeeded when I walked into the room and Mary and John had all cares completed, and Mary was playing on the floor mat with Sarah." Families transition from apprehension to excitement and anticipation about going home. This is part of what tells team members that the transfer of responsibility has occurred successfully, with a key characteristic identified by the social worker: "I knew they were ready to go home when they spoke about home with excitement."

LEARNINGS, CHALLENGES, AND CONSIDERATIONS

The interdisciplinary team members involved in Sarah's care (i.e., case management, social work, respiratory therapy, nursing, physical and occupational therapy) shared several common lessons they learned from working with Sarah and her family. In this section of the chapter, we review challenges identified by them and discuss considerations for practice changes based on their learned lessons. Further, Sarah's parents share their insights and make recommendations for teams to consider when delivering care to children with complex healthcare needs and preparing families for the transition to home.

Team members shared the importance of not passing judgment and avoiding preconceived expectations regarding a family's reaction in this situation of learning to care for a child dependent on technology. They commented on the importance of expressing compassion, empathy, respect, and understanding toward the family and the situation they were facing. As aptly described by Sarah's physical therapist, team members learned that to successfully support families in achieving the goals required for transition to home, they need to "appreciate the fear, anxiety, and stress the parents may be experiencing as they learn how to cope and care for a child with complex health-care needs." Developing plans of care considering the family's perspective is critical for goal achievement, as is adjusting the plan as necessary based on the needs of the family, rather than focusing primarily on the team member's agenda and goals. The physical therapist further commented:

My practice has matured over time. I used to come into a patient's room with my list of things that I needed to teach the parent. I had one hour to accomplish my list. I have come to appreciate that the parents of children with complex health conditions can be overwhelmed with not only what they need to learn but all the feelings they have as they try to cope with this new reality.

The respiratory therapist shared:

Most parents do not expect to have a child born with complex healthcare needs. Recognize the sense of loss of the "perfect" baby and help parents accomplish goals more in line with the "new normal." Listen to parents' concerns, dreams and desires. Acknowledge their loss. Help parents come up with ideas and solutions to adjust their dreams to meet goals for the developing child and the "new normal." Help parents see beauty in the new normal.

I've learned the importance of collaboration with the team to help meet a new normal for parents. We need to work with the team that will work with the family at home and build relationships. We need to make sure everyone is keeping up to date and informed. We need to make sure all team members have the same understanding of the plan of care, goals, outcomes, and have set some expectations for the family.

Sarah's primary nurse stated:

I now take more time when I come into a patient's room to listen to the parents, assess how they are doing and what they need from me today. I may change my approach completely that day, depending on what I find. I also don't take for granted that, just because a parent has been with us for three months, they are any less or more overwhelmed than a parent of a child that has been with us for a day.

As discussed earlier, Kirk et al. (2005) found that parents of children with complex health conditions fear they are causing pain or harming their child when they are performing necessary care (e.g., changing tracheostomy or gastrostomy tubes). Team members working with families can anticipate this fear, acknowledge it and name it as normal, explain the whys as well as the whats of the care, while helping families learn how to incorporate comfort measures along with the technical aspects of the care. Sarah's physical therapist realized that:

> I often took routine care for granted, such as tracheostomy care or moving a child with a tracheostomy and on a ventilator onto a play mat for normal developmental play time. I now appreciate, when teaching families, that these "routine" actions can cause significant fear for a parent. I now take time before I do any activity with the child, or guide the parent through the activity, to describe (a) what we are going to be doing, (b) why we are doing it, (c) how their child may react, and (d) how important the activity is to help their child.

This thoughtful approach helps to ease the parent's fears and reframes the temporary discomfort some activities may cause a child, so that it may be seen in terms of the positive impact these activities will ultimately have for the child. Team members were developing their own competencies around being with the other (i.e., the parents), knowing and relating to the other, communicating and engaging with the other in ways which were mindful and respectful of the parents' need to nurture and protect their child.

The team members identified the importance of maximizing every educational opportunity to support the parents' and child's smooth transition home. As Sarah's respiratory therapist described it, "Every moment should be a teaching moment." The team members discussed the importance of involving the parents in every aspect of care, adjusting the type of teaching based on the needs of the parents, and taking into consideration the condition of the child—all important considerations when engaged in transferring responsibility for caregiving. For example, Sarah's mother commented:

> It would have been helpful when therapies were cancelled because Sarah had a "bad night," if someone would have shared with us why they made that decision. What did a "bad night" look like, and why would they use such harsh words? What was Sarah looking like that made them think the therapy needed to be cancelled? Having someone help us understand their decision making would have helped us to learn about the things that we would need to consider when we make decisions at home for Sarah's activity.

Engaging the parents in the assessment process, asking the parents questions such as "What do you notice about your child today?" and guiding them through the team member's decision-making process supports the development of the parents' knowledge, critical thinking, and problem-solving skills, which leads to building the parents' confidence in caring for their child (Kirk & Glendinning, 2002). The physical therapist captured the team's increasing awareness of the following:

> I did not realize the impact that I had on parents when I cancelled their child's therapy without explaining why. I am now more careful with the words I use. I avoid using judgmental phrases when I describe their child's condition, like I heard the child had a "good" sleep or "bad" night. Instead I now take the extra time to explain and describe in detail why I am changing the therapy plan based on their child's condition.

The case manager commented that "With how complex these children are, and how much a parent needs to learn, we should never miss a learning opportunity." Sarah's mother also recommended that team members try to be as consistent as possible.

> It took time to develop trust with Sarah's team. Once I trusted the team member, I was more able to trust that they knew what I was capable of doing. When they told me that I could do something like Sarah's tracheostomy care, I believed them. That trust helped to build our confidence.

Further, Sarah's parents recommended that staff encourage parents to participate in 24-hour care sessions as often as feasible—not just shortly before discharge—as a way to better prepare parents for what is ahead. As identified by Mary, "Being present helped me to learn Sarah's cares, and it also helped me to pick up on her cues." Sarah's father cautioned, however, to:

> . . . understand that parents may not be able to be at the hospital as much as they or the team would like. The parent may have home or work responsibilities that pull them away from the hospital, or they just need to get away to a "normal" life for awhile. It is important to respect that, too.

The team members identified the importance of regularly updating and communicating the patient's plan of care with the parents and all other members of the care team in an effort to support the parents' and child's progress toward an efficient and effective transition to home. With excellent communication, each person interacting with the child and the parents has an opportunity to support the parents and child in achieving the goals outlined in the plan of care. The team members suggested using a multifaceted approach to communicate the plan of care, including activities such as (a) verbal discussion of the plan of care at daily patient and family-centered care planning rounds, (b) interdisciplinary care conferences, and (c) change of shift handoff report. In addition, as the patient moves from one unit to another or care changes from one team member to another, it helps both family and team members if the plan is visually displayed in the patient's room and documented within the patient's electronic health record.

The team members recognized they often made assumptions about parents' progress toward achieving the goals in the care plan based on the length of time a child had been hospitalized. Sarah's primary nurse commented:

> If a parent had been with us for several months, I assumed the parent was comfortable with what they know and what they can do. I realize [now] that is not true. Some families can be with us for two weeks and are able to verbalize and demonstrate all the skills necessary for going home. Other families may be with us for months and still require our guidance as they learn to care for their child.

Consistent with guided participation practice, clinicians can continue to communicate with parents, engage them in discussions about their child, and ask provocative questions to expand parents' critical thinking and problem-solving skills. For example, while observing a parent perform a tracheostomy tube change, team members might ask them, "What would you do at home right now, if the electricity went out, and you had no light?"

The team members also identified the importance of simulating the home environment in the child's hospital room as soon as feasible to further support the development of parents' care competencies and problem-solving skills. The room design should support the delivery of safe and efficient care and also support the developmental needs of the child (Williams, 2016). The team members in collaboration with the child's parents can consider locations of items such as room furniture, medical equipment and supplies, medication, oxygen, play mats, and toys, placing the items in a location similar to where they would be in the child's home space. This simulation provides parents with an opportunity to identify challenges they may face while delivering care in the home environment, and with guidance from the child's team members, problem solve the issues together (Williams, 2016). Consistent with guided participation practice, this process of simulation, identification of challenges, and problem solving together supports the development of parents' critical thinking skills and supports confidence building, as parents learn to be successful in this simulated environment.

Significant challenges to a smooth transition home identified by team members included the inability to locate (a) durable medical equipment (DME) vendors to provide the necessary equipment and supplies, and (b) qualified home health nurses to provide in-home care. The team members learned the importance of beginning work to locate a DME vendor and home healthcare agency willing and able to take the child's case, as soon as it is known that the child will have home care needs. Sarah's case manager commented, "If we know on the day of admission that the child will be going home with needs, we start the process to locate the DME vendor and qualified home healthcare nurses at the time of admission or shortly thereafter." She also shared:

> It is extremely important over time to cultivate and develop relationships with the DME vendors and home care agencies. I have come to appreciate that these

staff are an essential member of the child's team. It is important to keep these individuals informed of the child's progress over time and help them to appreciate the importance of their role in helping the child and family reach the goal of successful transition to home. Even after discharge [with family's permission] I continue to provide updates to this staff after a child's clinic visit.

CONCLUSION

In summary, interdisciplinary team members and families caring for a child with complex care needs encounter many challenges and opportunities. It is essential for team members to effectively collaborate and communicate with families and each other as the child's care plan is developed, implemented, evaluated, and adjusted based on the needs of the family and child. Teams applying a thoughtful approach consistent with guided participation practice will optimize the family's and the child's success in achieving a safe and smooth transition to home.

REFERENCES

American Hospital Association. (2013). Reconfiguring the bedside care team of the future. Retrieved from http://www.aha.org/content/13/beds-whitepapergen.pdf

Bowles, J. D., Jnah, A. J., Newberry, D. M., Hubbard, C. A., & Roberston, T. (2016). Infants with technology dependence: Facilitating the road to home. *Advances in Neonatal Care, 16*(6), 424–429. doi:10.1097/ANC.0000000000000310

Brenner, M., Larkin, P. J., Hilliard, C., Cawley, D., Howlin, F., & Connolly, M. (2015). Parents' perspectives of the transition to home when a child has complex technological health care needs. *International Journal of Integrated Care, 15*(29), 1–9.

Callans, B. M., Bleiler, C., Flanagan, J., & Carroll, D. L. (2016). The transitional experience of family caregiving for their child with a tracheostomy. *Journal of Pediatric Nursing, 31*(4), 397–403.

Cooper, L. G., Gooding, J. S., Galager, J., Sternesky, L., Ledsky, R., & Berns, S. D. (2007). Impact of a family-centered care initiative on NICU care, staff and families. *Journal of Perinatology, 27*(Suppl. 2), S32–S37. doi:10.1038/sj.jp.7211840

Deterding, R. R. (2010). Infants and young children with children's interstitial lung disease. *Pediatric Allergy, Immunology, and Pulmonology, 23*(1), (25–31). doi:10.1089/ped76.2010.0011

Elias, E. R., Murphy, N. A., & the Council on Children with Disabilities. (2012). Home care of children and youth with complex health care needs and technology dependencies. *Pediatrics, 129*, (996–1005). doi:10.1542/peds.2012-0606

Graf, J. M., Montagnino, B. A., Hueckel, R., & McPherson, M. L. (2008). Children with new tracheostomies: Planning for family education and common impediments to discharge. *Pediatric Pulmonology, 43*(8), (788–794). doi:10.1002/ppul.20867

Joseph, R. A. (2011). Tracheostomy in infants: Parent education for home care. *Neonatal Network, 30*(4), (231–242). doi:10.1891/0730-0832.30.4.231

Kirk, S., & Glendinning, C. (2002). Supporting "expert" parents: Professional support and families caring for a child with complex health care needs in the community. *International Journal of Nursing Studies, 39*(6), (625–635). doi:10.1016/S0020-7489(01)00069-4

Kirk, S., Glendinning, C., & Callery, P. (2005). Parent or nurse? The experience of being the parent of a technology-dependent child. *Journal of Advanced Nursing, 51*(5), (456–464). doi:10.1111/j.1365-2648.2005.03522.x

Nelson, K. E., & Mahant, S. (2014). Shared decision-making about assistive technology for the child with severe neurologic impairment. *Pediatric Clinics of North America, 61*(4), (641–652). doi:10.1016/j.pcl.2014.04.001

Pridham, K. F. (1993). Anticipatory guidance of parents of new infants: Potential contribution of the internal working model construct. *Image, 25*(1), (49–56).

Rogoff, B., Mejia-Arauz, R., & Correa-Chavez, M. (2015). A cultural paradigm—Learning by observing and pitching in. *Advances in Child Development and Behavior, 49*, (1–22).

Swartwout, E., Drenkard, K., McGuinn, K., Grant, S., & El-Zein, A. (2016). Patient and family engagement summit: Needed changes in clinical practice. *Journal of Nursing Administration, 46*(3S), S11–S18. doi:10.1097/NNA.0000000000000317

Taylor, A., Lizzi, M., Marx, A., Chilkatowsky, M., Trachtenberg, S. W., & Taylor, O. S. (2013). Implementing a care coordination program for children with special healthcare needs: Partnering with families and providers. *Journal for Healthcare Quality, 35*, (70–77).

Williams, L. (2016). Using technology in the transition of children from hospital to home. *AACN Advanced Critical Care, 27*(1), (24–28).

Zanello, E., Calugi, S., Rucci, P., Pieri, G., Vandini, S., Faldella, G., & Fantini, M.P. (2015). Continuity of care in children with special healthcare needs: A qualitative study of family's perspectives. *Italian Journal of Pediatrics, 41*, (7–15). doi:10.1186/s13052-015-0114-x

12

Supporting a School-Age Child With Complex Healthcare Needs

Kyle Landry, Kathleen Mussatto, and Karen Pridham

This chapter brings guided participation (GP) into view at the intersection of healthcare and school in coordinated work with children who have a complex chronic health condition and their families. The functions of nurses, in hospital or community, are highlighted within this cross-disciplinary and across-setting team. These functions put nurses in a position to develop and maintain GP through multiple phases of the child's development and changes in the health condition and schooling. Our aim, in this chapter, is to illustrate GP processes in operation for relationship development and teaching and learning for navigation of some of the issues that may be relevant for school-age children and adolescents who are transitioning from hospital to home, community living, and school. We illustrate the functions of nurse and other members of the child's healthcare and school team with a case example of an adolescent who anticipated and experienced a heart transplant. The chapter offers a longitudinal study of transferring responsibility as well as other GP processes.

Case Example 12.1

Adam developed heart failure when he was a junior in high school after years of living a relatively healthy life with hypoplastic left heart syndrome, a complex congenital heart condition. He had undergone multiple surgeries as an infant and young child. Hypoplastic left heart syndrome cannot be "fixed." The surgeries redirect blood flow so the condition is palliated, but the circulation is never normal. Adam was healthy for many years and went to school with his same-aged peers. At age 16, he became acutely ill. His heart was failing and it became clear he would need a heart transplant to survive. Throughout the next months he was in and out of school due to many heart-related complications.

At the beginning of his senior year, Adam had a ventricular assist device (VAD) placed in an attempt to stabilize his condition while waiting for a new heart. (There is a significantly longer wait time the older a patient gets.) The VAD procedure was very successful: Adam was able to attend school regularly and continue working toward completing his course requirements. A few months later, in January of his senior year, Adam got a new heart. During the transplant process he lost significant oxygen to his brain and suffered a stroke. Recovery was slow; regaining his balance, strength, and the ability to walk without assistance was frustrating at times, but the hospital had a very comprehensive plan of therapies in place.

At 18 years old, and stuck in inpatient care, Adam became anxious to return to his normal life. Hospital staff closely monitored Adam's progress and began incorporating some school work back into his daily routine as soon as he was ready. Upon discharge, the hospital and school intervention specialist arranged for a homebound tutor and a plan to attend all of his normal classes via Skype from his home. Adam could see his teachers, hear his classmates, and ask and answer questions as needed.

After the 3-month mandatory quarantine period postdischarge after transplant ended, hospital personnel, the school intervention specialist, and Adam's family met with school staff to explain Adam's medical needs, monitoring requirements, and limitations; establish updated accommodations; and select a reasonable class schedule to complete the school year. In May, Adam returned to school daily, following a schedule that covered all of his core content classes while allowing for flexible attendance and breaks as needed. In June of the same school year, Adam walked across the stage at high school graduation with his classmates.

Thereafter, Adam continued his education at a local college. The healthcare team spent a great deal of time collaborating with the college's Accessibility Resource Center to create a plan tailored to Adam's specific learning needs, including communication of cardiac emergency care with various campus staff members. The effort has paid off! Adam is both motivated and excited; his parents are thrilled; and I am so very, very proud of him!

CHILDREN WITH A COMPLEX CHRONIC CONDITION AND THEIR SCHOOLING

A large portion of a child's daily life is spent at school. Children with chronic health conditions often experience school disruptions due to health complications and hospitalizations (Gabbay, Cowie, Kerr, & Purdy,

2000). This chapter brings GP into view at the level of healthcare and school in coordinated work with children who have a complex chronic health problem and their families. The functions of nurses, in the hospital or community setting, are highlighted within this cross-disciplinary and cross-setting team. These functions put nurses in a position to develop and maintain GP through multiple phases of the health problem and its intersection with schooling. The nurse's work, however, in particular GP, must be carefully linked and attuned to the work of other team members. School Intervention specialists are relatively new members of the team and have functions in the hospital and community that can enhance a nurse's objectives for aiding transfer of responsibility for the inter-digitated health and education plan of care.

Many medical conditions secondarily impact brain development and functioning, which affect the child's ability to learn, comprehend, and retain information. Children with chronic health conditions often require academic accommodations, modifications, and special education services to provide them with the same access to learning as their healthy peers (Allen, Cristofalo, & Kim, 2011). Research shows that school support and comprehensive academic planning are critical for recovery, improved medical outcomes, and quality of life for children with complex health needs (Brosig et al., 2014; Rubens et al., 2016; Weil, Rodgers, & Rubovits, 2006).

Achieving optimal outcomes for children with complex health conditions requires healthcare clinicians to provide comprehensive care to patients and their families beyond their traditional medical or nursing roles. It is not enough to treat a condition; rather, attention must be paid to the whole child and family. GP can be useful in helping children and families become competent in skills that are personally, socially, and clinically relevant practices of everyday life (Bradley & Caldwell, 1995; Pridham, Limbo, Schroeder, Thoyre, & Van Riper, 1998). Healthcare clinicians, through GP, promote optimal recovery goals by co-creating with the child and family expectations for success for health, school performance, and reintegration into everyday life following hospitalization (Katz, Varni, Rubenstein, Blew, & Hubert, 1992). Along with the family and school personnel, healthcare clinicians are critical members of the child's care team.

Optimal outcomes are achieved through proactive collaboration among all care team members by trusting other team members' expertise and engaging in open communication about the health and educational needs of the child (Katz et al., 1992; Ratnapalan, Rayar, & Crawley, 2009). By engaging in academic planning prior to hospitalization, or as soon as possible after the child is admitted and participation in school activities is considered appropriate, healthcare clinicians can assist children and families in managing the inpatient recovery process and promoting successful reintegration into school after treatment (Katz et al., 1992; Weil et al., 2006).

The GP process of transferring responsibility is an essential part of the work done by the healthcare team together with the child and family in the dynamic process of moving from hospital to community and back again to the hospital. Transferring responsibility from hospital to family when the child goes home indicates that primary responsibility for guiding the child's healthcare, including deciding on the amount of academic content that can be tolerated, medication management, need for assistance, and evaluation of how well things are working, rests now with the child and family. Through work with members of the care team and access to GP, the child and family develop competencies needed to become central to the child's care. With competencies in emotion regulation, the child and the child's parents feel confident, able to do the problem solving inherent in all tasks associated with the child's care, feel capable of effectively communicating with healthcare team members, and if all has gone well, they know and are known by a community of caregivers. The relationship competencies of "being with" and "knowing and relating" that GP facilitated for Adam are punctuated with the statement of the school intervention specialist, "I am so proud of him."

NURSE-LED FUNCTIONS FOR GP PRACTICE WITH FAMILY, HEALTHCARE TEAM, AND SCHOOL

Although this chapter documents GP in the practice of the healthcare team in articulation with the school team, nurses are brought forward to the center of GP. Wherever the location of employment—hospital, school, or clinic—nurses are likely to have functions in respect to both health and school teams. Nurses interface with the child and family during hospitalization and during stays at home and attendance of school. The nurses comprehensively engage with families in (a) co-creating expectations, (b) coordinating care, (c) garnering authoritative healthcare information, (d) communicating medical and health needs to the appropriate recipient, (e) planning with the family for future hospitalizations and school transitions, and (f) providing GP leadership for issues requiring a guide (see Chapter 1, Figure 1.1). Nurses have many opportunities to practice GP as they work to nurture, protect, relate to, and support the learning that children and their families need to do to optimize quality of life (Pridham et al., 1998).

Many issues accompany a child's complex, chronic health condition in the context of schooling. These issues include re-entry into the child's classroom after a period of absence due to hospitalization; the requirement of special accommodations, aids, and resources; and the co-creating of developmentally supportive expectations. These expectations include timely assuming of self-care, consistent with the child's development; judiciously taking risks when health and social benefits must be balanced; and engaging in medically encouraged physical activity and self-limiting it when signs or symptoms indicate the need to do so.

Nurse leadership of GP is discussed here for the issue of judicious taking of risks when balancing health and social benefits. Starting with the issue of re-entry into the community classroom after a hospitalization, we assume a relationship with a school nurse is getting established with the support of the child's primary nurse at the hospital and the hospital team, including the hospital teacher. First, education for children with a chronic health condition is briefly reviewed, and the healthcare school team is introduced. Discussion of the issue of physical activity for these children follows. An overview of school education of children with a chronic health condition and school healthcare is discussed more fully in Chapter 13 of this book.

Education for Children With a Chronic Health Condition

Access to appropriate education is a right of every child. The Individuals with Disabilities Education Act (IDEA, 2004) and the Rehabilitation Act of 1973 (Section 504, 1973) mandate accommodations be made for children with special learning needs. For children with chronic health conditions, needs may be obvious (e.g., a wheelchair for a child with muscular dystrophy), or they may be subtle (e.g., when mild learning delays or attention-deficit issues require aids) and for children with congenital heart disease (Mussatto et al., 2014).

GP for the child with a chronic health condition is scaffolded in large part by the health and school plans and regulations (Bransford, Brown, & Cocking, 2000). In addition, documents that function as printed reminders or guides to problem solving or decision making may be made available to the child, parents, and school staff. When a child has a chronic health condition, healthcare clinicians, school staff (e.g., teachers, nurses, unlicensed assistive personnel), and parents form an essential partnership that provides integrated healthcare for the child. This team develops a consistent, jointly agreed-upon plan of care. The healthcare clinicians, as part of the medical and health plan, structure guidance concerning the child's activity participation and opportunities for development. The clinicians set guidelines for the classroom teacher to understand what types of signs, symptoms, or concerns warrant contacting the nurse or parent. A plan for intervention for common health problems may be created, including what signs or symptoms require a phone call to the parents and when 9-1-1 should be called (Katz et al., 1992). These guidelines, tailored to a child's health condition, developmental abilities, and family circumstances provide structure for GP that is ongoing, oriented to the needs and activities of a child and parents, facilitative of updating with developmental and health changes, and sensitive and responsive to the family's culture.

A healthcare clinician, perhaps the child's physician or nurse in a primary care clinic or tertiary setting, guides parents and child through school recommendations for educational arrangements and explains potential resources and risks. The GP process of structuring proceeds to bridging and connecting. At the point of hospital discharge, or when a child is medically cleared to return to school, healthcare clinicians, including a nurse, can give parents a teaching sheet of recommendations to facilitate the child's return (Ratnapalan et al., 2009). This sheet could be written to be shared with the child's teachers. Healthcare clinicians can prepare a document for the child's school that outlines activity recommendations and restrictions (Katz et al., 1992) with the intent of encouraging activity of a type and level that supports recovery and development. The sheet of recommendations and the letter concerning recommended activity could be starting points for the GP processes of getting and staying connected and of joining and maintaining attention. The nurse who is working with the child and parents, in whatever setting, can learn from them what they understand concerning the recommendations and the messages about activity. These GP discussions may support bridging processes, including reflecting and making connections. The discussions may need to include the teachers on occasion for sharing of understandings about the child's condition, challenges, prospects, and possibilities.

The processes of GP that focus on getting and staying connected, joining and maintaining attention, sharing understanding, bridging/connecting, and transferring responsibility will be useful for the child, family, and educators as they navigate the complex journey (Bradley & Caldwell, 1995; Pridham, Limbo, Schroeder, Thoyre, & Van Riper, 1998; Pridham et al., 2006).The relationship that a nurse forms with the child and parents with the understanding of its ongoing, continuous nature may be critical to engaging effectively in these GP processes. A nurse in the child's school may begin the process of getting and staying connected by exploring with the child and parents what the school re-entry challenges are for them, keeping in mind anticipated absences due to regularly scheduled clinic visits, medical complications and emergencies, and planned rehospitalizations (Ratnapalan et al., 2009). This chapter continues with GP in relation to the issues that express what the child and/or parent are working on—co-creating expectations, fostering independence, and defining and practicing safe risk-taking.

Co-Creating Expectations

After a family has received a diagnosis of a chronic health condition for their child, it is often very difficult to transition back to what life had been for them. It can be expected that a family will feel protective of their child and act defensively to keep the child safe from physical, emotional, and social challenges (Rempel, Blythe, Rogers, & Ravindran, 2012; Rempel, Ravindran, Rogers, & Magill-Evans, 2013). Planning for hospital discharge and eventual school reintegration ideally begins on admission. GP at the time of illness diagnosis or readmission to hospital offers an important opportunity to join and maintain attention with the child and parents. It is at these points of transition that GP may be effective in aiding the parents and child in clarifying and refining goals and, with the parents and child, co-creating or re-constructing expectations concerning issues of managing illness care. These issues include the child's development of independence and collaborative responsibility with parents, teachers, and the healthcare team in managing illness care, engaging in physical activity, with and without peers, and participation in everyday activities.

Fostering Independence

Fostering the child's independence is likely to be an issue experienced with intense interest, concern, and emotion by the parents and the child with a complex, chronic health condition. Facets of fostering independence include encouraging safe risk-taking, supporting the child in and limiting activities as physical signs and symptoms indicate the need to do so, addressing school staff's apprehensions about caring for a child with a complex chronic disease or disability, and establishing consistently set, appropriately high expectations for recovery and academic performance. Transferring responsibility from the healthcare providers to the parents, the child, and, ultimately, to the school system is an important process of GP that nurses and other clinicians can facilitate (Katz et al., 1992; Pridham et al., 1998; Ratnapalan et al., 2009; Weil et al., 2006). Developing competencies involving knowledge, judgment, skill, resolve, and action for engaging in education and managing health and healthcare are necessary, everyday practices for the family of a child who has a complex chronic health condition, such as complex congenital heart disease (Pridham et al., 1998).

Defining and Practicing Safe Risk-Taking

When a child with a complex chronic health condition is ready to reintegrate into school, most families have mixed emotions. They are relieved that their child is well enough to return to the usual, expected routine, but at the same time there is fear and apprehension about whether this is the best decision for their child. Although often frightening, many of the risks or challenges that are feared by parents and children are a part of every child's life (Erikson, 1963). While parents intend to protect their child, they may need guidance in carrying out this intention in ways that support the competencies the child is developing and that give protection that is consistent with the child's safely dealing with risky or challenging situations (Katz et al., 1992). GP processes can be used to help children and families bridge stressful health-related events and school expectations (Anderson, 2009; Bradley & Caldwell, 1995; Brosig, et al., 2014; Limbo, Petersen, & Pridham, 2003; Pridham et al., 2006; Rempel, Harrison, & Williamson, 2009).

Safe risk-taking is intended to support a child's competencies in making developmentally attuned choices or decisions within an environment that is regulated for developmentally adequate safety and protection. Parental monitoring with criteria of boundaries co-defined with the child's healthcare team is supported by GP in which parent and child learn to work together to manage and anticipate risk. Risk itself is an important part of child development; however, it takes thoughtful, intentional parental modeling and encouragement to help a child develop competencies for identifying and evaluating the physical, emotional, and social risks of an action, activity, or behavior (Limbo et al., 2003).

Through GP, parents and children can learn ways of anticipating threats to safety, assessing risk of situations and activities, and managing challenges to safety. Role-play, joint problem solving using simulated or real situations, nurse-modelled conversation, and discussion of situations that are actually risky or perceived as risky are some of the bridge-building and connecting strategies that can be structured through GP for learning to manage risks as safely as possible. Competencies that could be the objective of GP include problem-solving competencies, among them assessing and responding to risks confronted by same aged, typically developing children as well as children with the same health problem. Parents and child could produce lists of risks potentially encountered in the child's environment for discussion with the nurse in bridging or connection-making sessions. The child and parents could keep a journal of risks and challenges experienced, the strength or intensity of the risk or challenge, how risks and challenges were handled, and with what outcomes. Through discussions together with the nurse, the parents and child may strengthen competencies for regulating emotions, including fear, frustration, anger, and sense of a need for constant caution or hypervigilance (Anderson, 2009). The child or parents may want specific examples of safe, developmentally appropriate risks for the child.

Many other issues could be identified for application of GP processes and development of competencies. Parents, child, teachers, and clinicians could be oriented to focusing on, identifying, and describing competencies in whatever opportunities are available to take stock of the overall plan for transitions, reintegration, and transfer of responsibility.

CONCLUSION

GP, with leadership provided by nursing, can support development of being with and relating to others (Schroeder & Pridham, 2006), caring for oneself, communicating, problem-solving, and emotion-regulating competencies in school-age children and adolescents who have a chronic health condition and their parents. GP processes of sharing understanding, bridging and connecting, and structuring the task or learning can be oriented and directed to the parents and child who are working on constructing expectations for physical activity that leads to recovery and developmental gain as well as to intentions for safe risk-taking behavior. GP may also be used with members of the healthcare team and the school team with the aim of defining and clarifying goals, strengthening consistency of plans and of expectations, and increasing competence in problem solving issues as they surface for the child. GP may support emotion regulation by reducing worry and fear that often accompany concern about inadequate competence and that may lead to restriction of physical activity that limits development. These ideas merit study for evidence on which to base practice.

Ideas touched on in this chapter to keep in mind for observation and reflection include the following:

- GP is oriented to the participation of learners through all of its processes.
- The goal is the child and parent developing competencies to take a central role in the child's care in collaboration with and with the guidance of healthcare clinicians and the school staff.
- GP can be constructed to keep the network of relationships the child and parents have with healthcare clinicians and school staff in mind to advance partnerships.
- Partnerships, from a guided partnership perspective, are attentive to the issues on the minds of the partners, to developing shared understandings, and to making connections, that is, building bridges from what is known to what is unknown.
- When a child has a complex chronic health condition, the GP practice has to be constructed for continuity of goals and relationships.

Adam's story illustrates the life experience of a child who required the support of a mechanical VAD to sustain life until an organ donor became available (Brosig et al., 2014; Weil et al., 2006). While the implantation of a VAD posed many risks of its own, Adam's healthcare team strongly believed that working toward returning to school with accommodations for his recent surgery and new medical needs would be more beneficial in the long run than requiring him to stay at home. While Adam was also eager to return to school, there were many elements of fear and doubt in the planning process. Ultimately, his parents agreed that keeping a normal routine and continuing to hold high expectations for their son would be best. In this situation, Adam returned to school following the implantation of his VAD and remained enrolled in all core curriculum classes that were required for high school graduation until his heart transplant procedure.

Parents who encourage expectations for physical activity and participation in care at home may have difficulty asking others, such as teachers, to support the child in following through on the expectations at school. The goal of returning to life as usual, often referred to by parents and children as "normal life," and expected routines is critical to a child's overall quality of life, but it needs consistent support across settings to be achieved. In general, parents have continuing responsibility for communicating with the school and hospital the expectations for the child's activity and care participation. The healthcare team has responsibility for defining and communicating expectations for maintenance of health with school administrators and for creating guidelines that promote physical, mental, social, and emotional development (Limbo et al., 2003; Weil et al., 2006).

Partnership relationships among health and school team members can be fostered through GP approaches focused on joining attention, sharing understanding, building bridges, and transferring responsibility in a systematic, clearly understood manner. Healthcare clinicians and school staff can, together, enhance for a child with a complex chronic condition competency in problem solving and decision making for engaging in physical activity that is self-limited and in risk-taking activities within the limits of safety. Goals of the child's health-education plan, advanced through GP practice, include addressing school staff apprehensions and establishing and consistently enacting expectations that provide challenge, stimulation, satisfaction, and a sense of achievement for the child (Katz et al., 1992).

REFERENCES

Allen, M. C., Cristofalo, E. A., & Kim, C. (2011). Outcomes of preterm infants: Morbidity replaces mortality. *Clinics in Perinatology, 38*, 441–454.

Anderson, L. S. (2009). Mothers of children with special health care needs: Documenting the experience of their children's care in the school setting. *The Journal of School Nursing: The Official Publication of the National Association of School Nurses, 25*, 342–351.

Bradley, R. H., & Caldwell, B. M. (1995). Caregiving and the regulation of child growth and development: Describing proximal aspects of caregiving systems. *Developmental Review, 15*, 38–85.

Bransford, J. D., Brown, A. L., & Cocking, R. R. (Eds.). (2000). *How people learn: Brain, mind, experience, and school*. Washington, DC: National Academy Press.

Brosig, C., Pai, A., Fairey, E., Krempien, J., McBride, M., & Lefkowitz, D. S. (2014). Child and family adjustment following pediatric solid organ transplantation: Factors to consider during the early years post-transplant. *Pediatric Transplantation, 18*, 559–567.

Erikson, E. (1963). *Childhood and society* (2nd ed.). New York, NY: Norton.

Gabbay, M. B., Cowie, V., Kerr, B., & Purdy, B. (2000). Too ill to learn: Double jeopardy in education for sick children. *Journal of the Royal Society of Medicine, 93*, 114–117.

IDEA. (2004). *Individuals with disabilities education act reauthorization*. Pub L no. 108–446, 118 stat 2647.

Katz, E. R., Varni, J. W., Rubenstein, C. L., Blew, A., & Hubert, N. (1992). Teacher, parent, and child evaluative ratings of a school reintegration intervention for children with newly diagnosed cancer. *Children's Health Care: Journal of the Association for the Care of Children's Health, 21*, 69–75.

Limbo, R., Petersen, W., & Pridham, K. F. (2003). Promoting safety of young children with guided participation processes. *Journal of Pediatric Health Care, 17*, 245–251.

Mussatto, K. A., Hoffmann, R. G., Hoffman, G. M., Tweddell, J. S., Bear, L., Cao, Y., & Brosig, C. (2014). Risk and prevalence of developmental delay in young children with congenital heart disease. *Pediatrics, 133*, e570–e577.

Pridham, K. F., Krolikowski, M. M., Limbo, R. K., Paradowski, J., Rudd, N., Meurer, J. R., . . . Henriques, J. B. (2006). Guiding mothers' management of health problems of very low birth-weight infants. *Public Health Nursing, 23*, 205–215. doi:10.1111/j.1525-1446.2006.230302.x

Pridham, K. F., Limbo, R., Schroeder, M., Thoyre, S., & Van Riper, M. (1998). Guided participation and development of care-giving competencies for families of low birth-weight infants. *Journal of Advanced Nursing, 28*, 948–958.

Ratnapalan, S., Rayar, M. S., & Crawley, M. (2009). Educational services for hospitalized children. *Paediatrics & Child Health, 14*, 433–436.

Rempel, G. R., Blythe, C., Rogers, L. G., & Ravindran, V. (2012). The process of family management when a baby is diagnosed with a lethal congenital condition. *Journal of Family Nursing, 18*, 35–64.

Rempel, G. R., Harrison, M. J., & Williamson, D. L. (2009). Is "treat your child normally" helpful advice for parents of survivors of treatment of hypoplastic left heart syndrome? *Cardiology in the Young, 19*, 135–144.

Rempel, G. R., Ravindran, V., Rogers, L. G., & Magill-Evans, J. (2013). Parenting under pressure: A grounded theory of parenting young children with life-threatening congenital heart disease. *Journal of Advanced Nursing, 69*, 619–630.

Rubens, S. L., Loucas, C. A., Morris, M., Manley, P. E., Ullrich, N. J., Muriel, A. C., . . . Northman, L. (2016). Parent-reported outcomes associated with utilization of a pediatric cancer school consultation program. *Clinical Practice in Pediatric Psychology, 4*, 383–395. doi:org/10.1037/cpp0000150

Schroeder, M., & Pridham, K. F. (2006). Development of relationship competencies through guided participation for mothers of preterm infants. *Journal of Obstetric, Gynecologic, & Neonatal Nursing, 35*, 358–368.

Section 504. (1973). *Rehabilitation Act of 1973*, 29 U.S.C. 701.

Weil, C. M., Rodgers, S., & Rubovits, S. (2006). School re-entry of the pediatric heart transplant recipient. *Pediatric Transplantation, 10*, 928–933.

13

Guided Participation Supporting Development of Competencies of School Staff Caring for Children With a Chronic Health Condition

Lori S. Anderson

School plays an important part in children's cognitive and social development. It is a place where they spend a great deal of time, on average around 1,000 hours per year (Desilver, 2014). As the primary place of learning for most children, the educational experience in the school setting has a profound influence on outcomes later in life. A child with a chronic health condition (CHC) presents challenges for those in the school setting. Federal law under the Individuals with Disabilities Education Improvement Act (IDEA, 2004) and Section 504 of the Rehabilitation Act of 1973 mandate that health-care services must be provided for students who qualify. School nurses are often the only healthcare provider in a school setting and, as such, play a pivotal role in attending to the healthcare needs of students with CHC. School nurses work to create access to healthcare for students and families, they help identify children with chronic conditions, and they assist students in learning to manage chronic illness. These efforts increase time in the classroom and decrease student absenteeism, resulting in cost savings to the school district and an increase in the overall academic success of the student (National Association of School Nurses [NASN], 2012).

BACKGROUND

Children With CHC

The term *children with CHC* relates to conditions lasting 12 months or longer. The conditions can be physical, developmental, behavioral, and/or emotional and include children with asthma, cystic fibrosis, obesity, developmental disabilities, cerebral palsy, consequences of low birth weight and prematurity, and mental illness. Children with CHC experience consequences because of their condition, including the need for or use of prescription medications and/or specialized therapies (McPherson et al., 1998).

The overall rate of CHC in the population has increased from 12.8% in 1994 (National Survey of Children with Special Health Care Needs [NS-CSHCN], 2001) to 26.6% in 2010 (NS-CSHCN, 2011; Van Cleave, Gortmaker, & Perrin, 2010). The rising rates for certain individual conditions are also noteworthy. New cases of diabetes have almost doubled in past 10 years (May, Kuklina & Yoon, 2012). From 1997 to 2007, food allergies have increased 18% in children younger than 18 (Branum & Lukacs, 2008). More than 10 million school days are missed each year due to asthma (CDC, 2015) and 45,000 children less than 15 years develop epilepsy each year (CDC, 2017). Rates of children who are medically complex because of premature birth are also increasing (Burns et al., 2010). At school age, children born preterm have higher rates of learning disability, grade retention, special education, attention deficit disorder (ADD), and social–emotional problems than babies born at term (Allen, Cristofalo, & Kim, 2011). From 2002 to 2008, the percentage of children in special education with chronic or acute health problems increased by 55% (National Center for Education Statistics [NCES], 2016). Finally, for the first time in nearly 30 years, the top five disabilities affecting U.S. children are mental health problems rather than physical problems (Halfon, Houtrow, Larson, & Newacheck, 2012), with one in five children and adolescents having a diagnosable mental health disorder in the course of a year (Slomski, 2012). School nurses report spending nearly a third of their time providing mental health services (Bohnenkamp, Stephan, & Bobo, 2015).

Impact of Chronic Illness on the Child and Family

Children's lives are influenced by the presence of a CHC. Children with CHC often require care that involves multiple services across community, healthcare, and educational systems with little coordination (Anderson, 2009). The lack of coordination is especially problematic for racial/ethnic minority families (Bloom, Jones, & Freeman, 2012) and rural families (Skinner & Slifkin, 2007). Children with CHC are three times more likely to miss substantial amounts of school and nearly three times as likely to repeat at least one grade in comparison to healthy children (Byrd, 2005). Children with CHC are less motivated to do well in school, exhibit more disruptive behaviors, are more frequently victims of bullying, and have lower academic achievement (Forrest, Bevans, Riley, Crespo, & Louis, 2011; Moricca et al., 2013; Rodriguez et al., 2013). Compared to their healthy peers, children who grew up having a chronic illness have lower odds of graduating from college and being employed and higher odds of receiving public assistance and having a lower mean income as adults (Maslow, Haydon, Ford, & Halpern, 2011).

The families of children with CHC are affected as well. Almost 24% of parents of children with CHC report having to reduce employment or stop employment altogether in order to take care of their children (NS-CSHCN, 2011). Mothers of children with CHC report difficulty communicating with the school and advocating for their child (Anderson, 2009). Parents find themselves participating on educational teams, advocating for their child, and being decisional experts about the healthcare and educational needs of their child. They report feeling unprepared for those responsibilities (Anderson, 2009). In minority families, these difficulties are magnified by language and cultural differences (Ngui & Flores, 2006). Rural children with CHC are less likely to be seen by a healthcare provider and more likely to have unmet healthcare needs than urban children. Rural families of children with CHC are more likely to report financial difficulties and more likely to provide care at home for their children than urban families (Skinner & Slifkin, 2007).

Cost of Chronic Conditions in Children

There are additional expenses involved in the care of children with CHC. A study by Miller, Coffield, Leroy, and Wallin (2016) found that an extra $1,400 to $9,000 annually were spent on medical expenses for children aged 0 to 18 years with asthma, diabetes, or epilepsy compared to children without these conditions. When children with CHC are well managed, healthcare utilization and costs are reduced (Modi et al., 2012). Schools are an ideal place to support the management of children with CHC, and within the schools the school nurse is the health professional situated to be a valued member of the healthcare team and provide care coordination. Wang and colleagues found that for every dollar invested in school nursing, society gains $2.20 in other savings (2014).

School Nurse Role

As defined by the NASN (2017), school nursing is a specialized practice of nursing that protects and promotes student health, facilitates optimal development, and advances academic success. School nurses bridge healthcare and education, provide care coordination, advocate for quality student-centered care, and collaborate to design systems that allow individuals and communities to develop their full potential. School nurses are concerned with the health, well-being, and academic success of students. In caring for children with CHC in the school setting, school nurses promote normal development, health, and safety of students. They manage health problems, provide case management, and collaborate with others to support students and families. There are about 77,000 school nurses in the United States (U.S. Department of Health and Human Services [USDHHS], 2010) caring for 50 million school students, of which over 14 million have CHC (NCES, 2012; Van Cleave et al., 2010). Sixty-seven percent of public schools in the United States have at least one full- or part-time school nurse, but only 40% of schools have a full-time school nurse (NCES, 2012). Both full- and part-time nurses often cover more than one school building.

Schools are mandated by federal legislation to provide services needed to support the education of all students (IDEA, 2004; Section 504 of the Rehabilitation Act, 1973). The amount, type, and quality of healthcare children with CHC receive in school is not well defined, despite evidence that the quality of care a child with a CHC receives in school affects school attendance and performance (Ireys, Salkever, Kolodner, & Bijur, 1996; Maughan, 2003).

Federal agencies have called upon school-based health professionals to monitor or treat chronic conditions (Lear, 2007) and there is evidence that school nurse delivery of healthcare to children with CHC in school improves child health outcomes. When school nurses were involved in managing care of students with asthma, there was improvement in quality of life, decrease in asthma symptoms, decrease in use of emergency departments, increase in knowledge of disease management, increased availability of medication at school, increased peak flow meter use at school, and decreased school absences (Engelke, Guttu, Warren, & Swanson, 2008; Gerald et al., 2009; Levy, Heffner, Stewart, & Beeman, 2006; Moricca et al., 2012; Taras, Wright, Brennan, Campana, & Lofgren, 2004). Targeting blood glucose management in school was associated with better detection of low blood glucose and improved glycemic control in children (Nguyen, Mason, Sanders, Yazdani & Heptulla, 2008). The availability of school nurses to work directly with students to assess symptoms and provide treatment has been found to increase students' time in the classroom and parents' time at work (Lineberry & Ickes, 2015).

It is clear that there are increasing numbers of children with CHC in schools. These children have healthcare needs that must be delivered in the school setting and, most often, the school nurse is the healthcare professional who is responsible for the delivery of the healthcare. While the needs of children with CHC are becoming increasingly complex, and despite the recommendation that every school should have a full-time nurse (American Academy of Pediatrics [AAP], 2016; NASN, 2016), resources to support the delivery of healthcare in schools are lacking. More than half of the school nurses in the United States are part time and many cover several school buildings. This requires school nurses to delegate healthcare tasks to unlicensed assistive personnel (UAP) in order to support the health and safety needs of students (Shannon & Kubelka, 2013).

Delegation of Care for Students With CHCs

Delegation is a valuable tool for meeting the healthcare needs of students in a resource-poor healthcare environment. Delegation is defined as the ability of the nurse to transfer the responsibility of a nursing task to an unlicensed person while the nurse continues to be accountable for the outcomes (American Nurses Association [ANA], 2012). Specific rules for delegation of care for students with CHC are subject to an individual state's nurse practice act and vary from state to state. In general, nursing delegation in the school setting is the assignment by the school nurse to a competent and willing UAP to perform a specific nursing task for an individual student. The school nurse is responsible for the training, evaluation, and ongoing supervision of the UAP (NASN, 2015). Examples of school personnel who may have nursing tasks delegated to them include classroom assistants and paraprofessionals, administrators, teachers, bus drivers, playground attendants, or office staff.

The school personnel most likely to be involved in delegation include office staff and teachers (Tetuan & Akagi, 2004). None of these personnel have healthcare backgrounds. Because a UAP works under the direction of the school nurse, the school nurse must train and supervise the UAP. The UAP must agree to function according to the written instructions of the school nurse. In order to protect the UAP, the school, and the health and safety of students, the school nurse must follow the scope and standards of school nursing and the regulations of their state's nurse practice act which sets boundaries within which UAP can safely and legally function (ANA, 2012). To facilitate a better understanding of the roles of the school nurse and the UAP and the safety of the student, communication is needed between school nurses, administrators, staff, and families, and trusting relationships should be established (Resha, 2010).

If after review the nurse deems that delegation is appropriate, an individualized healthcare plan (IHP) should be developed that indicates which nursing tasks can and cannot be delegated. The nurse will also need to establish a process of evaluation to ensure that the delegated task is completed properly and produces the desired outcome (NASN, 2014). An important consideration in the process of delegation is the training of the UAP. The practice of guided participation (GP) may be useful for school nurses in teaching UAPs how to competently care for children with CHC by providing expertise and working alongside the learner.

GP SUPPORTING DEVELOPMENT OF COMPETENCIES OF SCHOOL STAFF CARING FOR CHILDREN WITH A CHC

GP is often undertaken in regards to the caregiving that others do on behalf of children. GP is a method of instruction in an everyday practice offered by someone who has expertise in the task to a less- or nonexperienced person. In this setting, the school nurse (teacher) is working alongside and instructing the UAP (learner) with the goal of helping them become competent in meeting children's healthcare needs while at school. The teaching and learning process is dynamic and occurs in the context of a relationship with an understanding of what the learner needs (see Chapter 1). Several processes are involved in the practice, including (a) getting and staying connected, (b) joining and maintaining attention, (c) sharing understanding, (d) bridging, (e) structuring the task/learning, and (f) transferring responsibility. This chapter offers examples for each process and discusses the use of technology to support GP practice.

Getting and Staying Connected

The underlying foundational process in GP is the connection between the school nurse and the UAP around a jointly held goal. Interpersonal communication, "Tell me what is on your mind," is a key feature of this process. To ensure safe and effective delegation, the school nurse needs to establish trusting relationships with all parties involved, including school administrators, the UAPs, the students, their families, and the healthcare providers. During this process, which takes some time, all parties come to understand the complexities of the delegation process and the responsibilities and roles of each partner in the process. These trusting relationships form the basis for safe and appropriate care of the student with CHC (Resha, 2010).

Joining and Maintaining Attention

Another step in the delegation process is assessment and planning. The school nurse assesses the specific needs of the student. When the nurse, parent, and healthcare provider determine that a child requires a procedure during the school day, the challenge is in answering specific questions to determine if delegation is appropriate and to whom the task should be delegated. The type of care must be identified along with details on whether the student has received the care before, for how long, and if there was a predictable response to the care. In addition, the nurse must assess the likelihood of an emergency or risk related to the provision of the care. The school nurse uses the gathered information to write an IHP and emergency care plan (Raible, 2012).

It is at this stage that the UAP is identified and a relationship begins to be established. The collaborative relationship starts with the more experienced school nurse listening to the UAP about what the learning means to them and what is relevant to them to become more skilled (see Chapter 1). Establishing an open communication process between all parties is vital. UAPs should have the opportunity to ask questions and to clarify expectations. Key to the delegation process is the willingness of the UAP to perform the task. The school nurse should be aware that anxiety might be a factor in the role of the UAP (Price, Dake, Murnan, & Telljohann, 2003). The school nurse can address this anxiety by asking questions to help make explicit the source of the anxiety. Knowing this allows the nurse and the UAP together to address the anxiety more effectively though a supportive relationship and through education specific to the UAP's needs.

The way in which a UAP is asked to perform care by the delegating school nurse influences the UAP's willingness to respond. The relationship between the school nurse and the UAP is a crucial factor. It is important that the school nurse and the UAP mutually recognize that both have valuable contributions to make to the care of the student with CHC. The quality of delegation is based on healthy interpersonal relationships, trust, and open communication. Effective delegation is based on both trust and an understanding of professional practice. Trust, a critical factor in relationships, is based on knowledge of one another's capabilities and confidence in these abilities (Weydt, 2010).

Sharing Understanding

With an established relationship in place, information can be organized and interpreted and processes established for delegation to occur. One way to organize information and establish a process for safe delegation of nursing tasks is to use the *Five Rights of Delegation* (National Council of State Boards of Nursing [NCSBN], 2016). These five rights consist of the right task, right circumstance, right person, right direction/communication, and right supervision/evaluation (Table 13.1).

A checklist based on these rights documents the school nurse's decision-making process in determining safe delegation. Considerations in determining the appropriateness of delegating a specific task to a UAP include safety, the needs and stability of the student, the complexity of the task, the competence of the UAP, the expected outcomes, and the needs of other students. Ultimately, school nurses are held accountable for delegating tasks appropriately and implementing them safely (Resha, 2010).

Bridging

The purpose of bridging is to support a learner in making connections between what is known, what is unknown, or what is misunderstood and in need of more information or clarification (see Chapter 1). Wondering with the learner is a strategy the school nurse may use to facilitate understanding. For instance, if a child is observed to be resistant to having a treatment or procedure, the nurse may wonder with the UAP why the student was behaving that way and explore how that made the UAP feel. The UAP may feel that the child does not trust or like them, when in fact, through mutual exploration, it may be determined that the child may want more privacy during the procedure.

TABLE 13.1 Five Rights of Delegation

Right Task	The activity falls within the school nurse's job description or is included as part of the established written policies and procedures of the school setting. ■ Is the task within the scope of the school nurse? ■ Is the task within the UAP's range of function? ■ Is the task performed according to an established protocol and similarly on all students?
Right Circumstance	The health condition of the student must be stable. If the student's condition changes, the school nurse must reassess the situation and the appropriateness of the delegation. ■ Has the school nurse assessed the student's needs prior to delegation?
Right Person	The school nurse, along with the school administrator and the UAP, is responsible for ensuring that the UAP possesses the appropriate skills and knowledge to perform the activity. ■ Does the UAP have the appropriate knowledge, skills, and abilities to accept the delegated task? ■ Does the ability of the UAP match the care needs of the student?
Right Directions and Communication	The school nurse is expected to communicate specific instructions for the delegated activity to the UAP. The UAP should ask for any clarification needed. The UAP must understand the terms of the delegation and must agree to accept the delegated activity. The school nurse should ensure that the UAP understands that she or he cannot make any decisions or changes in carrying out the activity without first consulting the school nurse. ■ Have school protocols for performing the task been communicated to the UAP? ■ Is there an established two-way communication process between the school nurse and UAP? ■ Has the UAP indicated his or her willingness to perform the delegated task? ■ Has the school nurse communicated his or her willingness and availability to support the UAP?
Right Supervision and Evaluation	The school nurse is responsible for monitoring the delegated activity, following up with the UAP at the completion of the activity, and evaluating student outcomes. The UAP is responsible for communicating student information to the school nurse during the delegation situation. The school nurse should be ready and available to intervene as necessary. The school nurse should ensure appropriate documentation of the activity is completed. ■ Is appropriate and timely supervision available for the UAP? ■ Was the delegated activity documented? ■ Was the delegation successful?

UAP, unlicensed assistive personnel.

Source: Association of Camp Nurses (ACN). (2017). Nursing delegation to unlicensed assistive personnel in day and resident camps: Practice guideline. Retrieved from https://s3.amazonaws.com/amo_hub_content/Association1124/files/Delegation%20PG%20March%202017.pdf; National Council of State Boards of Nursing (NCSBN). (2016). National guidelines for nursing delegation. *Journal of Nursing Regulation, 7*(1), 5–14.

Many strategies can be used in the process of bridging, but the goal is to advance the UAP's understanding and competencies with guidance. The school nurse observes and assesses what the UAP already knows and uses it to achieve the desired competence: safe care (see Chapter 1).

Structuring the Task/Learning

Procedure skills checklists can reduce the risks of delegation by outlining the processes for demonstrating accountability and competence of both school nurses and UAPs. They can reflect the student's specific healthcare needs while ensuring some uniformity across students and UAPs. They also provide an outline of step-by-step actions for reference and reinforcement of proper techniques (Shannon & Kubelka, 2013). The school nurse may want to give a family member of the student an opportunity to demonstrate the procedure for the school nurse. This may (a) identify differences from best practice and provide teaching opportunities for the school nurse to correct or improve the techniques applied in the home, (b) provide valuable information regarding home caregiving routines or techniques familiar to the child, and (c) give an opportunity for the family member and the school nurse to together develop routines for caregiving specific to the school setting. The school nurse also has an opportunity to return the demonstration of skills to the family member, which can instill confidence and trust in the school staff's ability to safely meet the student's needs at school (Shannon & Kubelka, 2013).

When GP is used for developing competencies in caregiving of children in the school setting, both the school nurse and the UAP are called to be with each other in ways that enhance sensitive responsiveness to the behavior of the other (see Chapter 1). Recognizing that UAPs are adult learners can help school nurses frame the learning activities to meet their specific needs and engage in a more effective learning experience.

Six factors are important for consideration with adult learners (Knowles, Holton & Swanson, 2005). They are the following:

- *Need to know.* Adult learners first need to know why it is important to learn what they are being taught.
- *Self-concept.* An adult's self-concept as a learner must be supported by the clear message that they are making decisions for which they will be held responsible.
- *Prior experience.* Adult learners bring their life experiences to the task of being a UAP and have their own learning styles and preferences.
- *Readiness to learn.* Adults learn in order to address their real-life situations.
- *Orientation to learning.* The role of the UAP can be framed as one involving problem solving and collaborating with the school nurse to ensure safety in the plan.
- *Motivation to learn.* Awareness of the impact of these affective factors on learning is important, although they are usually not included in task-oriented procedure skills checklists.

Transferring Responsibility

GP practice provides the structure and processes that support the UAP in achieving competence and confidence. As part of that, the responsibility for teaching and learning is passed to the UAP. The school nurse can explore with the UAP ways that they can impact the quality of care provided. For instance, the UAP could discuss with the child's classroom teacher the optimum time for the student to come to the health office for a procedure.

Because the relationship between the school nurse and the UAP is a legal one under a particular state's nurse practice act, further structure is needed to ensure that legal responsibilities are documented and the competence of the UAP is established. The use of procedure skills checklists that include demonstration and return demonstration can reduce the risks of delegation by demonstrating accountability and competence of both school nurses and UAPs (Shannon & Kubelka, 2013). In addition, a system of surveillance and supervision needs to be established. The school nurse communicates that they are ultimately responsible for the care provided to the student and as such the UAP needs to understand that the nurse will stop by to observe. The nurse can let the UAP know that they will not be able to provide care on their own until the school nurse is comfortable with what they are doing and the UAP is comfortable with what they are doing. Documentation in the form of records and logs will be reviewed and the health of the student will be periodically assessed. If necessary, the school nurse needs to be ready to intervene if problems arise or concerns develop, such as the task repeatedly not completed in a timely manner, an unexpected change in the student's condition, or if the UAP has difficulty performing the task (Resha, 2010).

These GP processes lend themselves to an effective and satisfying teaching and learning process for both the learner (UAP) and the guide (school nurse). The use of technology can facilitate the teaching processes for the school nurse. An example of that technology is discussed next.

USE OF TECHNOLOGY TO SUPPORT PRACTICE AND ONE-ON-ONE TRAINING OF SCHOOL STAFF

Technology and Education Needs of School Nurses

School nurses have access to the Internet and use it to find answers to practice challenges. Mobile technology offers one way for school nurses to access the needed information and resources to support their delivery of healthcare to children with CHC. There has been an increase in the use of mobile technology to deliver information to nurses, including nurses in community settings (Kidd, 2011). Characteristics that school nurses value in technology-based educational resources include portability, a clear benefit, quick access, convenience, ease of use, reliability, and conciseness (Anderson & Enge, 2012).

eSchoolCare: An Innovative Model for Supporting Healthcare Delivery in Schools

The eSchoolCare project was developed to assist school nurses in the delivery of care to children with CHC in the school setting and to support the training of UAPs (Anderson, 2013). eSchoolCare is a web-based, mobile resource that provides school nurses with expert-reviewed, evidence-based, up-to-date resources on student CHC. Content supports school-based care of students with chronic conditions such as allergies, asthma, cancer, diabetes, epilepsy, and gastrointestinal and mental health disorders and includes updated, reviewed, and organized materials and resources, which can be used as a just-in-time resource or for more in-depth professional development. Materials include videos for training and educating school staff, students, and families and a set of sample forms and checklists that can be used for training and school-based care.

Case Example 13.1

Javier, Alicia, and their family live in a small rural community in an upper Midwest state. Miguel is a 5-year-old with cystic fibrosis. He went through preschool screening when he was 3. As a result of the screening, he was sent for further testing and was eventually diagnosed with higher functioning autism spectrum disorder (ASD). He has been receiving early childhood services through the local public school system. Over the past year, he had been getting sick frequently and having eating issues. As a result, he had a gastrostomy tube (g-tube) placed. Miguel will soon be entering kindergarten.

The public school district that Miguel will attend is in a rural area. There is a full-time school nurse for the district but she is responsible for five school buildings and 4,000 children, and there are others who have CHC. Miguel's school employs a UAP, Loretta, to be in the health office for most of the school day. Loretta has not had any experience with g-tubes and she is very nervous about the situation. As the school nurse reflects on the situation, she realizes the book on GP she recently read might be useful in her practice. She asks herself:

- When and with whom would she initiate GP?
- What are the issues that she would need to address?
- What would GP offer in this situation? What makes it suited, as an approach to teaching and learning, for this UAP?
- What are potential challenges in implementing GP with this UAP?

The school nurse is meeting with Loretta to talk about Miguel, who will be enrolling in several weeks. Prior to the meeting, the school nurse has met with Miguel's family and his healthcare provider and established and documented, using the Five Rights of Delegation, that delegation is appropriate in this situation. She has developed an IHP and an emergency plan for Miguel. In her first meeting with Loretta, she encourages her to talk about her expectations, including her fears about the process. After some discussion, Loretta is interested in hearing more and being trained to provide feedings to Miguel via his g-tube. What should the next steps be for the school nurse? How might she want to prepare her teaching, being mindful that Loretta is an adult learner? How might she bridge and provide support for Loretta during this process? How can she ensure that Loretta learns the steps of the process and fells confident with the care she is providing? What resources might assist the nurse in providing the training for Loretta?

CONCLUSION

GP is a practice that school nurses can use when working with UAP who are providing care to children with chronic conditions in the school setting. The teaching and learning process is dynamic and occurs in the context of a relationship with an understanding of what the UAP needs. The processes of getting and staying connected, joining and maintaining attention, sharing understanding, bridging, structuring the task/learning, and transferring responsibility provide a structure through which the school nurse works alongside and instructs the UAP. The practice of GP may be useful for school nurses in teaching UAPs how to competently care for children with CHC by providing expertise and working alongside the learner.

REFERENCES

Allen, M. C., Cristofalo, E. A., & Kim, C. (2011). Outcomes of preterm infants: Morbidity replaces mortality. *Clinical Perinatology, 38*(3), 441–454.

American Academy of Pediatrics, Council on School Health. (2016). Policy statement role of the school nurse in providing school health services. *Pediatrics, 137*(6).

American Nurses Association. (2012). *Principles for delegation by registered nurses to unlicensed assistive personnel (UAP)*. Silver Spring, MD: Nursesbooks.org.

Anderson, L. S. (2009). Mothers of children with special health care needs: Documenting the experience of their children's care in the school setting. *Journal of School Nursing, 25*(5), 342–351.

Anderson, L. S. (2013). The development and implementation of eSchoolCare: A novel health care support system for school nurses. *Advances in Nursing Science, 36*(4), 289–303.

Anderson, L. S., & Enge, K. (2012). Continuing educational needs of school nurses: What technology supported resources meet their needs? *Journal of School Nursing, 28*(5), 358–369.

Association of Camp Nurses. (2017). Nursing delegation to unlicensed assistive personnel in day and resident camps: Practice guideline. Retrieved from https://s3.amazonaws.com/amo_hub_content/Association1124/files/Delegation%20PG%20March%202017.pdf

Bloom, B., Jones, L. I., & Freeman, G. (2012). Summary health statistics for U.S. children: National Health Interview Survey, 2012. *Vital Health Statistics, 10*(258), 1–72.

Bohnenkamp, J. H., Stephan, S. H., & Bobo, N. (2015). Supporting student mental health: The role of the school nurse in coordinated school mental health care. *Psychology in the Schools, 52*(7), 714–727.

Branum, A. M. & Lukacs, S. L. (2008). Food allergy among U.S. children: Trends in prevalence and hospitalizations. *NCHS Data Brief, 10*, 1–8.

Burns, K. H., Casey, P. H., Lyle, R. E., Bird, T. M., Fussell, J. J., & Robbins, J. M. (2010). Increasing prevalence of medically complex children in U.S. hospitals. *Pediatrics, 126*(4), 638–646.

Byrd, R. S. (2005). School failure: Assessment, intervention, and prevention in primary pediatric care. *Pediatric Review, 26,* 233–243.

Centers for Disease Control and Prevention (CDC). (2015). Asthma-related missed school days among children aged 5–17 years. AsthmaStats. Retrieved from https://www.cdc.gov/asthma/asthma_stats/missing_days.htm

Centers fof Disease Control and Prevention (CDC). (2017). Epilepsy fast facts. Retrieved from www.cdc.gov/epilepsy/basics/fast-facts.htm.

Desilver, D. (2014). School days: How the U.S. compares with other countries. Pew Research Center. Retrieved from http://www.pewresearch.org/fact-tank/2014/09/02/school-days-how-the-u-s-compares-with-other-countries

Engelke, M. K., Guttu, M., Warren, M. B., & Swanson, M. (2008). School nurse case management for children with chronic illness: Health, academic, and quality of life outcomes. *Journal of School Nursing, 24,* 205–214.

Forrest, C., Bevans, K., Riley, A., Crespo, R., & Louis, T. (2011). School outcomes of children with special health care needs. *Pediatrics, 128*(2), 303–312.

Gerald, L. B., McClure, L. A., Mangan, J. M., Harrington, K. F., Gibson, L. Erwin, S., . . . Grad, R. (2009). Increasing adherence to inhaled steroid therapy among schoolchildren: Randomized, controlled trial of school-based supervised asthma therapy. *Pediatrics, 123*(2), 466–474.

Halfon, N., Houtrow, A., Larson, K., & Newacheck, P. W. (2012). The changing landscape of disability in childhood. *Future Child, 22*(1), 13–42.

Individuals with Disabilities Education Improvement Act (IDEA). (2004). PL 108–446.

Ireys, H. T., Salkever, D. S., Kolodner, K. B., & Bijur, P. E. (1996). Schooling, employment, and idleness in young adults with serious physical health conditions: Effects of age, disability status, and parental education. *Journal of Adolescent Health, 19*(1), 25–33.

Kidd, R. (2011). Benefits of mobile working for community nurse prescribers. *Nursing Standard, 25*(42), 56–60.

Knowles, M. S., Holton, E. F., & Swanson, R. A. (2005). *The adult learner: The definitive classic in adult education and human resource development* (6th ed.). St. Louis, MO: Elsevier.

Lear, J. G. (2007). Health at school: A hidden health care system emerges from the shadows. *Health Affairs, 26*(2), 409–419.

Levy, M., Heffner, B., Stewart, T., & Beeman, G. (2006). The efficacy of asthma case management in an urban school district in reducing school absences and hospitalizations for asthma. *Journal of School Health, 76,* 320–324.

Lineberry, M. J., & Ickes, M. J. (2015). The role and impact of nurses in American elementary schools: A systematic review of the research. *Journal of School Nursing, 31*(1), 22–23.

Maslow, G. R., Haydon, A. A., Ford, C. A., & Halpern, C. T. (2011). Young adult outcomes of children growing up with chronic illness. *Archives of Pediatric Adolescent Medicine, 165*(3), 256–261.

Maughan, E. (2003). The impact of school nursing on school performance: A research synthesis. *Journal of School Nursing, 19*(3), 163–171.

May, A. L., Kuklina, E. V., & Yoon, P. W. (2012). Prevalence of cardiovascular disease risk factors among U.S. adolescents, 1999-2008. *Pediatrics, 129*(6), 1035–1041.

McPherson, M., Arango, P., Fox, H., Lauver, C., McManus, M., Newacheck, P. W., . . . Strickland, B. (1998). A new definition of children with special health care needs. *Pediatrics, 102*(1), 137–139.

Miller, G. F., Coffield, E., Leroy, S., & Wallin, R. (2016). Prevalence and costs of five chronic conditions in children. *Journal of School Nursing, 32*(5), 357–364.

Modi, A. C., Pai, A. L., Hommel, K. A., Hood, K. K., Cortina, S., Hilliard, M. E., . . . Drotar, D. (2012). Pediatric self-management: A framework for research, practice, and policy. *Pediatrics, 129,* e473–e485.

Moricca, M. L., Grasska, M. A., BMarthaler, M., Morphew, T., Weismuller, P. C., & Galant, S. P. (2013). School asthma screening and case management attendance and learning outcomes. *The Journal of School Nursing, 29,* 104–112.

National Association of School Nurses (NASN). (2012). Chronic health conditions managed by school nurses. Retrieved from https://schoolnursenet.nasn.org/blogs/nasn-profile/2017/03/13/chronic-health-conditions-managed-by-school-nurses

National Association of School Nurses (NASN). (2014). Nursing delegation to unlicensed assistive personnel in the school setting. Retrieved from https://schoolnursenet.nasn.org/blogs/nasn-profile/2017/03/13/delegation-nursing-delegation-to-unlicensed-assistive-personnel-in-the-school-setting

National Association of School Nurses (NASN). (2015). Nursing delegation in the school setting. Retrieved from www.nasn.org/nasn/nasn-resources/professional-topics/delegation

National Association of School Nurses (NASN). (2016). The role of the 21st century school nurse (Position Statement). Retrieved from https://schoolnursenet.nasn.org/blogs/nasn-profile/2017/03/13/the-role-of-the-21st-century-school-nurse

National Association of School Nurses (NASN). (2017). Definition of school nursing. Retrieved from www.nasn.org/nasn/about-nasn/about

National Council of State Boards of Nursing (NCSBN). (2016). National guidelines for nursing delegation. *Journal of Nursing Regulation, 7*(1), 5–14.

National Survey of Children with Special Health Care Needs 2001 (NS-CSHCN). (2001). Data query from the Child and Adolescent Health Measurement Initiative, Data Resource Center for Child and Adolescent Health website. Retrieved from www.childhealthdata.org

National Survey of Children with Special Health Care Needs 2009/10 (NS-CSHCN). (2011). Data query from the Child and Adolescent Health Measurement Initiative, Data Resource Center for Child and Adolescent Health website. Retrieved from www.childhealthdata.org

Ngui, E. M., & Flores, G. (2006). Satisfaction with care and ease of using health care services among parents of children with special health care needs: The roles of race/ethnicity, insurance, language, and adequacy of family-centered care. *Pediatrics, 117,* 1184–1196.

Nguyen, T. M., Mason, K. J., Sanders, C. G., Yazdani, P., & Heptulla, R. A. (2008). Targeting blood glucose management in school improves glycemic control in children with poorly controlled type 1 diabetes mellitus. *Journal of Pediatrics, 153*(4), 575–578.

Price, J. H., Dake, J. A., Murnan, J., & Telljohann, S. K. (2003). Elementary school secretaries' experiences and perceptions of administering prescription medication. *Journal of School Health, 73*(10), 373–379.

Raible, C. L. (2012). Training UAP to care for special needs students in the classroom. *NASN School Nurse, 27*(4), 187–188.

Resha, C. (2010). Delegation in the school setting: Is it a safe practice? *The Online Journal of Issues in Nursing, 15*(2), Manuscript 5.

Rodriguez, E., Rivera, D. A., Perlroth, D., Becker, E., Wang, N. E., & Landau, M. (2013). School nurses' role in asthma management, school absenteeism, and cost savings: A demonstration project. *Journal of School Health, 83,* 842–850.

Section 504, Rehabilitation Act of 1973, 29 U.S.C. § 701 (1973).

Shannon, R., & Kubelka, S. (2013). Reducing the risks of delegation: Use of procedure skills checklists for unlicensed assistive personnel in schools, part 1. *NASN School Nurse, 28*(4), 178–181.

Skinner, A. C., & Slifkin, R. T. (2007). Rural/urban differences in barriers to and burden of care for children with special health care needs. *Journal of Rural Health, 23*(2), 150–157.

Slomski, A. (2012). Chronic mental health issues in children now loom larger than physical problems. *Journal of the American Medical Association, 308*(3), 223–225.

Taras, H., Wright, S., Brennan, J., Campana, J., & Lofgren, R. (2004). Impact of school nurse case management on students with asthma. *Journal of School Health, 74*(6), 213–219.

Tetuan, T. M., & Akagi, C. G. (2004). The effects of budget, delegation, and other variables on the future of school nursing. *Journal of School Nursing, 20,* 352–358.

U.S. Department of Education; Institute of Education Sciences, National Center for Education Statistics (NCES). (2016). Elementary and secondary education. In Digest of Education statistics: 2016 (Chapter 2). Retrieved from https://nces.ed.gov/pubs2016/2016014_2.pdf

U.S. Department of Education, National Center for Education Statistics (NCES). (2012). Schools and staffing survey (SASS), public and private school data files, 2011–2012. Retrieved from https://nces.ed.gov/surveys/sass

U.S. Department of Health and Human Services (USDHHS), Health Resources and Services Administration (2010). The registered nurse population: Findings from the 2008 National Sample Survey of Registered Nurses. Retrieved from https://bhw.hrsa.gov/sites/default/files/bhw/nchwa/rnsurveyfinal.pdf

Van Cleave, J., Gortmaker, S. L., & Perrin, J. M. (2010). Dynamics of obesity and chronic health conditions among children and youth. *Journal of the American Medical Association, 303*(7), 623–630.

Weydt, A. (2010). Developing delegation skills. *Online Journal of Issues in Nursing, 15*(2), Manuscript 1.

14

Guided Participation and the Family Strength–Oriented Therapeutic Conversations Intervention: Supporting Families of Children With Cancer

Erla Kolbrun Svavarsdottir

Parents of children and adolescents newly diagnosed with cancer face many new tasks and responsibilities. Interventions designed to assist families in making short- and long-term adjustments to the chronic cancer experience focus on reducing parents' stress, enhancing coping, improving physical and psychological states, and supporting family and interpersonal functioning (Svavarsdottir, Sigurdardottir, & Tryggvadottir, 2014). The author and her research team developed the Family Strength–Oriented Therapeutic Conversations intervention (FAM-SOTC intervention) to aid family development of competencies for caregiving and navigation of life tasks. The researchers used deductive analyses from a knowledge translation research project (see Svavarsdottir et al., 2015) to create the FAM-SOTC intervention for both research and clinical practice. The FAM-SOTC intervention is based in the Illness Belief Model (Wright & Bell, 2009), the Calgary Family Assessment and Intervention models (Wright & Leahey, 2013), and the resiliency and hardiness components of the Resiliency Model of Stress Adjustment and Adaptation (McCubbin, Thompson, & McCubbin, 1996).

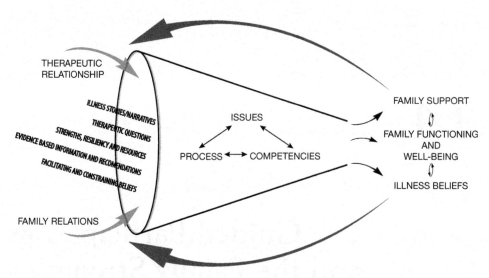

FIGURE 14.1 The GP framework of practice integrated into the Family Strength–Oriented Therapeutic intervention.

GP, guided participation.

FAM-SOTC intervention processes are focused on families' responses and adaptations to stressors due to illness.

The purpose of this chapter is to explore the integration of guided participation (GP) practice components—issues, processes, and competencies—with the FAM-SOTC model. The goal of this integration is to contribute to the operational features of the intervention. The FAM-SOTC model with the addition of GP components is shown in Figure 14.1.

THE STRUCTURE AND PROCEDURE OF THE FAM-SOTC INTERVENTION

The relationship-based model focuses on change in cognitive, affective, and behavioral domains of family functioning. The intervention is conducted in two sessions ranging from 45 to 90 minutes with an expected duration of 60 minutes. Change, framed as healing, occurs in these domains through the interaction of the nurse and family in relation to responses and adaptation to illness-related stressors. The effect of intervention is observed in the support that family members offer, the quality of the illness beliefs, and the adequacy of family functioning and well-being. Nurse practitioners use reflective questions contained within the FAM-SOTC assessment protocol to assess family functioning. The questions support family members by (a) focusing on the illness experiences and (b) bringing family strengths and resiliency into their awareness.

Family resiliency refers to internal resources that individuals draw on to motivate, enable, or drive themselves to cope with and learn from stressful life experiences (Grafton, Gillespie, & Henderson, 2010). Focusing on changing constraining illness beliefs that constrain behavior may lead to discovery of new meanings and may have an impact on family well-being. The structure and content of the first and second therapeutic conversations have been applied in research studies with parents of children with asthma, diabetes, and cancer. Similar to the FAM-SOTC intervention, the GP intervention focuses on relational practice between a nurse and a family member.

GP WITHIN THE FAM-SOTC INTERVENTION

GP strengthens the FAM-SOTC by bringing teaching–learning components into the structure and process of the intervention. GP is implemented through the working relationship formed by a guide, a pediatric nurse practitioner, subsequently referred to as "nurse," and novices or learners, a parent or parents. GP relies on joint attention of nurse and parent to the same issue with shared understanding of its cognitive and emotional meaning and of its importance from family, child, and clinical perspectives. Making connections and establishing a relationship of trust are important processes in developing caregiving competencies as the GP outcomes of interest.

In the subsequent clinical case, I offered two sessions of a GP FAM-SOTC intervention to a mother, Lena, with a 10-year-old son, Frank, newly diagnosed with acute lymphoblastic leukemia (ALL). I intended to use GP to support the mother in supporting her child in handling difficult treatments. What the mother and I would work on together was the issue of reconstructing her parenting functioning. Our jointly held goal was to aid Lena in developing competencies in supporting her son in dealing with illness treatment. That is, the mother needed to be competent in being with her son and caring for and protecting him through difficult treatment protocols. In addition, the mother needed to observe side effects, communicate with healthcare clinicians, engage in problem solving, and make difficult decisions regarding the following: (a) side effects of the treatment (e.g., giving effective doses of pain medications), (b) family life, and (c) her work.

Case Example 14.1

GP–FAM-SOTC INTERVENTION OFFERED IN TWO SESSIONS TO FRANK'S FAMILY

Background

In early June, Frank, who had just turned 10 years old, traveled to Reykjavik, Iceland, to spend his summer vacation with his grandparents. His parents were going to visit Iceland a little later in the summer. Frank was going to do a lot of exciting activities with his grandparents. One of these activities was going fishing with them, a sport Frank loved. Lena, Frank's mother, was on a business trip in Montreal when Frank traveled alone to Iceland. Shortly after Frank arrived in Iceland, his grandmother, Michele, noticed that Frank was not like he used to be. He was tired, acted as if he were not interested in anything, his face was pale, and his lips were not red anymore. Frank's grandparents took him on a fishing trip with them. Frank was tired and sleepy all the time they were on the trip, and his energy level was low. When Frank and his grandparents returned to Reyjavik, Michele read on the Internet about the signs and symptoms that she observed in Frank. Michele, fearing that something was seriously wrong with her grandchild, took him to see a physician. Blood samples were drawn at the clinic. Michele did not want to frighten Lena. Lena had come to Iceland as planned several days after Frank and his grandparents returned from their fishing trip and Frank had been seen by the physician.

Diagnosis

The morning Lena arrived, Michele told her daughter that she was going to take Frank to the physician to learn the results of the blood tests taken earlier. Lena thought her son had a bad flu. Frank went with his grandmother to the emergency department at the Children's Hospital at the Landspitali University Hospital. Not long after arriving there, Michele called her daughter and asked her to come to the emergency department. When Lena arrived at the parking lot in front of the emergency department, she was met by her mother. Michele told her daughter that Frank had ALL. This was shocking news to Lena. She had never ever expected that Frank had cancer or that he was indeed so sick. Lena reacted by breaking down at the parking lot. She reported that she had "cried and cried—I felt like my feet had given way beneath me."

Lena called her husband, Peter, Frank's father, right away, who was at the time at their home in Vancouver, still asleep in the very early hours of the morning. Lena and Peter had moved there 8 years earlier with their two children, Frank and Sara, now 20 years old, to take new jobs. Immediately, Peter booked a flight to Iceland for Sara and himself. The next day, they were able to be at the Children's Hospital where Frank had been admitted. Lena was staying with him.

Aftermath of the Diagnosis

Over the next days, things were very strange for the family. Their home was in Canada, and they were guests in Iceland, where their son was critically ill. The first few days after the diagnosis, Lena thought she would never ever smile again. That bright day in June, which was the brightest of the year in Iceland, the world was all of a sudden turned upside down for the family, and Lena found her emotions difficult to handle. Lena was concerned about

Frank's future and his health. She expected, with Frank having cancer, this was now the "brave new world" or the "new normal" that the family faced.

Over the first few weeks after the diagnosis, there were many decisions that the family needed to make, keeping the goal in mind of making the days ahead the best for Frank while he was being treated. The uncertainty, however, of how the treatment would affect Frank was very nerve-racking for Lena and Peter. In order to cope with the situation, Frank's parents started to celebrate the little things that were, nonetheless, huge in their minds. They celebrated when Frank took his pills "like a champion" and when he was no longer afraid to have medication injected by needle. Lena and Peter celebrated when Frank showed he had an appetite and ate better. Frank's parents celebrated when he calmly woke up after the anesthesia and when he was patient, strong, and optimistic. The family was convinced that they would get through this with the help of their family and friends, but they needed to take 1 day at a time.

Introducing GP

I met Lena for the first time 6 weeks after Frank had been diagnosed. She was interested in participating in our research and wanted to learn as much as possible regarding the illness and how to deal with it. I offered Lena two sessions of the GP intervention. The first session lasted 90 minutes and the second session lasted 50 minutes. The second session took place 2 weeks after the first session. The interviews were conducted in an interview room at the Children's Hospital. Peter was with his son at the cancer unit while Lena participated in the interviews. I learned that Frank's family (see Figure 14.2) was a very close and caring family. His family wanted to do everything they could do for Frank. Frank was closely connected to his parents and his sister as well as to his grandparents. The nuclear family, living abroad, had developed close relationships among each other.

The components of GP practice (see Chapter 1, Figure 1.1) structured our intervention sessions. The specific issues, processes, and competencies that we focused on were as follows: (a) issues: guiding and protecting Frank through the treatment; (b) competencies: being with and caring for Frank (e.g., supporting him in handling the side effects of the medications and accompanying him to the analgesia room) communicating, problem solving, and regulating emotions; and (c) processes: joining attention, sharing understanding, structuring the task and learning, building bridges, and transferring responsibility. We emphasized several competencies, among them communicating and engaging with others and regulating emotions.

The First Session of GP

In the first session, the process of building bridges was structured by drawing a family tree with Lena. As the family tree was constructed, I got to

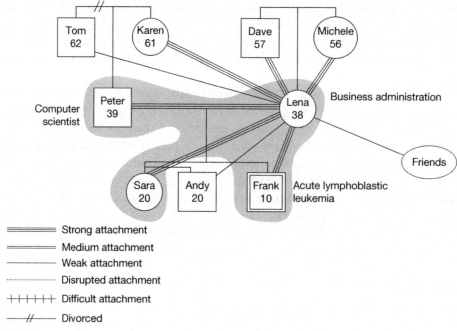

FIGURE 14.2 Frank's family tree and support network.

know the family by asking about the family support network and learning about the family relationships. Lena was then given the opportunity to tell her story concerning Frank's illness. I asked Lena to tell me about the day that Frank was diagnosed with ALL and her reaction to the diagnosis. She explained who in the family the ALL diagnosis had impacted the most, and who was suffering the most. Lena took a long time telling me about the day when Frank was diagnosed and about how difficult and scary it was for her and her husband to learn about the diagnosis. Emotionally, this was very difficult to accept. Frank's parents felt vulnerable and helpless, and worried about how the illness would develop. They had been having many sleepless nights.

When I asked Lena what had been the most helpful thing she and her husband had received from the healthcare clinicians, she immediately responded that it concerned getting to know about the etiology of the illness and the prognosis and the treatment of ALL. Then Lena said that it had also been helpful for her and her husband to talk to the priest who was a specialist in posttraumatic counseling. The priest gave them simple but important information about taking care of themselves, including taking turns in staying with Frank at the hospital at night, having good and healthy nutrition, and being available for each other. Lena said the entire family was suffering because of Frank's ALL diagnosis and treatment. Lena identified her support network, which included Frank's grandparents and Lena's and Peter's friends.

Therapeutic Communication Intervention

As the first session of the GP intervention continued, I asked Lena questions drawn from the therapeutic conversation protocol. These questions included the following: (a) What was least helpful about Frank's hospitalization and treatment at this time? (b) What beliefs did they have about Frank's illness? (c) What beliefs did they have about finding the most helpful clinicians to rely on concerning the ALL treatment? (d) What did they believe the future held for their family following the ALL diagnosis and treatment? Lena's answers to these questions expressed her motivations, goals, expectations, and intentions concerning her caregiving responsibilities and activities in relation to her son's illness.

Lena told me that she had not found it helpful when she was scheduled to have an appointment with a psychologist at the Children's Hospital the day after she and Peter had scheduled themselves for time away from the hospital, feeling the need for a break from the hospital after a 15-day stay there. Rather Lena indicated that looking ahead to the next 5- to 7-day block of treatment, she preferred to schedule meetings with healthcare clinicians while staying in the hospital. Also, she said that it was helpful for her when she and her husband took turns staying at the hospital nights and when they were using their support network to help them go through their emotional experiences. Lena believed that the next 2½ years would be the most difficult years they would ever have and that their son would grow up very quickly because of his experience with the ALL treatment. Lena also strongly indicated that she believed her son would be cured.

Lena's responses to the therapeutic conversation intervention questions were highly important to naming, specifying, and clarifying issues; to selecting, creating, scaffolding, and sequencing processes for bridging; and to transferring learning and applying competencies. The GP component of the intervention brought the FAM-SOTC intervention into patient and family-oriented operation.

Evaluation of the caregiving competencies that Frank's family were demonstrating showed that the family was nurturing and protecting Frank as well as being with him throughout the hospital stay. In addition, Frank's parents and his sister were caring for him, communicating with healthcare clinicians, problem-solving issues at hand, and regulating their own and Frank's emotions. They were also structuring the caregiving tasks and activities at hand and making connections with healthcare clinicians, family members, and friends. Throughout the interview, I described the competencies I had observed to give the parents a frame of reference and language with which to assess their contributions to Frank's well-being. I also brought forward the family strengths. For example, I let Lena know how lucky Frank was having his family to support him through this difficult experience. The family was doing everything they could for him by being available and supporting him in handling the treatment and its side effects. Lena wept when she received this information. It was difficult for her to hear that she was doing the best that she could do for

Frank in this situation by always being there for him. She, however, responded quickly, saying, "This is a difficult project that we as a family need to finish."

Two weeks before our first intervention session, Lena had learned that Frank did not respond very well to the treatment and that the ALL illness was more aggressive than they had at first thought. The family was offered a family interview with the physician to learn about the treatment protocol ahead. The news of Frank's poor response to treatment was shocking to Lena and her husband. They had learned that only 20% of children with ALL had the more aggressive type. About 80% of children with ALL had the type that did not need an aggressive treatment protocol. When I asked Lena how she and Peter as a couple would be using their strength and resiliency to handle the ALL treatment ahead of them, she indicated that they were not alone in this. She perceived themselves to have very good support people around them who were ready to help them. She and Peter would need to use their support network to go through this experience. For Lena and her family, the support received through having and achieving hope was important, and was an indicator of the family's use of their strengths and resilience to handle and cope with their situation. Lena believed they were a strong family that would work on the tasks associated with Frank's cancer and overcome it.

Toward the end of our first intervention session, I asked Lena about what gave her life meaning and purpose these days, another question from the FAM-SOTC intervention protocol. Lena responded that the expectation that her son would be healthy again and the intention to celebrate the small successes in treatment gave her life purpose and meaning. Lena and I then scheduled the second interview for a time 2 weeks later.

The Second GP Session

When I arrived at the Children's Hospital to meet Lena for the second session, I received a text message from her. She told me that she could not meet me because Frank was very ill, he was in a lot of pain and needed his mother at his side. I called Lena and asked if she wanted to schedule a new time. She asked me to contact her at the same time the next day. When I talked to Lena the next day, she wanted to meet. Frank was doing somewhat better than he had been doing the day before. I waited for Lena in the interview room. When she arrived a little late, she appeared sad and withdrawn. She had been crying. I realized that something had happened.

After Lena sat down, I asked her how things were going. She responded that things were going very badly. She and her husband had just learned a few minutes ago that the treatment was not going well. Frank needed a bone marrow transplant at the Karolinska Institute in Stockholm, Sweden. We both sat there quiet for a while. Lena cried. She continued and told me that she and her family never got any good news from the physicians. They only got bad news regarding the illness. Then she cried inconsolably.

When her sobbing had ceased enough to converse with me, I asked her what she needed the most at this time. Lena said that she did not know.

She did not know anything about the bone marrow procedure, stem cell replacement, and what they would be going through and where they would be living in Stockholm or how long they would be there for treatment. She rallied and said that what would be the most helpful was to meet another family going through a course of treatment similar to what they were going through now. I told Lena that the treatment at the Karolinska Institute was considered to be one of the best that a child could have. The University Hospital in Reykjavik had a long history of sending children with ALL to the Karolinska Institute for treatment, and she and her family would be in good hands.

Lena, now much calmer, told me about how the past 2 weeks had been going. She had learned a few days ago that Frank would not be able to have children following a bone marrow transplant. She also told me how quickly things were developing regarding the illness. She and her family had moved out of her parents' home and were now living in an apartment owned by the Icelandic Cancer Association and located close to the Children's Hospital.

Our conversation moved to how much of a roller-coaster ride this journey was for the family, and how difficult it was to absorb all this within such a short period of time. Lena cried while she was telling me about her fears and feelings, and I noticed how vulnerable and sad she was. I told her that Frank was very lucky to have her as a mother and how supportive she and her husband were to their son. Frank had a high need for their support now. Lena nodded her head, and told me that this was a project they needed to finish. They needed to finish the treatment. They did not have any choice.

I then asked Lena about the support the family was receiving from the healthcare clinicians. She responded that everyone was very good to them and that the service was excellent, but they had participated in only one family meeting together as a couple with the physician. Now things were developing so quickly that she felt another family meeting with the physician was needed. After discussion of how this might be accomplished and my communication of that scheduling a family meeting with the physician could be arranged, I sensed that Lena was feeling a little better. She had regulated her emotion through her discussion with me.

Lena emphatically stated the conclusions she had made about communicating with healthcare clinicians. When one's life is turned upside down and your family does not have any control over its situation, a plan to meet with healthcare clinicians regularly and a plan for being informed about bad news would be good to have. Parents, Lena stated, should meet with healthcare clinicians without having the child present. Parents needed scheduled and follow-up meetings with a psychologist and priests. Frank should be offered posttraumatic counseling sessions alone with a psychologist or a priest for discussion of the psychological effect of the treatment on him.

Reflecting with Lena on the intervention session, I concluded that our conversation had helped Lena to express her worries and fears. I perceived that Lena showed relief, gained through talking about her experience. In addition to competence in emotion regulating with my support, Lena revealed competencies in goal-setting and problem solving for herself and for Frank. She showed increased competence in using the interview as a resource to make specific plans and to regulate her emotions through expressing them in words. These competencies contributed to greater resilience through the relationship she had with me, formed as the basis of GP.

We ended the session by my wishing Lena and her family all the best regarding the bone marrow transplant at the Karolinska Institute in Stockholm. After the session was over, I informed the head nurse at the children's cancer unit about Lena's concerns and wishes to meet another family that had experienced bone marrow transplant at the Karolinska Institute and to have another family meeting with the physicians. Lena had a plan of action that she had participated in making to accomplish her goal of finishing the task of being a good support person for her son. After our sessions, Lena may also have had greater confidence in her competence to be helpful to Frank and to other members of her family.

CONCLUSION

The GP perspective and components of its practice were integrated into a family therapeutic conversations intervention, the FAM-SOC, for the purpose of strengthening its capacity to structure and implement teaching–learning practice with families of children with a chronic illness. In this chapter, the case study showed the depth and breadth of the teaching–learning that was engaged through the relationship-based therapeutic conversation. The FAM-SOC intervention protocol provided a structure for GP processes that facilitated ongoing nurse–parent management of teaching–learning for the parents' support of their son's learning to manage stressors. Conversational interventions that have teaching–learning goals could draw on the GP methods for undertaking teaching–learning and behavioral change aims.

An issue that may be prominent for many parents of children with a chronic illness concerns supporting the child in responding to and adapting to stressors. Parental development of competencies in supporting a child with a chronic illness, such as ALL, to go through a difficult cancer treatment program is likely to require focused attention to teaching–learning processes. These GP processes intersect with the inputs and outputs of the FAM-SOTC intervention. This intersection offers parents an opportunity to develop competencies in communicating, engaging together in providing care, and regulating emotions. These competencies and the efforts to develop them through the participatory experiences of GP can create a trusting environment between parents and a pediatric nurse.

Svavarsdottir and Sigurdardottir (2013) suggested that in therapeutic conversations between nurses and parents of children newly diagnosed with cancer, parents can be provided with the opportunity to reflect on their experiences and to talk openly about how they are handling their situation. Reflection on experience can decrease isolation, increase connectedness, and empower families. The findings from the GP intervention that Frank's family was offered indicates that GP can be a meaningful healthcare service for families dealing with pediatric cancer. The results from Frank's clinical case regarding how his family was dealing with the ALL diagnosis and treatment support the benefit of GP integrated with FAM-SOTC intervention in clinical settings.

- GP in the context of the family strength–oriented conversation opened up the space for Frank's mother to reflect on difficult emotions and feelings.
- Frank's mother learned through discussions that drew on GP principles about how important a support person she was for her son while he was going through cancer treatment.
- Pediatric nurses can use GP processes to help parents develop competencies that ease or soften difficult feelings like those Lena experienced through the diagnostic and treatment procedures her son had to undergo.
- Pediatric nurses can also use GP processes to facilitate families' use of their emotion-regulating competencies in handling the "bad news" that families constantly receive.

GP in the context of the family strength–oriented therapeutic conversations intervention focused on giving Lena the opportunity to tell her illness stories and, with the advanced practice nurse, reflect on her strength for supporting her family and the competencies she viewed herself as needing to develop. Lena was empowered by this experience. GP was valuable to Lena, and she indicated that it would be helpful, in her opinion, to offer it on a regular basis to families dealing with ALL in a child. Further study of clinical cases could be the source of the types of issues families of a child with a chronic illness, such as ALL, are likely to encounter and that could be addressed by GP in the context of family strength–oriented therapeutic conversation.

REFERENCES

Grafton, E., Gillespie, B., & Henderson, S. (2010). Experiences of parents with caring for their child after a cancer diagnosis. *Journal of Pediatric Oncology Nursing, 28*(3), 143–153.

McCubbin, H. I., Thompson, A. I., & McCubbin, M. A. (1996). *Family assessment: Resiliency, coping and adaptation: Inventories for research and practice*. Madison, WI: University of Wisconsin–Madison, Center for Excellence in Family Studies.

Svavarsdottir, E. K., & Sigurdardottir, A. O. (2013). Benefits of a brief therapeutic conversation intervention for families of children and adolescents in active cancer treatment. *Oncology Nursing Forum, 40*, E346–E357. doi:10.1188/13

Svavarsdottir, E. K., Sigurdardottir, A. O., Konradsdottir, E., Stefansdottir, A., Sveinbjarnardottir, E. K., Ketilsdottir, A., . . . Guðmundsdottir, H. (2015). The process of translating family nursing knowledge into clinical practice. *Journal of Nursing Scholarship, 47*, 5–15. doi:10.1111/jnu.12108

Svavarsdottir, E. K., Sigurdardottir, A. O., & Tryggvadottir, G. B. (2014). Strengths-oriented therapeutic conversations for families of children with chronic illnesses: Findings from the Landspitali University Hospital Family Nursing Implementation Project. *Journal of Family Nursing, 20,* 13–50. doi:10.1177/1074840713520345

Wright, L. M., & Bell, J. M. (2009). *Beliefs and illness: A model for healing.* Calgary, Alberta, Canada: 4th Floor Press.

Wright, L. M., & Leahey, M. (2013). *Nurses and families: A guide to family assessment and intervention.* Philadelphia, PA: F. A. Davis.

Section IV

GUIDED PARTICIPATION IN MENTAL AND BEHAVIORAL HEALTH OF CHILDREN AND FAMILIES

15

Providing Spiritual Care to Children and Families

Darryl I. Owens and Hadley Kifner

Spiritual care for families of infants and young children is a topic not often written about in the literature. In fact, many healthcare professionals and parents themselves may not think of newborns or infants living lives with spiritual dimensions. The purpose of this chapter is to show how Bowlby's (1988) caregiving theory and guided participation ([GP]; Pridham, Limbo, Schroeder, Thoyre, & Van Riper, 1998) can be used as models for teaching and learning about spiritual needs in young children and their families.

INTRODUCING RACHEL AND HER FAMILY

Baby Rachel was born at 39 weeks of age with an acute respiratory depression and multiple congenital anomalies. Her parents were not legally married but were committed to each other and had been in relationship with each other for 5 years. In addition to baby Rachel, they had two other young children together. Although Rachel's parents expressed feeling intimidated by the medical language of the doctors and rarely asked questions directly to the primary attending physician, they felt comfortable articulating their needs and sharing concerns with Rachel's primary nurse at the bedside. Access to a dependable car and money for gas were both obstacles for them in getting to the bedside in the neonatal critical care center (NCCC), yet they were creative about ways to support baby Rachel from afar and when they were present, they were caring, loving, and wanted to be actively involved in her care as much as possible. The NCCC team recognized the difficulty of Rachel and her family's circumstances and wanted to encourage bonding and comfort as fully as possible. Given that baby Rachel's life will be shortened due to her diagnosis, how can the bedside nurse and medical team work together, with Rachel and her family as partners, to best utilize practical and clinical tools, all with the goal toward spiritual and emotional wholeness for baby and family? We invite you to consider these questions throughout this first section as we explore spiritual care in the context of caregiving, with GP principles consistently in the background.

Spiritual care, in the healthcare setting, can take on different meanings for patients, especially when the concept of spirituality is connected to religion. Grossoehme et al. (2011) noted that through religion, people can "regain a sense of mastery or efficacy in the midst of chaotic times" (p. 424). To provide effective spiritual care to patients, it is important for them to be able to define their spirituality and have it addressed in those terms, with special consideration of the context of the chaos in which they find themselves (Koenig, 2015; Puchalski & Romer, 2000). When a patient understands the concept of spirituality, recognizes how their own spirituality adds meaning to their experience of life, and articulates how spirituality may be used as therapeutic coping resources during a hospitalization, chaplains and spiritual care providers can respond directly by offering resources and care. But what happens when a patient is not able to articulate their own spirituality? What if their concept of spirituality is shifting because a chaotic moment has overwhelmed the patient and the family greatly? Finally, what if a patient is too young (developmentally and/or verbally) to use words to name their spiritual beliefs and places of need? None of these hypothetical, yet common scenarios excuse the chaplain or spiritual caregiver from giving quality spiritual care to the patient. Rather, the chaplain or caregiver is called to more deeply investigate other channels of communication and ways of gathering helpful information from the patient in order to provide the most effective, personal, and appropriate spiritual care.

Given this understanding, spiritual care to children requires a creative, generous, curious, and committed approach. As we provide brief information on the major stages of childhood developmental needs, we will use this working definition of spiritual care: "recognizing and responding to" (NHS Education for Scotland, 2010, p. 4).

Let us look for a moment at the particular spiritual needs of a newborn baby. The connectedness of a baby to his or her mother in utero is interrupted when the baby is born and reconnectedness has to take place after birth (Burkhardt, 1991). That reconnectedness with the mother and connectedness to others is assessed by adults based on external signs of the infants (Burkhardt, 1991). The manifestations of infant spirituality or connectedness are love, presence and connection, wonder and meaning, and faith (Surr, 2012). The spirituality is based on how the infant experiences life and being in relationship with others. Infants are spiritual beings, as all human beings are spiritual beings, but even for the most emotionally aware and sensitive adults, it can be very easy to overlook, dismiss, neglect to nurture, or struggle to recognize and understand an infant's spirituality (Mueller, 2010).

The spirituality of a toddler is focused on being within the context of the family and how the toddler is loved and cared for; while a preschooler can learn the religious belief of the parents and, to some extent, assume them as well as the practices associated with them as their own, and a school-age child's spirituality is tied to more abstract thinking (Burkhardt, 1991; Elkins & Cavendish, 2004).

In addition to the prenatal, newborn (sensorimotor), and toddler stages, according to Piaget (as cited in Shelly, 1982) and Erikson (as cited in Shelly, 1982), there are a few other major stages of cognitive and spiritual development: the preoperational stage (ages 2–7 years); the concrete operational stage (ages 7–12); and the formal abstract operational stage (older than age 12; Shelly, 1982). The main components of each of these stages include maturation of self-awareness, self-identity, autonomy and independence, and differentiation and assimilation. As Piaget and Erikson's professional work proved, as a child moves in and out and through these various stages, maturation can be somewhat predicted based on age-appropriate cognitive and developmental milestones. However, as family dynamics and life experiences naturally occur as well, the maturation process happens relative to the uniqueness and individuality of each child. Thus, spiritual development is relative to the individual person, occurring in its own time and intensity.

No matter what the numerical or developmental age of a child, the most effective and holistic spiritual care for a child understands the fundamental importance of spiritual caregiving for the entire family unit. In other words, caring for the spirit of a child, ideally, must also include caring for the spirits of all of the adults in that child's life. As the hospitalization of a child is indeed a "chaotic time" and the child's spirit may need extra care in order to maintain wholeness, so too must the collective spirit of the family (Grossoehme et al., 2011). The authors stated, "Hospitalized children represent a threatened future to parents" (p. 423). In order to do effective caregiving with these parents, it is important to determine how parents utilize their spirituality/religion when their child is a patient (Grossoehme et al., 2013).

When assessing the spiritual needs of the family unit, it is necessary to gather necessary information from the infant's caregivers or the children themselves if they are able to answer the question. Chaplains or spiritual caregivers are not the only ones responsible for getting this information. Puchalski and Romer (2000) identified the importance of physicians taking spiritual inventories of their patients for better assessing how to treat them. Toward this end, Puchalski created the FICA assessment tool (*F*aith or Beliefs, *I*mportance and *I*nfluence, *C*ommunity, and *A*ddress). It is important to note that this tool, as well as other spiritual assessment tools, are not to be used with religious patients and families only; this tool is used best as a standard of practice, respecting and valuing that all human beings are spiritual beings, regardless of how they recognize, express, and/or practice their spirituality (Cadge, Ecklund, & Short, 2009; de Jager Meezenbroek et al., 2012;

Elkins & Cavendish, 2004). (Note: Puchalski's is one of many spiritual assessment tools and it is the one used primarily for discussion in this chapter.)

After completing the spiritual assessment, the chaplain clarifies the spiritual needs with the patient and/or family and then comes up with prescriptive plans to meet those needs. Plans of pastoral care can include general ways to offer emotional support to a patient and/or family, as well as specific spiritual interventions such as prayer, spiritual counsel, listening, providing prayer beads and rugs, and rituals at bedside (Koenig, 2014). All of these spiritual interventions are offered to the patient and/or parent with respect, understanding, and explanation of the significance and benefits.

PARENTING/CAREGIVING AS A SPIRITUAL EXPERIENCE

Psychiatrists Donald Winnicott (2016) and John Bowlby (1988) both noted in their writings that parenting is the earliest and likely most important form of caregiving that humans experience (Caldwell & Robinson, 2017). Additionally, parenting is a creative process in that each parent expresses his or her identity as a caregiver to a child in a unique, ever-evolving, and deeply personal way. Like putting paint on a canvas, words on a page, or notes into the air, the experience of being a parent is difficult to explain and one authentic interaction between parent and child might be nearly impossible to replicate in a future moment. There is no one set or prescribed approach to best nurture, protect, encourage, challenge, and support a young person. Values, experiences, relationships, personality type, priorities, and resources all affect how an adult lives into a parental role. The personality and needs of the child may also inform how a parent responds. Some new mothers and fathers might look to older generations and respected family members as models for how to parent well; other new parents interact with their child(ren) in ways that are intentionally different than what they grew up with because they think an alternative approach would be better. Some look to articles, blogs, or books for advice on how to parent, whereas others still believe that their own individual intuition is the best source of insight.

No matter where the motivation, inspiration, or instruction comes from, parenting can be understood as a creative process in that it is, according to author–teacher Julia Cameron, like art, a spiritual transaction (Cameron, 2002). When a touch, conversation, glance, or mundane or significant moment is shared between one person and another, no matter their ages, there is transaction or a passing of energies between them. Some argue that these kinds of transactions or shared experiences between a child and a parent are sacred and holy and need to be recognized and respected as such. The early moments of bonding between a newborn baby and a parent can be deeply spiritual experiences. Recalling the moment when her brand-new baby was placed on her chest immediately after being born, many mothers share a sentiment of euphoria, as if something within her all along had at once been awakened and now, as a parent, she feels very alive and with a deep peace. Others might recognize that becoming a parent awakens a dormant spirituality within them. Something about accepting the responsibility of raising and mentoring a human being throughout the early years of life often inspires new parents to search for deeper connection to those around them and to seek the wisdom of a higher power (Fuchs, 1996).

Mother and podcaster Krista Tippett says, "The experience of parenting tends to raise spiritual questions anew. We sense that there is a spiritual aspect to our children's natures and wonder how to support and nurture that" (onbeing.org/programs/sandy-eisenberg-sasso-the-spirituality-of-parenting). Tippett goes on to introduce the guest for the podcast, Sandy Eisenberg Sasso, a rabbi, mother, and grandmother, who suggests that "the spiritual life begins not in abstractions, but in concrete everyday experiences." Concrete everyday experiences for a newborn in the NCCC include lots of touch—changing of diaper, feeding of milk or medicine, moving to chest for kangaroo care. These encounters, when offered with gentleness and respect, can potentially lead to an experience of safety, care, and well-being for a child. That in turn can lead to an experience of trust and gratitude for a parent, and fulfillment and helpfulness for a clinical caregiver. These, each and all, can be interpreted as significant emotional and spiritual experiences.

Sasso adds, "We want our children to be gracious and grateful. We want them to have courage in difficult times. We want them to have a sense of joy and purpose. That's what it means to nurture their spiritual lives" (Sasso, 2010). Countless times at the bedside of an acutely ill baby in the NCCC, parents utter similar desires to meet the spiritual needs of their children. Perhaps especially in the midst of a trying time, a crisis, parents want some measure of certainty that their child is not suffering and, in fact, may even be experiencing whole, purposeful, and insightful living. *If only, she could know that I love her. Do you think he can hear me encouraging him to rest? Is it silly to want to tell my baby that I am proud of her? Even in his pain, I want him to know that he is loved and we believe in him.* This kind of spiritual depth can be experienced and witnessed even though the body proves to be unwell, motionless, and failing.

The parental response to having a child with special needs, a serious medical condition, or terminal prognosis varies greatly. Seligman and Darling (2007) present several ways that families may view having a child with a diagnosis of any kind and suggest that personal, familial, cultural, and religious beliefs play a role in influencing how a parent will step into this unexpected role. Some may feel that their child's life is a blessing and makes them feel specially designated for the role of parenting; others may view the child's prognosis as a crisis and experience great distress in thinking about the future; still others may interpret it to be some sort of punishment or trial, a consequence for earlier behaviors or mistakes or a test to see if they will respond faithfully.

Now that we have laid a foundation for the spiritual care of children, in general, we look to a specific child and family to further describe how GP can be a reliable and effective way to provide spiritual care, as well as ongoing assessment of emotional and spiritual needs. We use cocreation.

Case Example 15.1

Rachel was born at 39 weeks of age with an acute respiratory depression and multiple congenital anomalies. Genetics, metabolic, neurology, pulmonology, and neuromuscular teams were consulted in coming up with goals of care and a treatment plan. During hospitalization, Rachel received mechanical ventilation and a nasogastric (NG) tube was placed for feeding. She was born to parents Maria and Johnny, who are not married but had been in a relationship together for over 5 years and had two other children together (ages 2 and 4). Maria was emotionally and spiritually connected to the baby and also physically, as she was recovering from a cesarean birth and her breasts were producing colostrum and milk. Johnny had been hesitant to connect with the baby throughout the pregnancy, fearing that if her prognosis was accurate, her life would be shortened. In an attempt to protect his heart from grief, he struggled to come to the unit to visit. Instead, Johnny focused on keeping the other two children at home on as normal a schedule as possible and providing emotional support to Maria.

Maria was unemployed and Johnny had begun a new job with a local engineering plant about 3 months prior to Rachel's birth. They lived about 1.5 hours away from the hospital and shared a car. They were new to the area and did not have many friends or neighbors yet on whom they could depend for support, meals, and child care for their other children.

Rachel's family was not currently connected with any particular religious group or community, but they did have spiritual beliefs and some level of desire for their spiritual connection with their baby to be acknowledged and incorporated into the plan of care. Johnny was raised a devout Catholic, but professed since he did not agree with some of the religious doctrine, he had not actively participated in any religious activities since his teenaged years. Maria identified as an agnostic who, given many life experiences of grief and trauma, had come to understand that there may be a God and there may not be, but she did not really mind not knowing for sure. She believed in angels and communicated with loved ones who had died, maintaining that even after death spiritual connections can remain intact. She found the voice of the sacred in nature and often looked to animals, the season, and lunar calendar for affirmation. Maria was not interested in explicit spiritual practices but was open to experimenting with different things. Johnny was reconsidering the practices of his childhood faith in an attempt to make meaning of their situation, and he would occasionally wear a rosary around his wrist when he visited the NCCC. Maria used spiritual language to express her emotions and process grief, mentioning angels, messengers, and confirmations from the universe and relationships with other loved ones who have died.

Rachel had two siblings—a 2-year-old brother and a 4-year-old sister. Her 2-year-old brother is often asleep in his stroller when they visit the unit and is too young to verbalize his connection to baby Rachel. Rachel's 4-year-old sister, however, is bright and energetic, emotionally expressive for her age, and felt very spiritually bonded to Rachel. She sang to her, asked to sit beside her isolette in the NCCC so she could hold her hand, and she would say things like "you were with the stars before you were born to us." Maria and Johnny had hoped that as Rachel grew and received care in the NCCC, her prognosis would improve and that resources, therapies, and treatments that could improve her life would be identified and utilized. They also understood that her congenital anomalies might be too much to overcome, requiring risky surgery after surgery without promise of benefit, and so hoped for a quality of life for her in the midst of her hospitalization. Their greatest fear, perhaps even greater than a possible death, was that Rachel would experience any kind of suffering or physical pain, and so they were wary of extreme or heroic medical procedures or medications.

Rachel's parents were unable to be at her bedside in the unit much of the time due to limited financial resources (the cost of gas to travel the more than 75 miles from their home to the hospital, as well as the cost of parking were prohibitive), her father's work schedule, and their commitment to maintaining a stable household for their other young children; however, they called multiple times a day to talk with the primary nurse, emailed a few times a week with the case manager, and visited as a family for an entire day every weekend. Although they expressed feeling intimidated by the medical language of the doctors and rarely asked questions directly to the primary attending physician, both Maria and Johnny articulated questions and needs easily to the nurse, social worker, family support specialist, and chaplain and utilized all resources available to them.

As we continue to explore this case study more specifically, consider how the issues, processes, competencies, and strategies shown in the caregiving infographic (see Figure 15.1) and GP triangle (see Chapter 1, Figure 1.1) relate to Rachel and her family. The issue at hand for Maria and Johnny is to connect as deeply as possible with baby Rachel, contributing to her quality of life, sharing hopes about her future, and maintaining a stable structure for their other children at home, while at the same time accepting the possible reality that Rachel may not experience life outside of the NCCC. Perhaps the biggest challenge for Maria and Johnny is to experience the time they share together as a family for what it is in the present moment without dwelling too much on the fact that Rachel's life may be short.

In order to connect with Rachel, Maria and Johnny need to identify ways to experience reciprocated relationship—giving love to her and either receiving the same from her or experiencing some sort of response to that love from her. As they learn how to be parents to her at her isolette bedside, they are also learning how to be medical caregivers, learning about

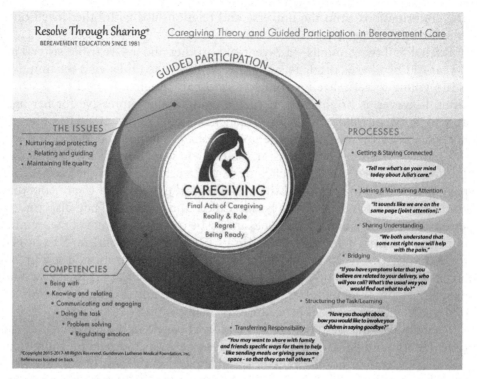

FIGURE 15.1 Caregiving infographic.

Copyright 2012–2017. Resolve Through Sharing. Gundersen Lutheran Medical Foundation. Used with permission.

Sources: Bowlby, J. (1969/1982). *Attachment and loss: Vol. I. Attachment*. New York, NY: Basic Books; Limbo, R., & Lathrop, A. (2014). Caregiving in mothers' narratives of perinatal hospice. *Illness, Crisis & Loss, 22*(1), 43–65; Pridham, K., Harrison, T., Brown, R., Krolikowski, M., Limbo, R., & Schroeder, M. (2012). Caregiving motivations and developmentally prompted transitions for mothers of prematurely born infants. *Advances in Nursing Science, 35*(3), E23–E41; Pridham, K., Limbo, R., Schroeder, M., Thoyre, S., & Van Riper, M. (1998). Guided participation and development of care-giving competencies for families of low birth-weight infants. *Journal of Advanced Nursing, 28*(5), 948–958.

medication times, preferred sleeping positions, how to change her diaper without jostling the feeding tube, and effective ways to soothe her. Together with the medical professionals, they are responsible for caring for her as a tiny human being as well as a patient. Such responsibility could inspire appropriate stress, anxiety, and feelings of being overwhelmed or aggrieved.

As they continue on in their role as parents–caregivers, Maria and Johnny are aware of competencies they need to work toward. Being present at Rachel's bedside, having presence, or "shows pleasure in being with the baby" (Pridham et al., 1998, p. 951) is one of these competencies. Since Maria and Johnny cannot be physically present for baby Rachel in every moment, it is important for them to understand other ways that they can relate to her, communicate with her, and connect with her. Beginning to understand and focusing on their spiritual connection with each other and to her—the ways in which they are bound to and in relationship with one other outside of being in the same place at the same time—may be relieving. This competency points back to the "transferring responsibility" in that Maria and Johnny trust that others may "have presence" with Rachel, too—the primary nurse, the attending physician, and/or even God or a divine power.

Some strategies they could employ to work toward these competencies, along with the help of the medical team, include what many chaplains and spiritual care providers call "meaning making" (Meert & Eggly, 2016). The goal of meaning making with the parents is to help Maria and Johnny cope with all that is happening medically and emotionally with Rachel (Grossoehme et al., 2011). The goal of processing these events through conversation with the chaplain or spiritual caregiver is for Maria and Johnny to connect with their own spirituality as a resource for themselves and then to have spiritual resources for them to continue to connect with Rachel (Sanders & Burke, 2014). This conversation can include GP strategies such as promoting reflection or providing information with Maria and Johnny. This GP process can include staying connected, maintaining attention, and bridging with Maria and Johnny. This conversation is also conducted in a consultative manner to enable them to use the GP competencies of knowing themselves spiritually, and regulating their emotions to be able to connect deeply with their daughter. As these parents are reflecting on their spirituality to provide internal strength for themselves and for Rachel, the chaplain or spiritual caregiver invites these parents to connect with their internal view of this event. How do they perceive what has happened and what is happening with Rachel? Are they looking at this illness as punishment or are they viewing it as something that happens in life. As they connect with their internal views of Rachel's condition (meaning making), Maria and Johnny can identify where they may need assistance in finding ways to shift their internal evaluations. Doing so may allow them to use other coping strategies to connect more deeply with Rachel, which is a spiritual goal as discussed earlier in this chapter.

Making meaning out of Rachel's life, and her parents' experience as a family with her, inspires reflective questions such as "What was our life like before her birth?" "What is our life like now that she is born and with us?" "If she dies, what will our life be like after that?" Other things they wonder may be, "Should/could we have done something different during the pregnancy that might have changed the current situation?" "Are we making the best decisions for her that we can, given what we know now?" "When we are done with this hospitalization, will we look back and have any regrets?" As Rachel's family attempts to offer her the best quality of life they can, while also aiming to experience as much quality of life as possible as a family, they are having a conversation with the past and the present and even wading into the future. Such processes involve bridging, a richly developed and often-used way of understanding and problem solving around relationships.

Another opportunity to use GP with this family presents itself in one of many conversations with Maria and Johnny, in which the chaplain or spiritual caregiver hears the need for Johnny to have tools to help quiet his anxieties, worries, and fears when visiting with Rachel (*problem to be solved*). He desires to be an example for the two older children to purposefully be fully present with Rachel for those weekend visits. The competencies can include *regulating emotion, being with Rachel,* and *relating to himself.* The chaplain or spiritual caregiver notices the rosary Johnny is wearing around his wrist and suggests prayer can be a possible effective tool for Johnny. The strategy can include *reflection on the significance of the rosary, making a suggestion about using prayers, and cocreating (chaplain and Johnny) ways the rosary can be used,.* The process can be *using the concept of prayer to bridge his movement from anxiety, worry, and fear to a place where he can make meaning of the hospital experience and his baby daughter's illness, gain control of his emotions or thoughts, and experience comfort or intimacy with God* (Grossoehme et al., 2011).

Challenges of GP in the Clinical Setting

Although GP in the clinical setting has mutual benefits for patients, families, and even staff, it is not always a straightforward and easy method to engage at the bedside. There are several challenges and many of them are common among all parents with a critically ill child. First, parents and families are often uncomfortable providing care at the bedside to their child. They may be first-time parents and do not feel confident in their role as parent yet, or they may have had other children who were healthy and had no need to be in a hospital and so the clinical setting is intimidating and foreign to them. Because of these feelings, they may be hesitant to engage directly with their baby in ways other than words of greeting and love; they may look to the bedside nurse or other clinical provider to invite them into care, providing special instruction.

Second, many fathers express concern over unintentionally harming or agitating their baby, assuming that they may not be able to be gentle enough to touch their baby. This anxiety keeps them from becoming engaged and they may tend to stay back, playing a more passive yet seemingly safer role. It can be difficult for parents to ask for help or affirmation when needed if they have put pressure on themselves to innately know how to bond with their baby or they assume that only clinical experts and professionals know best. In these instances, it is imperative for clinical caregivers to encourage parental involvement; provide education on best practices; recognize and affirm the important and unique role of parental involvement; and create a nonjudgmental, relaxed, and welcoming atmosphere at the bedside (Hollywood & Hollywood, 2011).

Another challenge is the practical ability to be present, available, and undistracted at the bedside. Families with a small child or baby in the hospital often have many other simultaneous stressors in their life in addition to or sometimes because of the hospitalization. Maintaining work hours in an effort to keep a paycheck, caring for other children at home, maximizing maternity leave, and juggling limited transportation resources (money for gas or parking, unreliable or restricted access to vehicle) are all factors to be considered. Along these lines, sometimes a mother and/or father will resist being at the bedside or actively involved in their child's hospitalization in an attempt to protect themselves from potential emotional distress. Many parents believe, implicitly or explicitly, that bonding opportunities and emotional/spiritual connection are directly proportionally related to each other. For example, the more opportunities for joining and maintaining a relationship, the deeper and more lasting the emotional/spiritual connections will be. However, bonding between a baby and a family is most often connected to quality, rather than quantity, of time together.

Language barriers can be a fourth challenge to GP within the healthcare setting, and the challenge can go in two different directions. The direction of the challenge can flow from parents to the healthcare team (Steinberg, Valenzuela-Araujo, Zickafoose, Kieffer, & DeCamp, 2016) and/or from the healthcare team to the parents (Turner, Chur-Hanson, & Winefield, 2014). In the Steinberg et al. study, parents described "the healthcare encounters as a battle" (p. 1320). These mothers preferred bilingual providers and had biases toward interpreted encounters, although some had never experienced anything negative in their encounters. Other themes in the Steinberg study were feeling they were getting by with limited language skills, a fear of being a burden because of the language differences, and experiences of stigma and humiliation because of the language barriers. With these stated themes, GP for these parents will be challenging due to all of the emotional struggles of the parents as learners/teachers and the staff as teachers/learners. The results from this study highlight the need to develop competencies in communicating for both providers and parents. The researchers also remind healthcare providers to focus on the relationship with the interpreter as a critical one among parents, baby, and care providers. Turner et al. (2014) also identified language barriers among staff and pediatric parents as problematic. In this study, nurses believed the language differences prevented them from establishing a supportive relationship with the parents. Because verbal skills are such an important component of the relationship, when the languages of the nurses and parents are different, communication is affected, making GP with the parents even more difficult.

Anticipatory grief is the grief experienced before the actual death of a loved one. In addition to anticipating the death of a child, as in this case, Maria and Johnny can experience anticipatory grief because Rachel is not "the idealized child" or the healthy child they expected at the beginning of the pregnancy, which can prevent them from bonding with Rachel early on (Siegel, Gardner, & Merenstein, 2002). When babies are born early or with a condition requiring admission to NICU, parents experience stress and anxiety (Martin, Fanaroff, & Walsh, 2010). In addition to the stress and anxiety, anticipatory grief affects people cognitively, physically, emotionally, and spiritually (Simon, 2008). If parents are experiencing these described effects of grief, it may be difficult for parents to participate with the staff in learning to accomplish new goals and in bonding with the baby if their grief is not addressed by the staff. Fathers and mothers can experience anticipatory grief and the medical staff not know it if they are not familiar with this type of grief (Valizadeh, Zamanzadeh, & Rahiminia, 2012). Should this lack of recognition occur, frustration could arise with the medical staff, assuming the parents are resistant to the learning process when in fact their learning capabilities are compromised by this grief. Frustration could also occur with parents not wanting to learn something new at the time. GP would then focus on helping parents and staff work together on developing the competency of emotion regulation.

The final challenge we want to highlight is when the medical team's spiritual/religious understanding and expressions differ from those of the patients and the parents. In this case study, Rachel's life will be shortened due to her diagnosis, and Johnny and Maria both have acknowledged their different expressions of spirituality. Toward the end of Rachel's life, if Johnny and/or Maria begin to use "miracle language" related to Rachel, which is not the spiritual language of her medical caregivers, this can cause moral distress, and inner conflict in some of the team members (Green, 2015). In one study of physicians and patients, results showed differences in religious affiliations and the general population of patients, which means the physicians and patients/families can hold very different religious views at end-of-life situations (Franzen, 2015). In another study with pediatricians and families, only 49% of the physicians talked with families about their spiritual and religious concerns, whereas only 13% of the pediatricians in the study ever received formal training on the role of spirituality and religion in healthcare (Cadge et al., 2009; Grossoehme et al., 2007). This challenge can affect whether Johnny and Maria feel understood or misunderstood. For Johnny to begin to rely on his Catholic upbringing, he may want to talk about hope and the possibility of miracles for Rachel. If this view is not held or honored by the team members, Johnny can feel alone in his wish or desire, especially since Maria does not share his same spiritual history. When changing hopes become the central focus for both parents and healthcare providers, spiritual principles become logical representations of a cocreated language.

These five challenges can be met with creative solutions and overcome, but this often requires extra patience and time from the clinical care providers. For example, in one NCCC, nurses have created a program for families who cannot consistently be at the bedside by coordinating audio and video phone calls that allow the staff to speak to the parents and show them how their precious baby is doing. Another unit hosts a weekly program for fathers that shares tips on how to pick up a premature baby in the most gentle and safe manner—an example of helping the parent develop the competency of "doing the task."

The key is to acknowledge the challenges that are present, rather than avoiding or ignoring them. Naming challenges to GP (e.g., communicating, being with the baby, or overall caregiving) allows a family to be known and cared for in ways that add benefit to the family as a whole; it also empowers the family to be the best care providers they can be within the context of their circumstances. This kind of assessment of needs and hopes, providing of resources, accepting of limitations, and celebrating of strengths, fosters open-ended communication and professional utilization of supportive care.

Teaching Insights

Because of the potential benefits of presence, touch, bonding, and shared love, utilizing the parental role at bedside as fully as possible is an important priority for Rachel's providers. When parents feel most healthily bonded and engaged with the care of the baby, no matter the outcome of the hospitalization, baby, family, and clinical caregiver experience decreased distress about the baby's experience of life (Flacking et al., 2012). Moreover, while the NCCC nurse practitioner is expert at dosing, determining most beneficial combinations and timing of medications, and advance planning decision making—of clinically caring for the infant patient—mother and father are experts at spiritually and emotionally caring for their child because they have participated in the creation of this baby and have a connection with each other that surpasses facts, predictions, and science. Said another way, the lives of the baby and family would be intertwined and dependent on each other whether or not the hospitalization had ever happened or not.

One role may be valued more subjectively than the other in certain situations. Generally, chaplains or clergy take the lead with spiritual practices. Parents and the chaplain have a relationship with the baby and with each other, creating a unique and intimate opportunity for the parents and clinician to explore and cocreate spiritual practices. Simply, any clinician has a particular purpose and role in relation to the child that complements that of the parents and the unique parent/child bond. The fact that those who care for the baby may engage in a special way with the child speaks to the power of relationship in human nature, sometimes, in this situation, referred to as liminality. This serves as the basis for the profound nature of caregiver suffering and grief, centered on both parents and child.

CONCLUSION

Given all of this, parents need not be seen as "visitors" at the bedside and "allowed" or "invited" to participate in the baby's care. Rather parents can be seen as "partners" and "supported and engaged" in caring for their baby in ways that are meaningful for patient and family. It is important then for clinical providers to be open to the idea that the family and child can teach as well and that the expert is not the only one who can participate as leader. Specific to GP, parents and care providers are both teachers and learners. An example of this would be learning about the baby's behaviors and features that serve to help both parents and professionals get to know the baby better (knowing and relating to the baby as a person).

There is no prognosticating tool for the health of the human spirit. Nor is there a clinical tool that can measure the strength or predict the resilience of the human spirit. The monitors and machines told the clinical story of how baby Rachel's organs and systems were responding to medicines and struggling to improve. But it was Rachel's unpredicted and mysterious responses to her family's touch and voice, linked to the invisible ways in which these responses inspired her family that told *her* story and *their* story.

RESOURCES

Note to readers: The following information includes resources for further reading and examples of prayers and other spiritual practices grounded in guided participation. We have included these to enhance the reader's spiritual practices and use of GP at the bedside.

American Holistic Nurses Association (AHNA). Founded in 1981, the AHNA "supports the concepts of holism: a state of harmony among body, mind, emotions, and spirit within an ever-changing environment." Retrieved from www.ahna.org

Barnes, L., Plotnikoff, G. A., Fox, K., & Pendleton, S. (2000). Spirituality, religion, and pediatrics: Intersecting worlds of healing. *Pediatrics*, *104*(6), 899–908. doi:10.1542/peds.106.4.S1.899

Carson, V. (1989). Spiritual developments across the life span. In V. Carson (Ed.), *Spiritual dimensions of nursing practice* (pp. 24–51). Philadelphia, PA: W. B. Saunders.

Carson, V. (1989). *Spiritual dimensions of nursing practice*. Philadelphia, PA: W. B. Saunders.

Coles, R. (1990). *The spiritual life of children*. Boston, MA: Houghton Mifflin.

D'Souza, R. (2007). The importance of spirituality in medicine and its application to clinical practice. *The Medical Journal of Australia*, *186*(Suppl. 10), S57–S59.

Heilferty, C. M. (2004). Spiritual development and the dying child: The pediatric nurse practitioner's role. *Journal of Pediatric Health Care*, *18*(6), 271–275. doi:10.1016/j.pedhc.2004.03.007

Limbo, R., & Kobler, K. (2013). *Meaningful moments: Ritual and reflection when a child dies*. La Crosse, WI: Gundersen Medical Foundation.

McDonough-Means, S. I., Kreitzer, M. J., & Bell, I. R. (2004). Fostering a healing presence and investigating its mediators. *Journal of Alternative and Complementary Medicine*, *10*(Suppl. 1), S25–S41.

Speck, P. (1998). The meaning of spirituality in illness. In M. Cobb & V. Robshaw (Eds.), *The spiritual challenge of healthcare*. London, UK: Churchill Livingstone.

REFERENCES

Bowlby, J. (1969/1982). *Attachment and loss: Vol, I Attachment*. New York, NY: Basic Books.

Bowlby, J. (1988). *A secure base: Parent-child attachment and healthy human development*. New York, NY: Basic Books.

Burkhardt, M. A. (1991). Spirituality and children: Nursing considerations. *Journal of Holistic Nursing*, *9*(2), 31–40.

Cadge, W., Ecklund, E. H., & Short, N. (2009). Religion and spirituality: A barrier and a bridge in the everyday professional work of pediatric physicians. *Social Problems*, *56*(4), 702–721. doi:10.1525/sp.2009.56.4.702

Caldwell, L., & Robinson, H. T. (Eds.). (2017). *The collected works of D. W. Winnicott*. Vol. 6. New York, NY: Oxford University Press.

Cameron, J. (2002). *The artist's way: A spiritual path to higher creativity*. New York, NY: Putnam.

de Jager Meezenbroek, E., Garssen, B., van den Berg, M., van Dierendonck, D., Visser, A., & Schaufeli, W. B. (2012). Measuring spirituality as a universal human expereince: A review of spirituality questionnaires. *Journal of Religion and Health*, *51*(2), 336–354.

Elkins, M., & Cavendish, R. (2004). Developing a plan for pediatric spiritual care. *Holistic Nursing Practice*, *18*(4), 179–184. doi:10.1097/00004650-200407000-00002

Flacking, R., Lehtonen, L., Thomson, G., Axelin, A., Ahlqvist, S., Moran, V. H., . . . The SCENE Group. (2012). Closeness and separation in neonatal intensive care. *Acta Paediatrica*, *101*(10), 1032–1037. doi:10.1111/j.1651-2227.2012.02787.x

Franzen, A. B. (2015). Physicians in the USA: Attendance, beliefs and patient interactions. *Journal of Religion and Health*, *54*(5), 1886–1900.

Fuchs, N. (1996). *Parenting as a spiritual journey: Deepening ordinary and extraordinary events into sacred occasions*. San Francisco, CA: Harper Collins.

Green, J. (2015). Living in hope and desperate for a miracle: NICU nurses perceptions of parental anguish. *Journal of Religion and Health*, 54(2), 731–744. doi:10.1007/s10943-014-9971-7

Grossoehme, D. H., Cotton, S., Ragsdale, J., Quittner, A. L., McPhail, G., & Seid, M. (2013). "I honestly believe God keeps me healthy so I can take care of my child": Parental use of faith related to treatment adherence. *Journal of Health Care Chaplaincy*, 19(2), 66–78. doi:10.1080/08854726.2013.779540

Grossoehme, D. H., Jacobson, C. J., Cotton, S., Ragsdale, J. R., VanDyke, R., & Seid, M. (2011). Written prayers and religious coping in a paediatric hospital setting. *Mental Health, Religion & Culture*, 14(5), 423–432. doi:10.1080/13674671003762693

Grossoehme, D. H., Ragsdale, J. R., McHenry, C. L., Thurston, C., DeWitt, T., & VandeCreek, L. (2007). Pediatrician characteristics associated with attention to spirituality and religion in clinical practice. *Pediatrics*, 119(1), 117–123. doi:10.1542/peds.2006-0642

Hollywood, M., & Hollywood, E. (2011). The lived experiences of fathers of a premature baby on a neonatal intensive care unit. *Journal of Neonatal Nursing*, 17(1), 32–40. doi:10.1016/j.jnn.2010.07.015

Koenig, H. G. (2014). The spiritual care team: Enabling the practice of whole person medicine. *Religions*, 5(4), 1161–1174. doi:10.3390/rel5041161

Koenig, H. G. (2015). Religion, spirituality, and health: A review and update. *Advances in Mind- Body Medicine*, 29(3), 19–26.

Limbo, R., & Lathrop, A. (2014). Caregiving in mothers' narratives of perinatal hospice. *Illness, Crisis & Loss*, 22(1), 43–65.

Martin, R. J., Fanaroff, A. A., & Walsh, M. C. (2010). *Fanaroff and Martin's neonatal-perinatal medicine*. St. Louis, MO: Elsevier.

Meert, K. L., & Eggly, S. (2016). Observed trauma in the PICU and parental meaning making. *Pediatric Critical Care Medicine*, 17(4), 375–376. doi:10.1097/PCC.0000000000000687

Miquel-Verges, F., Donohue, P. K., & Boss, R. D. (2011). Discharge of infants from NICU to Latino families with limited English proficiency. *Journal of Immigrant Minority Health*, 13(2), 309–314. doi:10.1007/s10903-010-9355-3.

Mueller, C. R. (2010). Spirituality in children: Understanding and developing interventions. *Pediatric Nursing*, 36(4), 197–203, 208.

NHS Education for Scotland. (2010). *Spiritual care matters: An introductory resource for all NHS Scotland staff*. Edinburgh, Scotland: NHS Education for Scotland.

Pridham, K. F., Harrison, T., Brown, R., Krolikowski, M., Limbo, R., & Schroeder, M. (2012). Caregiving motivations and developmentally prompted transitions for mothers of prematurely born infants. *Advances in Nursing Science*, 35(3), E23–E41.

Pridham, K. F., Limbo, R., Schroeder, M., Thoyre, S., & Van Riper, M. (1998). Guided participation and development of care-giving competencies for families of low birth-weight infants. *Journal of Advanced Nursing*, 28(5), 948–958. doi:10.1046/j.1365-2648.1998.00814.x

Puchalski, C., & Romer, A. L. (2000). Taking a spiritual history allows clinicians to understand patients more fully. *Journal of Palliative Medicine*, 3(1), 129–137. doi:10.1089/jpm.2000.3.129

Sanders, M. R., & Burke, K. (2014). The "hidden" technology of effective parent consultation: A guided participation model for promoting change in families. *Journal of Child and Family Studies*, 23(7), 1289–1297. doi:10.1007/s10826-013-9827-x

Sasso, S. E. (2010, June 17). *The spirituality of parenting* [Audio podcast]. K. Tippett, Trans, Minneapolis, MN.

Seligman, M., & Darling, R. B. (2007). *Ordinary families, special children*. New York, NY: Guilford Press.

Shelly, J. A. (1982). *The spiritual needs of children: A guide for nurses, parents, and teachers*. Downers Grove, IL: InterVarsity Press.

Siegel, R., Gardner, S. L., & Merenstein, G. B. (2002). Psychosocial aspects of neonatal care—families in crisis: Theoretic and practical considerations. In G. B. Merenstein, & S. L. Gardner (Eds.), *Handbook of neonatal intensive care* (pp. 725–753). St. Louis, MO: Mosby.

Simon, J. L. (2008). Anticipatory grief: Recognition and coping. *Journal of Palliative Medicine*, 11(9), 1280–1281. doi:10.1089/jpm.2008.9824

Steinberg, E. M., Valenzuela-Araujo, D., Zickafoose, J. S., Kieffer, E., & DeCamp, L. R. (2016). The "battle" of managing language barriers in health care. *Clinical Pediatrics*, 55(14), 1318–1327. doi:10.1177/0009922816629760

Surr, J. (2012). Peering into the clouds of glory: Explorations of a newborn child's spirituality. *International Journal of Children's Spirituality*, 17(1), 77–87. doi:10.1080/1364436x.2012.677810

Turner, M., Chur-Hansen, A., & Winefield, H. (2014). The neonatal nurses' view of their role in emotional support of parents and its complexities. *Journal of Clinical Nursing, 23*(21–22), 3156–3165. doi:10.1111/jocn.12558

Valizadeh, L., Zamanzadeh, V., & Rahiminia, E. (2012). Comparison of anticipatory grief reaction between fathers and mothers of premature infants in neonatal intensive care unit. *Scandinavian Journal of Caring Sciences, 27*(4), 921–926. doi:10.1111/scs./2005

16

Supporting Parent–Child Relationships, Toddler Autonomy, and Adherence to Medical Care

Audrey Tluczek

This chapter illustrates the application of guided participation (GP; Pridham, Limbo, Schroeder, Thoyre, & Van Riper, 1998) to enhance parents' competencies in the care of their toddler with a serious chronic health condition, such as cystic fibrosis (CF). This case is conceptualized within a model of person-, family-, and culture-centered care that requires clinicians to assess the family within the multiple contexts of the child's development, parent–child relationship, and the family's psychosocial–cultural milieus (Lor, Crooks, & Tluczek, 2016). Although this chapter focuses on toddlers, these principles may apply to caregiving for children of any age with serious health concerns.

TODDLERHOOD

Toddlerhood is typically considered to extend from 12 to 36 months (Davies, 2011), a phase marked by a surge in physical growth, motor skills, and language acquisition. These children are now able to walk, run, jump, climb, turn knobs, and throw balls. As keen observers of their environments and masters of imitation, they are rapidly learning new behaviors. By two, their vocabularies can range from 60 to 500 words with a mean of 300 words.

Three-year-olds have the capacity to share their internal worlds through the narratives of their verbal stories and their symbolic play (Davies, 2011).

According to Erik Erikson, this stage of psychosocial development is characterized by a mastery of autonomy over shame and self-doubt (Miller, 2011). The emergence of "no" in the vocabulary around the age of 15 months personifies this phenomenon of seeking some degree of independence from parental caregivers. Mahler and colleagues (1975) describe this stage as a time during which the child begins to separate and individuate from the primary caregiver. As young children become increasingly mobile and physically capable of moving away from their parents, they also begin to recognize themselves as beings who are separate from their parents. Toddlers typically engage in rapprochement behavior (Mahler, Pine, & Bergman, 1975) by tentatively wandering off to explore their little worlds while maintaining a sense of connection to their parents through eye contact. Another example of this individuation process is illustrated by the child's appropriate use of the pronouns "I," "me," and "mine." Tantrums can also be a way the child communicates frustration when his or her level of competencies do not match those that are required for the successful completion of a particular task (Lieberman, 1993).

PARENT–CHILD RELATIONSHIP

The shift from complete physical dependency on parents to more autonomous behavior can also affect the parent–child relationship. The ethological perspective about child development posits that human beings are genetically and biologically programed to develop attachments (Bowlby, 1988; Miller, 2011). By toddlerhood, internal working models of relationships are still developing, behavioral attachment systems are becoming established, and parent–child interactions are fairly well synchronized. Thus, the parent and child tend to respond to each other's cues in systematically predictable ways. Securely attached toddlers use their newfound motor skills to comfortably separate from parents in exploration of their environments, occasionally seeking parental proximity through visual contact, returning to the proximity of the parent, or seeking physical contact with a quick hug (Landy, 2002). Their attachment systems are roused by threatening situations (e.g., the presence of strangers) or physical discomfort (e.g., fatigue or illness). When distressed, securely attached toddlers are also able to make use of parental comforting to calm themselves. Insecurely attached toddlers either anxiously cling to parents without exploring environments or they wander off on their own without consideration of the parent's whereabouts. Insecurely attached children can also become easily emotionally dysregulated or develop behavioral problems (Landy, 2002). Lieberman (1993) describes the parent–child relationship as a partnership in which the parent helps the child internalize the external protections provided by the parent through empathy, encouragement, and limit-setting within a physically and psychologically safe environment.

These dynamic changes in children's physical growth and psychosocial development can pose many challenges to new parents. For example, it is not unusual for parents to misinterpret a toddler's constant use of "no" as oppositional behavior. The child who once willingly cuddled in the parent's arms now prefers mobile activities. It is easy to see how some parents might consider such developments to be negative reflections on their parenting competencies and/or relationship with the child. Such worries can be compounded when the child has a serious health condition, such as CF, that requires modification of many aspects of everyday life.

CF OVERVIEW

As one of the most common life-shortening inherited conditions in the United States, CF can serve as an exemplar for addressing the needs of families who have a child with a serious chronic health problem. Although symptom severity depends on a combination of genetic and environmental factors, CF typically affects multiple physiological systems. Most children with CF have frequent lung infections, difficulty digesting certain foods, and excessive salt in their sweat (Cystic Fibrosis Foundation, n.d.). Early diagnosis and intervention resulting from newborn screening offers hope for prevention of long-term complications (Montgomery & Howenstine, 2009). The translation of genetic research into precision medicine and the application of evidence-based guidelines to care have significantly improved the quality of life and increased the longevity of individuals with CF (Davies, Ebdon, & Orchard, 2014; Schechter & Gutierrez, 2010). The Cystic Fibrosis Foundation reports, "the life expectancy for a baby born with CF in 2016 is 47 years of age" (Marshall, 2017).

Affected families face a number of issues in managing their children's health. Parents are responsible for time-consuming home care, such as aerosolized treatments, chest therapy, nutritional supplements, and medications that must be administered throughout the day. Parents must monitor their children for signs of medical complications and avoid environmental risks, such as individuals with respiratory infections and conditions associated with poor air quality. Research has shown that the diagnosis of CF early in life is associated with mothers choosing bottle-feeding over breastfeeding (Tluczek, Clark, McKechnie, Orland, & Brown, 2010), perceptions of their children as being vulnerable to illness (Tluczek, McKechnie, & Brown, 2011), and parental depressive symptoms (Glasscoe, Lancaster, Smyth, & Hill, 2007; Tluczek, Clark, Kosick, & Farrell, 2005). Maternal depression can adversely affect mothers' capacities to provide their infants with sensitive and responsive caregiving (Goodman, 2007), which is essential to infants forming secure attachments with their parents and close interpersonal relationships later in life (DeKlyen & Greenberg, 2008). Toddlers diagnosed with CF in early infancy (based on CF symptoms, rather than newborn screening) have been found to have higher rates of insecure infant–mother attachments than children diagnosed with CF later in infancy (Simmons, Goldberg, Washington, Fischer-Fay, & Maclusky, 1995). There is also evidence of disruptive mealtime behavior and nonadherence with respiratory therapies in toddlers and preschool-age children with CF (Ernst, Johnson, & Stark, 2010). Thus, the combination of normative developmental transitions, demands of CF-related home care, and emotional burden of the child's condition can create unique parenting challenges and potentially negative consequences to the child's physical and mental health, parents' coping capacities, and family functioning.

Case Example 16.1

Although the following case is based on a real family, many details have been changed and pseudonyms are used to protect their confidentiality. Wendy (age 26) and Mark (age 30), a Caucasian middle-class couple, are the proud parents of 19-month-old Jeremy, their only child, diagnosed with CF at 2 weeks of age as the result of an abnormal newborn screen. Although he was healthy at the time, the screening test identified two gene mutations associated with CF. The diagnosis was confirmed by the results of a sweat test and physical assessment conducted at a CF center. The family was referred to a clinic that specializes in parent–infant mental health. The reason for the referral was nonadherence to chest therapy and feeding problems (i.e., food refusal and disruptive mealtime behavior).

Family Assessment

The assessment involved a combination of family interview, standardized measures of parents' mental health, and observations of parent–child interactions. Given Jeremy's diagnosis and with permission from his parents, the assessment also included a review of his health records. During the interview, the parents expressed their frustrations about the child refusing to sit still during chest therapy that usually resulted in them just giving up and not completing the procedure. They also described mealtimes as a "battle of the wills"—a battle the parents acknowledged they usually lost. They explained that sometimes they "had to force him to take his enzymes (oral medication) before meals." They also described Jeremy as a "picky eater" with very strong food dislikes and preferences. The problem behavior began when he was about 8 months and continued to worsen, particularly around the age of 14 months "when he began saying 'no' to everything." An assessment of the child's domains of functioning revealed a normal perinatal history, no problems with sleep, and toilet training had not yet begun. During the interview, Jeremy was observed to be a pleasant, socially engaging, and active toddler. He enjoyed exploring his new environment while occasionally returning to his mother with a toy that he tried to name. She responded by accepting the toy and either repeated the name he uttered or offered a name when he could not.

A review of Jeremy's medical records indicated that Jeremy received regular care through his primary care provider as well as the CF center. Despite the CF diagnosis, he showed steady growth with a height and weight above the 50th percentile and his chest x-rays were normal. He had never been hospitalized. Prescribed treatment includes enzyme supplements with all meals, daily vitamin supplements, a calorically dense diet, and chest therapy twice daily. His parents had been cautioned to avoid exposing him to anyone with respiratory infections. His overall development was appraised to be appropriate for age and he was up to date with his immunizations. There was also documentation of frequent telephone communications between mother and healthcare providers regarding questions she had about what was normal for a child with CF at various ages.

The parents reported a family history of anxiety and depression on both sides but no other serious mental health problems. They described the devastating shock they experienced when they learned about the abnormal newborn screen and the subsequent "emotional roller coaster" related to the diagnosis and adaptation to life with a child who has special healthcare needs. They knew of no family history of CF and had never heard of it before their child's birth—which added to their surprise when informed about the diagnosis. Although both parents were actually involved in the assessment, the remainder of this case includes only mother and child information, partly for parsimony in writing and partly because she was the primary caregiver.

Based on mother's completion of the Center for Epidemiologic Studies Depression Scale (Radloff, 1977), she was experiencing mild depressive symptoms. The Parenting Stress Index (Abidin, 1986) suggested a low sense of competence in parenting, social isolation, and that she viewed parenting Jeremy as demanding. The assessment also suggested a supportive spousal relationship that was confirmed during the interview. The Parent–Child Early Relational Assessment (Clark, 1985, 2006) was used to assess the affective and behavioral quality of interactions between Wendy and Jeremy during a snack, free play, and structured task. Assessment of these 5-minute vignettes was divided into parent, infant, and dyadic domains. Observations of Jeremy showed him to have wide affective range; he made good eye contact with his mother, his verbal and nonverbal messages were easy to read, and his play and activity levels were age appropriate. Additionally, his behavior suggested a strong will; for example, he cried easily when he did not get his way. However, he soothed easily when distressed, usually after his mother gave in to his demands. Observations of Wendy showed her to have a limited range in affect, appearing tense most of the time. The video also illustrated how she was unwittingly reinforcing his refusal behavior. Her approach to feeding was oriented more toward accomplishing the task of getting Jeremy to ingest food, than any social aspect of a shared mealtime. To accomplish her goal, she seemed to either misread or ignore his cues. By contrast, during the play interaction and structured task, she was warm and nurturing. She showed a capacity to mirror his affect and sensitively respond to his social initiative. She also appeared to be comfortable with him not completing those tasks.

Video Playback

A video playback session (Clark, 1985, 2006) was conducted with Wendy for the purpose of gathering additional information about the meaning that she ascribed to Jeremy, his diagnosis, and his behavior. It also served as an intervention by collaborating with Wendy to develop goals for the intervention plan, to amplify and build upon existing family strengths, and identify areas of concerns or parenting challenges. During that session, Wendy discussed her concerns about Jeremy's CF diagnosis, her sense of guilt for "giving him defective genes," and an urgency to "keep him healthy." She tearfully recounted her reaction to the initial diagnosis as a "death sentence." She also noted that, over time, seeing Jeremy's growth and development has helped her feel more hopeful. She explained how she remains ever vigilant for signs of respiratory illness and committed to providing him "lots of calories" as recommended by the CF experts who reportedly emphasized "that is the best way to keep him healthy." When Jeremy refused foods she offered, she reported that she also felt like he was rejecting her. She confided that she and her husband have no one to talk with about their situation. She explained that friends and relatives try to be supportive "but no one really understands." They knew no other families affected by CF. Furthermore, their attempts to prevent Jeremy's exposure to respiratory infections led them to limiting how much they socialized with other people. Thus, she felt isolated.

On the videotape, they observed how, when he refused to eat, she tried harder to cajole him, which led to even more vehement refusal behavior from Jeremy. Together the clinician and Wendy discussed their shared observations of how he became increasingly emotionally dysregulated and behaviorally disruptive while she looked increasingly frustrated and anxious. She commented that such behavior caused her to feel like a "failure" because, as she stated, "a good parent should know how to feed her own child and his health and future depend on it." They also viewed the interactions with Jeremy during play and the structured task of building blocks. She agreed that the two of them were much more relaxed. She commented about how much she enjoyed just playing with Jeremy—something she rarely had time to do. This session provided an opportunity to point out how Jeremy's facial expression brightened to her smile, eye contact, and warm tone of voice. They both noted how much more cooperative he was during those segments.

Intervention

The clinician and Wendy jointly developed intervention goals based on assessment information gleaned from the interview, parent self-reports, videotaped observations, and video playback sessions (Clark, Tluczek, & Gallagher, 2004). These goals included (a) support Jeremy's development of age-appropriate autonomy, (b) increase Wendy's problem-solving competencies and self-confidence in parenting, (c) enhance the quality of the parent–child relationship, and (d) promote Wendy's coping capacities.

To accomplish these goals, the intervention incorporated GP, described as "[an experienced] guide helping another person become competent enough to engage in a socially important activity by providing expertise and working alongside the learner" (Chapter 1). Examples of various components of GP, illustrated in Chapter 1, Figure 1.1, are noted in parentheses in the following text. The clinician served as the guide for Wendy, the learner. GP, as a relation-based method of teaching and learning, presumes trust between the guide and learner (getting and staying connected). Therefore, the clinician used a parallel process in her relationship with Wendy to model the sensitive responsiveness she was helping Wendy to learn (joining, bridging). For example, the clinician tried to remain attuned to Wendy's expressions of emotion and responded empathically to Wendy's cues by naming the emotion as well as the content of Wendy's communications. In response to Wendy's account of Jeremy's uncooperative behavior, the clinician stated, "It sounds like Jeremy's resistance to your efforts are really frustrating for you. You recognize how important eating and chest therapy are and when things do not go as you wish, you become worried about the effects on Jeremy's health and you feel bad about your parenting. Is that right?" Such conversations afforded opportunities for clarifying the clinician's appraisal of Wendy's concerns (sharing understanding) and normalizing this mother's experience.

Interventions for this family were based on the conceptualization that they had many competencies, which Wendy and the clinician used as a foundation upon which to work together in scaffolding to help Wendy build new competencies. Foundational competencies included the following:

- *Being with:* Wendy's capacity for warm gentle interactions with Jeremy
- *Knowing and relating to Jeremy as a unique person and emotion regulation:* Wendy's motivation to meet his psychosocial as well as his health needs
- *Communicating and engaging, knowing and being with:* a supportive marital relationship
- *Doing the task:* Jeremy's normative development
- *Emotion regulation:* Jeremy's cheerful demeanor
- *Knowing and relating, being with, emotion regulation:* Jeremy's mix of exploratory and secure-base proximity-seeking behavior suggesting a secure attachment to his mother

Competency development focused on Wendy's struggle to understand and accommodate the normative development of her child's strivings for autonomy while adhering to recommended CF care, which the child still depended upon her to provide (doing the task, problem solving, decision making). This clash between the child's developmentally driven behavior and mother's caregiving goals contributed to her self-doubt about her competency as a parent. Her self-doubt was exacerbated by her misinterpretation of her child's behavior as "rejecting" her (mother's emotion regulation, knowing, and relating). She also appeared to still be grieving the loss associated with the CF diagnosis and she was obviously very worried about her son's future (mother's emotion regulation). Her attempts to protect Jeremy from infections prevented her from receiving much-needed social support (problem solving, communicating). Her self-doubts, grief, anxiety, and social isolation most likely contributed to her depressive symptoms (mother's emotion regulation).

ANTICIPATORY GUIDANCE TO SUPPORT TODDLER AUTONOMY

Some sessions combined nonjudgmental developmental, anticipatory guidance (Pridham, 1993) with GP. Information about child development was blended with evidence in support of Wendy's competent parenting (communicating and engaging). For example, the clinician helped Wendy reframe her understanding of Jeremy's use of "no" and refusal behaviors as the normal developmental transition from infancy to toddlerhood. Such strong-willed, goal-directed behavior indicated that he was becoming his own person, wanting to learn new things and become more independent. The clinician emphasized that, while challenging, these are desirable milestones and a credit to Wendy's responsive and nurturing parenting, particularly during his first year of life. After consulting with the CF center experts, the clinician also reviewed the child's growth charts with the mother and pointed out the steady healthy growth pattern that reflected her effectiveness in providing her child adequate nutrition. They discussed eating patterns that are typical of toddlers and preschool children, such as food jags (e.g., only wanting to eat a certain food, neophobia [dislike of new foods]). Wendy received written materials with tips about feeding toddlers, was directed to website that address these issues, and was encouraged to discuss her concerns with the nutritionist at the CF center (bridging, joining, and maintaining attention). Suggestions included offering a variety of healthy food options and a recognizing a toddler's need for autonomy in wanting to feed himself. Therefore, finger foods that Jeremy can easily eat by himself are optimal. The clinician/guide suggested that Wendy make mealtime an enjoyable family event and avoid focusing on Jeremy not eating. The clinician also suggested that Wendy let Jeremy be messy. The sensory pleasures of playing with food might increase his interest in eating it. To parents of infants and toddlers, this idea may be new and go against the parent's own experiences of being parented (e.g., parental messages she received as a child such as "Don't play with your food"). Photos of young children with food in their hair, smiling broadly or hands in their food dish may serve as examples of what is possible (bridging from the known to the new). Reviewing the videotape of Jeremy eating solid food also provided in-the-moment examples of the enjoyment and developmental pleasure he derives from feeding himself. As Wendy came to understand and adopt such eating practices, the GP process of transferring responsibility from guide to learner was effective.

Content also focused on helping Wendy understand the principles of social learning theory (Miller, 2011) that she could apply to any child behavior including, but not limited to, mealtime and chest therapy. The ABCs of child behavior modification include Antecedent→ Behavior → Consequences (bridging). Antecedents are things that come before and therefore influence the identified behavior. Parents can help the child be successful by providing antecedents that encourage cooperative behavior. Antecedents can include consistency, giving clear directions, foreshadowing transitions from one activity to the next (e.g., from play to chest therapy; from chest therapy to mealtime; from mealtime to play). Consequences are the things that happen afterward and can also influence the child's behavior. Negative as well as positive reinforcements can cause problem behavior to persist. For example, cajoling or pleading with a child to eat is a form of negative reinforcement because these behaviors are a kind of parental attention. Therefore, it is wise to avoid cajoling, pleading, bribing, or force-feeding. Wendy was also encouraged to remember grandma's rule, "You can have dessert after you have eaten your vegetables or food." She was taught that it is more effective to ignore minor problem behavior (e.g., food refusal) and notice the child's cooperative behavior with praise and encouragement.

GP TO ENHANCE PARENTAL COMPETENCIES AND QUALITY OF PARENT–CHILD RELATIONSHIP

GP (Pridham et al., 1998) was used to enhance parental competencies and the quality of the parent–child relationship. Interventions focused on specific domains to help Wendy (a) be with Jeremy in a mutually enjoyable way and gain insights about who he is as a person and (b) problem solve challenging parenting situations. The GP was accomplished by using a technique called "bug in the ear." Parent and child were situated by themselves in the clinic playroom. Wendy was given an ear piece that allowed her to receive verbal communications from the clinician who could observe the dyad from behind a mirrored window but could not be seen by the parent or child. The clinician used a phone to communicate suggestions that guided the mother in her interactions with her child. The clinician made a strategic decision to begin building competencies that centered around mother and child being together in mutually enjoyable ways, thus, increasing the reinforcement value of the interactions for each member of the dyad (structuring the task/learning → competencies).

During the first GP sessions, the clinician introduced Wendy and Jeremy to "floor time" (Greenspan & Wiedner, 1998), sometimes referred to as "special play." Floor time involves about 15 minutes of one-on-one playtime between parent and the child. Typically, the parent gets down on the floor and follows the child's lead in play. Parents are encouraged to carefully "tune into" what the child is doing, using a warm tone of voice to describe what the child is doing and unobtrusively imitating the child's play. In so doing, the parent encourages shared attention, two-way communication, and the child's expression of feelings and ideas. It also allows the child to experience the parent as being fully present, emotionally as well as physically, just for him. During these sessions, the clinician offered Wendy suggestions about what to notice about Jeremy's play (e.g., his enjoyment of putting toys in and out of containers, his gleeful surprise with pop-up toys). She verbally guided Wendy to mirror affect. Mirroring affect includes such responses as expressing surprise when Jeremy shows surprise. The clinician also assisted Wendy in monitoring her facial expressions, tone of voice, and gestures so she could respond to Jeremy's play initiatives in a reciprocal manner (getting and staying connected, joining and maintaining attention, sharing understanding → being with, knowing and relating, communicating and engaging). Wendy was advised to engage in floor time with Jeremy at home at least three times per week (transferring responsibility → doing the task). Upon perfecting this technique, Wendy commented that floor time provided her a better appreciation of Jeremy's likes and dislikes, his personality, who he is, rather than her imposing an image of who she might want him to be or become.

Subsequent GP sessions focused on helping Wendy build competencies in the application of the social learning principles to the contexts of mealtime and chest therapy. Sessions were structured to replicate situations the dyad would likely experience at home (structuring the task/learning → problem solving). The clinician encouraged Wendy to bring foods she would typically offer him at home and the equipment she used for chest therapy. Separate sessions were devoted to each context. The "bug in the ear" technique was also used. For example, during mealtime, the clinician guided Wendy in what to say and how to talk with Jeremy during mealtime. She was encouraged to take a similar approach as with floor time by simply using a warm "mommyese" tone of voice to describe what she observed in Jeremy, for example, "You really like feeding yourself, don't you?" and "That was a big bite of carrot you took." Occasionally, Jeremy would offer her a bite of his food. Wendy was encouraged to accept the food with a warm "thank you" and reciprocate with an offer of something from her plate with "Do you want a taste of Mommy's fruit?" When his attention turned to other objects in the room (e.g., lights in the ceiling), she was guided to notice the switch and verbally reflect it, stating, "You see those bright lights?" The clinician helped her recognize and sensitively respond to Jeremy's cues indicating that he had reached satiety and wanted no more to eat, though he had not finished all the food on his plate. She used phrases such as "Looks like you are all done. Are you all done?" She was coached in using specific praise at the end of the meal in a way that recognized his autonomy: "You did such a nice job of eating all by yourself!"

The chest therapy sessions were similar in the use of GP and application of social learning principles. There were several notable differences.

These sessions involved helping Wendy identify playful distractions that would make the chest therapy more enjoyable and hold Jeremy's interest. Examples included singing child-friendly songs, giving him a stuffed animal to hug or imitate mother doing chest therapy, telling him stories, and blowing bubbles together when he needed to take deep breaths. These sessions also involved helping Wendy recognize the limitation of his ability to sit still. Just *before* he was likely to begin protesting, she was coached to interrupt the therapy, have them both stand up, and do jumping jacks or some fun physical activity for just a few minutes before returning to complete the chest therapy. After several sessions, Wendy reported much improvement in Jeremy's cooperation (transferring responsibility → doing the task).

SUPPORT OF PARENTAL COPING CAPACITIES

The clinician also directly addressed Wendy's coping needs. For example, Wendy was prone to "catastrophize" situations. When she observed a change in Jeremy (e.g., nasal sniffle), she thought about the worst-case scenario, which understandably increased her anxiety. The clinician helped her to recognize when such thoughts entered her mind and to use self-talk to "stop" them and examine the evidence for the scenario. Wendy was encouraged to consider what actions she could take to prevent negative outcomes. The point of this exercise was to help her recognize that she had agency in controlling her thoughts and related anxieties as well as to influence potential outcomes. The clinician also encouraged Wendy to consider using mindfulness exercises (e.g., daily meditation for 5 minutes) to help her relax, stay focused, and manage her own emotions. The clinician used GP to assist Wendy in acquiring these skills (joining and maintaining attention, structuring task/learning → emotional regulation, doing the task). Finally, the clinician collaborated with the CF center to assist Wendy in connecting with other parents who had children around the same age as Jeremy as sources of mutual social support (bridging and transferring responsibility → emotional regulation). Upon completion of a series of sessions, Wendy reported much improvement in her mood and decreased depressive symptoms.

CONCLUSION

This relationally based intervention combined theories of child development, emotion regulation, and strategies from GP to effectively address the psychosocial development and healthcare needs of a toddler with a serious health condition, increase parental problem-solving competencies and self-confidence, enhance the parent–child relationship, and improve parental coping capacities. This case underscores the value of addressing the parents' personal issues as well as the child's needs, amplifying family strengths, and collaborating with the parent/family throughout the intervention process.

REFERENCES

Abidin, R. R. (1983). *Parenting stress index: Manual, administration booklet, [and] research update.* Charlottesville, VA: Pediatric Psychology Press.

Bowlby, J. (1988). *A secure base: Parent-child attachment and healthy human development.* New York, NY: Basic Books.

Clark, R. (1985, 2006). *The parent-child early relational assessment.* Unpublished instrument. Madison, WI: Department of Psychiatry, University of Wisconsin Medical School.

Clark, R., Tluczek, A., & Gallagher, K. C. (2004). Assessment of parent-child early relational disturbances. In R. Del Carmen-Wiggins & A. Carter (Eds.), *Assessment of mental health disorders in infants and toddlers* (pp. 25–60). New York, NY: Oxford University Press.

Cystic Fibrosis Foundation. (n.d.). Retrieved March 28, 2018 https://www.cff.org/What-is-CF/About-Cystic-Fibrosis

Davies, D. (2011). *Child development: A practitioner's guide* (3rd ed.). New York, NY: Guilford Press.

Davies, J. C., Ebdon, A., & Orchard, C. (2014). Recent advances in the management of cystic fibrosis. *Archives of Disease in Childhood, 99*(11), 1033–1036.

DeKlyen, M., & Greenberg, M. T. (2008). Attachment and psychopathology in childhood. In J. Cassidy & P. R. Shaver (Eds.), *Handbook of attachment: Theory, research, and clinical applications* (2nd ed., pp. 637–665). New York, NY: Guilford Press.

Ernst, M. M., Johnson, M. C., & Stark, L. J. (2010). Developmental and psychosocial issues in CF. *Child and Adolescent Psychiatric Clinics of North America, 19*(2), 263–283.

Glasscoe, C., Lancaster, G. A., Smyth, R. L., & Hill, J. (2007). Parental depression following the early diagnosis of cystic fibrosis: A matched, prospective study. *Journal of Pediatrics, 150*(2), 185–191.

Goodman, S. H. (2007). Depression in mothers. *The Annual Review of Clinical Psychology, 3,* 107–135.

Greenspan, S. I, & Wiedner, S. (1998). *The child with special needs: Encouraging intellectual and emotional growth.* Reading, MA: Addison-Wesley Longman, Inc.

Landy, S. (2002). *Pathways to competence: Encouraging healthy social and emotional development in young children.* Baltimore, MD: Paul H. Brookes Publishing.

Lieberman, A. (1993). *The emotional life of the toddler.* New York, NY: Free Press.

Lor, M., Crooks, N., & Tluczek, A. (2016). A proposed model of person-, family-, and culture-centered nursing care. *Nursing Outlook, 64*(4), 352–366. doi:10.1016/j.outlook.2016.02.006

Mahler, M. S., Pine, F., & Bergman, A. (1975). *The psychological birth of the infant: Symbiosis and individuation.* New York, NY: Basic Books.

Marshall, B. C. (2017). Survival trending upward but what does this really mean? Cystic Fibrosis Foundation. Retrieved March 28, 2018 from https://www.cff.org/CF-Community-Blog/Posts/2017/Survival-Trending-Upward-but-What-Does-This-Really-Mean

Miller, P. H. (2011). *Theories of developmental psychology.* New York, NY: Worth Publishing.

Montgomery, G. S., & Howenstine, M. (2009). Cystic fibrosis. *Pediatrics in Review, 30*(8), 302–309. doi:10.1542/pir.30-8-302 quiz 310

Pridham, K. F. (1993). Anticipatory guidance of parents of newborns: Potential contribution of the internal working model construct. *Journal of Nursing Scholarship, 25*(1), 49–56.

Pridham, K. F., Limbo, R., Schroeder, M., Thoyre, S., & Van Riper, M. (1998). Guided participation and development of care-giving competencies for families of low birth-weight infants. *Journal of Advanced Nursing, 28*(5), 948–958.

Radloff, L. S. (1977). The CES-D Scale: A self-report depression scale for research in the general population. *Applied Psychological Measurement, 1*(3), 385–401.

Schechter, M. S., & Gutierrez, H. H. (2010). Improving the quality of care for patients with cystic fibrosis. *Current Opinion in Pediatrics, 22*(3), 296–301.

Simmons, R., Goldberg, S., Washington, J., Fischer-Fay, A., & Maclusky, I. (1995). Infant–mother attachment and nutrition in children with cystic fibrosis. *Journal of Developmental and Behavioral Pediatrics, 16*(3), 183–186.

Tluczek, A., Clark, R., Kosick, R. L., & Farrell, P. M. (2005). Mother–infant relationship in the context of neonatal CF diagnosis: Preliminary findings. *Pediatric Pulmonology, 28,* 179–180.

Tluczek, A., Clark, R., McKechnie, A. C., Orland, K. M., & Brown, R. L. (2010). Task-oriented and bottle feeding adversely affect the quality of mother–infant interactions after abnormal newborn screens. *Journal of Developmental and Behavioral Pediatrics, 31*(5), 414–426.

Tluczek, A., McKechnie, A. C., & Brown, R. L. (2011). Factors associated with parental perception of child vulnerability 12 months after abnormal newborn screening results. *Research Nursing Health, 34*(5), 389–400.

17

Guided Participation in Public Health Nursing Practice

Jill Paradowski, Polly Belcher, Mary McCarron, and Karen Pridham

Guided participation (GP) used by public health nurses (PHNs) with families of infants highly vulnerable to morbidity and growth and developmental deficits functions to promote health and prevent illness and to aid parents of vulnerable infants to access and link with clinical care. All of these GP functions target major aims of public health nursing (Bekemeier, Zahner, Kulbok, Merrill, & Kub, 2016; Swider, Krothe, Reyes, & Cravetz, 2013; Swider, Levin, & Reising, 2017). How GP can be used by PHNs to promote health and prevent illness is described in this chapter and is based on the experiences of five PHNs and their nurse supervisor. The knowledge and skills these PHNs developed for GP practice were supported through participation in two sequential pilot programs (Pridham, Krolikowski, et al., 2006; Pridham, Limbo, Schroeder, Krolikowski, & Henriques, 2006).

The GP processes highlighted in this chapter include transferring responsibility from NICU nurses to a PHN and from PHN to mother; joining and maintaining attention, which entails sharing understanding; making connections or bridging understandings for development of new or different ways of caregiving and of working with the infant's clinicians; and structuring partnership relationships of the mother, PHN, and primary care clinicians. All of the infants in this report were premature and very low birth weight (VLBW). The following case example is used to illustrate typical challenges encountered by PHNs as well as opportunities to effectively engage families in addressing caregiving issues using GP methods. We revisit this case throughout the chapter.

Myla sits on the edge of her single bed in her bedroom of her family's home, holding her 1-month-old prematurely born, VLBW infant, Nadia. The PHN has come to visit concerning Nadia's nutritional intake, growth, and developmental progress as well as her health status in general. Nadia's growth has been less than expected, and her formula intake has been less than her doctor advised Nadia's mother to aim for. Myla is preparing to feed Nadia a bottle of formula while simultaneously adjusting the television station to a soap opera she watches every day. Nadia is making smacking sounds with her lips while trying to suck on her hands. She is receiving supplemental oxygen for chronic lung disease through a nasal cannula. Her 2-year-old brother is playing in a corner near the bed with a toy the PHN has brought in her bag. Nadia eagerly accepts the nipple and gazes at her mother's face. Myla, soon after the feeding has begun, however, turns her gaze to the soap opera. Nadia loses her grasp of the nipple and her gaze changes to a half-lidded, drowsy appearance. In about a minute, Myla notices that Nadia has zoned out of the feeding. She rubs her face in frustration mixed with anxiety.

PUBLIC HEALTH NURSING AND GP IN THE HOME

Public health nursing is a unique practice requiring nurses to use many skills independently as they provide care in a variety of settings (Wald, 1934). Homes have become the main location for public health nursing visits because they provide a family setting for comprehensive assessment and intervention—for the most part, educational—generally not feasible in clinical environments. Home visiting of families during pregnancy and infancy by PHNs has shown enduring, positive health effects (Kitzman et al., 2010; Olds et al., 2014). Visiting families in their homes provides PHNs an opportunity to be with parents in a locale where they are not only in control of activities but also left on their own to care for their infant. Often families have little support. Frequent home visits allow for a PHN to form enduring relationships within the family.

GP processes and the competencies it aims to support are consistent with educational functions of public health nursing to equip families for autonomous and collaborative caring for members who have or are vulnerable to health deficits (Swider et al., 2017). For the population of families with a prematurely born VLBW infant, vulnerable to health, growth, and developmental deficits, PHNs are oriented to the participation and autonomy of the family and its individual members, all hallmarks of GP. Within the family environment, PHNs are primed for GP by the opportunity to witness caregiving issues and to observe family members interacting about them and revealing their caregiving compentencies. In addition, PHNs are in a position to identify structures and scaffolding provided within the family to support caregiving competencies.

PHNs are in a good position to assess GP outcomes and consequences of naturally occurring events supportive of GP over time. Furthermore, family goals and needs for health-related teaching–learning—prerequisite knowledge for GP—may be more discernible and recognizable when observed through conversation in the home. In sum, GP fits right into home visiting practice, particularly for parental caregiving of VLBW prematurely born infants. In the Midwestern urban setting of this chapter, we examine GP for teaching–learning\parents what they need for infant caregiving—feeding, in particular, monitoring infant health status, and responding to changes in status with good judgment.

A PLAN TO ADDRESS FAMILY NEEDS TO DEVELOP COMPETENCIES FOR CAREGIVING OF VLBW INFANTS

PHNs working in a large urban health department often have many roles to fill as they serve their community. Commonly funded from many sources, the position description of PHNs is often linked to the objectives of that funding, thus limiting flexibility in home visiting. The PHNs whose work is described in this study were engaged in a health department program structured for frequent visits to families of VLBW infants made at appointed times within a 3-year period of time for each family.

Historically, serving at-risk populations has been a major part of a PHN's work. Beginning in the last decade of the 20th century, the rate of preterm infant births in the city often reached 10% of the total births, an estimated 1,000 infants each year. Health department policy determined that selected PHNs would give priority for home visits to families of VLBW infants born very prematurely. Many of these infants required assessment of health status as often as every week after coming home from the hospital. Only infants most at risk and born most prematurely and with low birth weight would receive this intensive follow-up.

A family program with comprehensive assessment processes was implemented to support the priority home visiting plan. An increased number of public health issues with fewer PHNs available to address them made it difficult for all of the families with VLBW infants who could have benefited from intensive nurse visits to receive them. Challenges presented to providing health promotional and preventive services to families of vulnerable infants included the complexity of the infant's medical condition and the family's limited resources, both of which at times made parent communication with the infant's healthcare clinicians tenuous, difficult, or uncertain.

As PHNs implemented the home visiting program to identify and respond to health-related needs of high-risk infants, a pilot program, funded by a foundation grant, was made available to PHNs and NICU nurses in the city. The program offered 12 months of classroom and clinical supervision in GP to PHNs and NICU nurses to support parents' competencies in caregiving of VLBW infants at home. This program included seven afternoons, totaling approximately 15 hours of classes interspersed with supervised GP. The supervised GP was given for one or two families selected from each nurse's own practice. Following the classroom time, each PHN had 9 months of GP practice facilitated in person or on the telephone by one of the three course instructors. A 1- to 1 1/2-hour session for reflective supervision (Fenichel, 1992; Ordway, Sadler, Dixon, & Slade, 2014) was held every other week at a public health district office. At the end of the course, PHNs received a certificate of completion from the University of Wisconsin–Madison Department of Continuing Education.

The GP course was designed to accomplish three major aims: (a) increase the competence of nurses regarding caregiving of the highly vulnerable VLBW infants, particularly their feeding and their early signs of physiologic change, instability, or decrements, that parents would need to handle, respond to, or contact the infant's clinician to manage; (b) increase NICU nurse and PHN competence in practice of GP and support its focused use with families of high-risk VLBW infants; and (c) develop, with NICU nurses and PHNs, collaborative patterns and competence for transfer of infant care responsibility to the family. A family service provider was available to work with the nurses and the families they served on social and resource issues. The description of the GP program and the work of PHNs that follows were contributed by PHN participants. Myla and her baby, Nadia, introduced at the beginning of this chapter, were one of the families served by a PHN using GP.

DEVELOPING GP PRACTICE

NICU Nurse–PHN Partnership: Platform for GP Practice

When we were asked to participate in the training for GP, we viewed the GP program as a good match for improving services to the at-risk infants and their families. Learning new skills to help mothers develop competencies in relating to, caring for, feeding, supporting growth and development, and monitoring health would make our public health nursing services more valuable to families and increase the benefit of visiting mothers just before or soon after bringing a prematurely born VLBW infant home from the NICU. Collaborating with NICU nurses to support mothers in taking responsibility for their infant's feeding through a transition that could be anxiety-laden and was often very scary could help us develop a relationship with families that put us in a better position to provide a useful service and to be welcomed into the home.

When a baby is born very early, the NICU staff is responsible for keeping the infant alive, growing, and developing. The infant's care requires many interventions from the nurse in charge of the infant, and parents' engagement in care of their infant may be discontinuous, disrupted, or confusing due to personal distress, the infant's condition, family conditions, or NICU opportunities (Aagaard, Uhrenfeldt, Spliid, & Fegran, 2015; Borghini et al., 2014; Brown, Griffin, Reyna, & Lewis, 2013; Park et al., 2016; Thoyre,

Hubbard, Park, Pridham, & McKechnie, 2016). Mothers shared stories with us (PHNs) when we home visited about their experiences when their babies were in the NICU. They reported often feeling like they had no control over what was going on or happening. PHNs spoke to NICU nurses to problem solve issues of infant care at discharge, but never really had a chance to connect with the NICU nurse prior to discharge. The GP program structured interaction of NICU nurses and PHNs prior to discharge. Both sets of nurses were able to establish relationships that were very important for mothers in gaining a sense of their caregiving competencies and in identifying what they needed to feel confident that they were expert in the care of their babies.

The GP program was designed to support a relationship between a NICU nurse and a PHN that would aid mothers in feeling more competent—and thus less anxious—in taking their babies home from the NICU. This relationship supported the expectation that a PHN needed an opportunity prior to the infant's NICU discharge to get acquainted with how comfortable the parents were in being with the baby, their competence in the techniques, strategies, and plans for care, their competence and assurance in problem solving with clinicians, and their steadiness and emotional resilience in dealing with difficulties. Knowledge of these competencies is the substance of transferring responsibility from NICU nurses to parents who would be followed by a PHN.

When we (PHNs) made visits, parents reflected with us about how frightening the technology of care in the NICU was, as well as the threat the NICU staff's attention to the details of infant feeding skill, nutrient intake, and growth presented to their confidence and sense of efficacy in caregiving. Their conversations with us about bringing the baby home from the hospital were laced with a sense of doubt in their capacity and competence in managing care. Mothers made clear their need for PHN GP to enlarge their competence in regulating emotion and in problem solving. A PHN commented on the mothers' experience in the NICU as follows:

> *The Parental Competencies for Infant Caregiving (**www.springerpub .com/pridham**, Chapter 1) provided a guide for charting gains mothers were making in caregiving competence.*

"It's not surprising that many moms feel less than confident in the NICU. It's a very complicated place, staffed by experts in medicine and technology. The nurses changed every shift, but there was only one mom. . . . Perhaps the most important thing that I would see happen over time while using guided participation with moms of preemies was that they would gradually become convinced they were the experts when it came to understanding their baby's cues and feeding needs."

A PHN described the GP program structure for collaboration of NICU nurses and PHNs:

"I spent time in the NICU meeting with families and nursing staff about the baby's anticipated needs at home. Then, when discharge was planned, the NICU nurse would arrange to see the family in the home with the goal of getting a clear sense of the baby's home-care environment and to figure out with parents how the baby's feedings would be done, and the sleep arrangements the parents had made for the baby."

After the infant had been at home for several weeks, the NICU nurse and PHN made a joint home visit to reassess the infant's health status, feeding and nutrient intake, growth, and development as well as family adaptation to the infant and to parenting and care. The deliberate steps the NICU nurse and PHN took to get acquainted with a family and infant in each other's setting of infant care was a unique part of the GP training. An assumption underlying this component of the GP program was that GP, as participatory teaching–learning, requires some knowledge of the life experience of the learners as a starting place for gaining joint attention and sharing understanding. Neither the families nor we as nurses had explicitly participated in this kind of practice arrangement prior to the GP program.

Learning and Practicing GP

The course work NICU nurses and PHNs had was designed to give them information about premature infants, their feeding, growth, and development, illness and health problems and response to them, development of relationships, and social services to support families. Concurrent with course work, GP program participants were identifying families with whom they were establishing a relationship for support of caregiving of a prematurely born VLBW infant. One of the three instructors/nurse guides worked with each nurse and the two or three families she worked with throughout the year of the program. GP practice was learned in the course of engaging in it with participation in guidance through personal interaction, joint home visits, and group input during reflective supervision. Nurse caregiving competencies were regularly assessed by nurses themselves and with faculty as a means of tracking progression in the course.

In addition to investing time in the classroom and being mentored and guided in GP, we had other tasks. We had to adapt our public health nursing practice in several ways. Not all of the GP program expectations were easy to accommodate. Fitting GP training into a very busy caseload with many and varied concurrent assignments was challenging. Often a plan to home visit a family with a VLBW infant was interrupted to cover a communicable disease outbreak, which always took priority. Continued home visiting to a family was difficult when the family was not home at the prearranged time.

 *The Nurse Caregiving Competency Assessment, accessible through this link: **www.springerpub.com/pridham**, Chapter 1, was a framework for nurses' periodic self-assessment.*

Reflective Supervision and Evaluation Research

Above and beyond the GP we were doing with specific families in our caseloads were the interactions with GP program instructors each of us had about our GP work and the reflective supervision sessions held every 2 weeks (Fenichel, 1992). The classroom, NICU, and home were settings where PHNs were mentored by nurses responsible for the GP program in a process parallel to what the PHNs were engaging in with parents. A goal for the nurse trainers was to help PHNs feel competent in practicing GP with parents so the parents could develop competence and confidence in caring for their infants.

In the reflective supervision sessions, we stepped back from direct work with families to reflect with the other PHNs in our group and two of the course instructors. Reflective supervision included discussion with the other PHNs and the NICU nurses training for and doing GP. The purpose of these sessions was to support development of our GP practice with specific families. We discussed what we were trying to accomplish, how it was going, how we were feeling about it, and how the relationships with the parents and family were developing. It was a safe place to express frustration, ineffectiveness, confusion, sadness, anger, and joy with insights and new understandings. The reflective supervision sessions required thinking through in advance what to share with the group and how to present it in an organized and clear way. Both the aims and format of reflective supervision were new to us, and we had to learn how to conceptualize a relationship and decipher its meaning in the behavior parents expressed in their interactions with us. We often reoriented our GP and saw new directions for GP with a family as a consequence of a reflective practice session.

The GP program required participation in evaluation research. Research is not often a component of a PHN's practice. PHNs engaged in three types of evidence gathering for program effectiveness: (a) regular assessment of GP practice competencies (Nurse Caregiving Competency Assessment, **www.springerpub .com/pridham**, Chapter 1); (b) problems developed from the situations of families with whom nurses were working; and (c) a survey of satisfaction with the program at the end of the year. The survey of nurse satisfaction is accessible through this link: **www.springerpub.com/pridham**, Chapter 17.

GP Processes in Relation to Infant Feeding: Structuring Video Recording and Playback With Myla

We had new practice processes to learn and use in homes. One of these processes was use of video recording of mother–infant interaction during feedings and spontaneous play followed by a semistructured conversation with the mother. This conversation was prompted and bounded by playback of selected segments of the recording. We will use the story of Myla and her baby daughter, Nadia, to illustrate the video-supported conversation about engagement in a caregiving (feeding) or play process. Myla had this conversation when her infant was 1 month old with the PHN who worked with her consistently through the year.

The PHN talked with Myla about how feedings usually went for her and Nadia, how this feeding was similar to or different from other recent feedings, and how she had decided to initiate and end the feeding. The PHN first stopped the video recording at the point when Nadia was gazing directly at her mother and eagerly taking formula from the bottle nipple while her mother returned the gaze. Myla commented spontaneously that Nadia was "real hungry, and wanted to feed." Myla intently watched the video as it played forward and frowned when Nadia pulled away from the nipple. The baby had half-lidded, drowsy-looking eyes that were no longer focused on her mother's face. Myla, herself, was focused on the soap opera on the television screen. The PHN stopped the video recording:

PHN: What is happening here for you and Nadia?
Myla: She knows I am not paying attention to her.
PHN: I wonder how that made you and Nadia feel?
Myla: She [Nadia] needs me to get someone else [Myla's mother or sister] to feed her when I know I am going to watch my soap.

Although Myla's response may have seemed to be an avoidance of responsibility, the PHN viewed this young mother as taking a step toward increased competence in assessing her baby's needs and her own capacity to meet them.

We learned that video recording, although it required some planning and change in usual visit procedure, could have an impact on a mother's feeding competencies when used with wondering about decision points and feelings to support a mother's reflection for making connections and learning.

Structuring GP for Learning and Practice in Public Health

Although GP training started with a curriculum for classroom instruction, much of the learning for GP practice occurred, in keeping with its participatory principles, while working with families to accomplish specific learning objectives concerning issues that mattered to them and their infant's health and well-being. To help define GP with families, a checklist of parent competencies, accessible through this link: **www.springerpub .com/pridham**, Chapter 1, was made available to PHNs taking the GP course to structure their practice, guide their observations, and aid follow-up and ongoing work with a family.

Methods for GP With Parents in the Home

PHNs need ways to identify parents' competencies in caring for their VLBW infant. Development of competencies and skills for GP involved structuring into home visits methods that had been developed in practice and research studies (Pridham, Limbo, Schroeder, Thoyre, & Van Riper, 1998).

Simulating Challenging Situations

One of the methods involved a PHN simulating situations a parent needed to problem solve. This method is illustrated in an article by Limbo, Peterson, and Pridham (2003). The participation of the parent was structured with questions that followed presentation of a challenging caregiving situation:

- What was going on? What did it mean for the baby and parent?
- What would the parent do?
- How would the parent know she had taken the right action?

Video Recording and Playback of Video Episodes

Processes of caregiving, particularly feeding, may be complex and difficult to recall. The goal was to obtain on video for later joint reflection a feeding as it naturally progressed, uninterrupted and not commented on by the PHN. Immediately following the feeding, viewing the video recording of the feeding was initiated with playback of specific, brief episodes of the feeding. These episodes had been noted by the PHN during the feeding to suggest the parent was problem solving, decision making, or expressing emotion or the infant was giving cues of need for a change in the feeding activity. The recording was stopped for brief, focused discussion with the parent of what was going on for the parent, the infant, or the feeding. Observation by PHN and parent of the same activity provided an opportunity for joining attention around tangible infant and parent feeding behavior and for the PHN to get a sense of the parent's understanding of infant cues for feeding needs. Recognizing, identifying, and responding sensitively to these cues are important competencies in feeding which the parents of a premature infant need to learn.

Watching a video recording with a mother of her feeding her infant and noting cues is a GP practice for developing feeding competencies. Mothers who watch their babies' feeding behavior for even a few brief 30-second to 1-minute video segments often get the idea of paying attention to infant signs of initiating, maintaining, or terminating a feeding or of needing to pause for breathing, fatigue, or other kinds of distress. Parents also learn to think through puzzling situations with questions such as What is going on here? What could explain what I am seeing? What can I do about it? What should I change? How will I know I did the right thing? The joint observation and the questions support a parent's development of feeding competencies.

One of the nurses shared this observation:

Watching for baby cues, like putting his hand toward his mouth, palm outward, helped his mother to recognize the baby's signs of needing a breather while eating. When I talked with the mother about this cue of needing a pause in feeding, she said: "I often see him doing that, and now I know why." When we were together the next time, she pointed out the cue the baby had given her. I praised her for watching her baby for cues while she fed him. Learning to think about infant behavior as cues of needs or agendas helped the mother to feel competent when feeding her baby.

Infants were not the only ones giving nonverbal cues during feedings. Often during a discussion, a mother would give a cue that she did not feel competent in what she was being asked to do. PHNs learned to stop and discuss what the mother was feeling.

Guidelines: A Vehicle for GP for Response to Health Problems

The Common Illness Guidelines, accessed through **www.springerpub .com/pridham**, Chapter 17, were written with input from parents to support a careful, informed, and effective response to a vulnerable infant's signs of acute illness or a common problem of infancy, for example, hard stools or "constipation" (Pridham, Krolikowski, et al., 2006). PHNs, along with a family service provider, in a feasibility study of the guidelines, explored their usefulness in helping parents problem solve how to respond to signs of illness, when to contact the infant's primary care provider, the information to give to the provider, and how to follow through in managing the illness or common infant health problems. One of the nurses reflected on the guidelines as follows:

> Often the mothers' confidence would dim when infants went home. Caring for their high risk babies without staff close by was tough, but when the baby got sick, it could be terrifying. Upper respiratory infections are especially dangerous for premature infants. The Guidelines helped mothers to problem solve with the baby's health care provider and then to decide with that provider what was the best course of action.

The guidelines provide information about illness and health problems that parents would need in order to recognize a problem and steps a parent could take before calling the baby's healthcare provider. When mothers who were participating with PHNs in the feasibility study brought their baby to a healthcare setting, they indicated they were more competent in their decision making and in sharing information with the provider when they used the guidelines. For PHNs, the guidelines were helpful in simulating illness situations and wondering with mothers about what they might do when the infant was ill. Often nurses role-played with a mother to help her feel competent when calling the doctor about the baby's signs of illness.

Nurse and Parent Caregiving Competencies

The competencies and skills we were learning to use in GP with parents coincided with the competencies and skills parents were learning through GP.

The competencies that we were developing, self-assessing, and reviewing with the course mentor, shown in the document Nurse Caregiving Competence Assessment—GP Process, indicated what to focus on in our GP practice. For both NICU nurses and PHNs, some competencies were new and some involved sharpening. Competencies for gaining joint attention to begin joint problem solving, for example, were novel for some nurses in respect to some conditions of infant feeding. Being with parents and sustaining a relationship, communicating with parents and the infant's clinicians about infant needs, problem-solving caregiving issues, and transferring responsibility to parents were at the core of the competencies we were developing through GP with the GP course instructors and, in particular, the course mentor who worked with specific PHNs throughout the year to reflect on the GP they were doing with parents and to review development of competencies.

The GP Program and Practice

Perhaps as important as developing competencies for direct GP practice with parents was developing competencies for a working relationship with NICU nurses to aid transfer of caregiving of the infant to parents in hospital and eventually at home. When reflecting on the GP program, the following comments were made by PHNs:

- GP was an important skill to use with families and the course work.
- Support, and interaction with the NICU nurses, was an experience that could be used as a model for application in other settings of nursing practice.
- Families certainly benefited from this training.
- The relationship with families, developed through frequent home visits, was credited with being a key factor in the success of GP practice over the long run of visits.
- The basics of GP, especially the focus on parents' development of competency in child caregiving, were key concepts for PHNs to learn and then use with families.

One nurse expressed her assessment of GP practice in this question:

What could be more critical for parents to learn than about their competence for caring for their at-risk infant and about their expertise in their babies' care?

Being with a parent was particularly important as PHNs interacted with parents, both inside the NICU and once they had taken the baby home. The mother was listened to and supported in viewing herself early on as having a part in her baby's care. The mother's having a goal and a plan helped the baby and the mother.

Another nurse observed:

> Guided participation is useful with mothers who are caring for a VLBW infant, but also with many other families. It becomes part of my relationship building and in helping whomever I am dealing with to feel more competent.

The structure of the course provided an opportunity for discussions between nurses from two very different practices of nursing. The interaction of nurses from both practices helped not only the family but also the nurses involved. Each practice of nursing was important for the success of the family. Contact with the NICU nurses benefited not only the families involved with the study but also improved the general communication between the NICU units and the health department. These relationships were important for these families as well as those to come. Two of the nurses involved in the study felt that the GP program provided an opportunity to appreciate what happens to families while their infant is hospitalized and also what is necessary to make a smooth transition to home possible.

When a PHN was asked what difference GP had made in her practice she said this:

> I have been using guided participation for so long that I am no longer conscious of it most of the time. But whether it's picking up cues from a client who might be in need, monitoring my own nonverbal cues so as not to interrupt a client, parenting my own children, even watching an audience when I'm teaching a class, I am forever grateful for having been schooled in guided participation.

CONCLUSION

Myla was home visited when Nadia was 1 year old. Now a toddler, Nadia sat on the floor "feeding" a baby doll with a tiny bottle and nipple. The PHN commented on how gently and attentively Nadia fed her doll and wondered with Myla how her child had learned to feed so responsively. Myla claimed not to know. The PHN continued talking with Myla about what had happened for her in feeding Nadia and, in particular, about her experience in periodically viewing the video recording of feeding through Nadia's first year. Myla responded, "I learned that I had to pay attention to my baby while she was feeding."

Reflections on GP in Public Health Nursing Practice

GP is consistent with the strong educational thrust of public health nursing practice. Reflecting on it, we want to share these points as we conclude the chapter:

- GP for public health nursing must be adaptable to the circumstances in which PHNs work and the family lives.

- PHNs generally have a concept of what healthy conditions are (e.g., they have set goals for the infant's care and desired outcomes at various ages and stages).
- Attention to what parents are working on and need to work on in light of health objectives and family and environmental challenges and resources is a place to start GP with parents of an infant, born very prematurely and with VLBW.
- GP practice derives from and operates in relation to what the infant's parents are working on in the context and constraints of a PHN's overall practice demands.
- GP often does not flow out of a structured curriculum, but has to flexibly issue from what is going on in the family and the time constraints for both PHN and family.
- The effectiveness of GP practice may be influenced by many factors, among them probably these: (a) PHN sensitivity and responsiveness to the parents' motivations for infant caregiving, parental orientation to caregiving (what they expect and intend to do), and what needs to take priority from the perspectives of both personal and public health and family culture; and (b) the support of the public health agency for the person/family-oriented competence that GP aims to develop over time.
- PHNs have responsibility in GP practice to keep in mind the knowledge parents need to have from health, developmental, and safety perspectives and to make it available to parents as learning is structured, connections are made, and responsibility for caregiving is transferred to parents. At the same time, PHNs keep in mind the issues that parents are working on and bring them into the larger health, safety, and developmental reality.
- For infants born very prematurely with VLBW, and likely other infants who have chronic or ongoing health vulnerabilities, PHNs may be in the best position to offer effective GP to a family if they can structure their GP to articulate with nurses in other sectors of the healthcare system, for example, in hospitals that provide secondary or tertiary care.
- Electronic means of communication and mobile apps may expedite transfer of responsibility between nurses, an aspect of GP in public health nursing that is yet to be explored.
- Reflective supervision is a facet of GP practice in public health nursing that shows promise of supporting new understandings. How it can be incorporated into very busy public health nursing units calls for ingenuity and persistence in bringing to bear reflectiveness, creativity, and regularity of PHN discussion.

Questions for Reflection

1. Imagine that you want to establish yourself as practicing GP with parents of high-risk infants. How would you introduce GP and your role as a guide to a family?

2. How would you structure moments of reflection, as described in Chapter 1, into your GP practice (a) with parents? (b) with other PHNs?
3. Identify a recent interaction with parents in which you were aware of a not-yet-confronted issue that was likely to be emotionally challenging yet needed to be discussed in order to make decisions. How would you wonder with the parents about how they viewed the issue? How would you start the discussion with the parents?

REFERENCES

Aagaard, H., Uhrenfeldt, L., Spliid, M., & Fegran, L. (2015). Parents' experiences of transition when their infants are discharged from the neonatal intensive care unit: A systematic review protocol. *JBI Database of Systematic Reviews and Implementation Reports, 13*(10), 123–132.

Bekemeier, B., Zahner, S. J., Julbok, P., Merrill, J., & Kub, J. (2016). Assuring a strong foundation for our nation's public health systems. *Nursing Outlook, 64,* 557–565. doi:10.1016/j.outlook.20016.05.013

Borghini, A., Habersaat, S., Forcada-Guex, M., Nessi, J., Pierrehumbert, B., Ansermet, F., & Muller-Nix, C. (2014). Effects of an early intervention on maternal post-traumatic stress symptoms and the quality of mother-infant interaction: The case of preterm birth. *Infant Behavior & Development, 37,* 624–631. doi:10.1016/j.infbeh.2014.08.003. Epub 2014 Sep 15.

Brown, L. F., Griffin, J., Reyna, B., & Lewis, M. (2013). The development of a mother's internal working model of feeding. *Journal of Specialists in Pediatric Nursing, 18,* 54–64. doi:10.1111/jspn.12011

Fenichel, E. (Ed.). (1992). *Learning through supervision and mentorship to support the development of infants, toddlers and their families: A source book.* Arlington, VA: Zero to Three.

Kitzman, H. J., Olds, D. L., Cole, R. E., Hanks, C. A., Anson, E. A., Arcoleo, K. J., & Holmberg, J. R. (2010). Enduring effects of prenatal and infancy home visiting by nurses: Follow-up of a randomized trial among children at age 12 years. *Archives of Pediatric & Adolescent Medicine, 164,* 412–418. doi:10.1001/archpediatrics.2010.76

Limbo, R., Petersen, W., & Pridham, K. F. (2003). Promoting safety of young children with guided participation processes. *Pediatric Health Care, 17,* 245–251. doi:10.1016/S0891-5245(02)88335-3

Olds, D. L., Kitzman, H., Knudtson, M. D., Anson, E., Smith, J. A., & Cole, R. (2014). Effect of home visiting by nurses on maternal and child mortality: Results of a two-decade follow-up of a randomized clinical trial. *Journal of the American Medical Association Pediatrics, 168,* 800–806. doi:10.1001/jamapediatrics.2014.472

Ordway, M. R., Sadler, L. S., Dixon, J., & Slade, A. (2014). Parental reflective functioning: Analysis and promotion of the concept for paediatric nursing. *Journal of Clinical Nursing, 23,* 3490–3500.

Park, J., Thoyre, S., Estrem, H., Pados, B. F., Knafl, G. J., & Brandon, D. (2016). Mothers' psychological distress and feeding of their preterm infants. *MCN. American Journal of Maternal Child Nursing, 41,* 221–229. doi:10.1097/NMC.0000000000000248

Pridham, K. F., Krolikowski, M. M., Limbo, R. K., Paradowski, J., Rudd, N., Meurer, J. R., . . . Henriques, J. B. (2006). Guiding mothers' management of health problems of very low birth-weight infants. *Public Health Nursing, 23,* 205–215. doi:PHN230302 [pii]

Pridham, K. F., Limbo, R., Schroeder, M., Krolikowski, M., & Henriques, J. (2006). A continuing education program for hospital and public health nurses to guide families of very low birth-weight infants in caregiving. *Journal of Continuing Education in Nursing, 37*(2), 74–85.

Swider, S. M., Krothe, J., Reyes, D., & Cravetz, M. (2013). The Quad Council practice competencies for public health nursing. *Public Health Nursing, 30,* 519–536. doi:10.1111/phn.12090

Swider, S. M., Levin, P. F., & Reising, V. (2017). Evidence of public health nursing effectiveness: A realist review. *Public Health Nursing, 34*(4), 324–334. doi:10.1111/phn.12320

Thoyre, S. M., Hubbard, C., Park, J., Pridham, K. F., & McKechnie, A. (2016). Implementing co-regulated feeding with mothers of preterm infants. *MCN. American Journal of Maternal and Child Nursing, 41,* 204–211. doi:10.1097/NMC.0000000000000245

Wald, L. (1934). *Windows on Henry Street.* Boston, MA: Little, Brown.

18

Guided Participation Practice for Pediatrics in a Community Hospital Setting

Michele M. Schroeder

Is it possible to make use of guided participation (GP) methods with nursing and interdisciplinary healthcare team members in a community hospital setting where care of children and families is part but not the focus of services offered in the organization? Can a clinical nurse specialist (CNS) take the GP methods described in working with children and families and apply them to working with team members as well—that is, engage in a parallel process that the CNS (guide) hopes in turn will be mirrored in team members' (learners) own clinical practice with children and families (see Chapter 1)? What results, if any, might be achieved by supporting nursing and interdisciplinary team members in this manner—those caring for children and families—and by extension, by supporting the children and families themselves? In this chapter, the practice of a pediatric CNS (the author) who uses GP processes to advance the care of children and families (not including infants and families in perinatal services) at a community hospital is explored, potential outcomes are identified, and questions for reflection are offered.

BACKGROUND

According to the American Hospital Association's 2015 Annual Survey (2017), 4,862 of the 5,564 registered hospitals in the United States are community hospitals. Of the remaining noncommunity hospitals, approximately 250 are children's hospitals (Children's Hospital Association, n.d.). While children's hospitals are geared to caring specifically for children of all ages with a wide range of acute and chronic health issues and their families (e.g., environment and supplies; primary and ancillary staff trained to care for children and families in developmentally and family-centered sensitive ways), community hospitals may or may not have access to, budgets for, and/or leadership support for specialized resources and education devoted exclusively to children and their families.

Nonetheless, clearly, there are many children and families coming to community hospitals for care. Staff may find themselves responsible for providing care to persons across the lifespan, from children of all ages (i.e., newborns, infants, toddlers, school agers, and adolescents) to very aged persons. Community hospitals and their staff are, by and large, very committed to providing the best care possible, with the resources available, to all those they serve, children and families included. However, community hospital staff do not always feel comfortable and confident in caring for children and families, often due to limited education and/or professional experiences specific to caring for children in a healthcare setting, which can be anxiety-inducing for staff.

Practice Site

The hospital is a nonprofit 448-bed community hospital, with a complete range of medical, surgical, and perinatal services, located in a Midwestern, midsized urban area. The service line emphasis is on adult and perinatal care specialties. There is a combined staff of approximately 3,500 employees. The hospital underwent a gradual realignment over a period of years in the scope of pediatric services offered outside of perinatal services as the local children's hospital expanded its depth and breadth of services available and local insurance companies adjusted coverage.

Over a period of approximately 25 years, inpatient pediatrics traveled from (a) its own floor unit—including several pediatric intensive unit (PICU) beds—staffed by pediatric-trained nurses who chose to care for children and families, to (b) semiprivate rooms at one end of the adult medical–surgical unit staffed by a combination of pediatric nurses and adult care nurses cross-trained to pediatrics, to (c) a three-room unit created within emergency services (following a similar model adopted by community hospitals on the east coast) staffed by emergency room nurses cross-trained to inpatient care, to (d) caring for older adolescent patients with routine conditions on the appropriate diagnosis-specific adult unit staffed by adult care nurses. For the most part, care offered here has been for children with common childhood conditions and illnesses, typically acute, self-limited health concerns. Children with more complex, life-threatening and/or chronic health conditions are typically cared for at the local children's hospital.

Staff Challenges

While healthcare clinicians are committed to providing the best care possible to all of their patients and families, sometimes they "don't know what they don't know." They may refer to and rely upon personal parenting experiences, values, and beliefs to guide the care offered, rather than systematic assessments incorporating evidence-based and developmentally grounded practices (Blake, Wright, & Waechter, 1970). Staff may be uncertain about, anxious, and/or afraid to take care of children, especially infants, toddlers, and preschoolers who are not yet able to communicate wants, needs, hurts, and fears in the typical, more familiar ways of older children and adults. For example, just like parents, staff may be worried about causing a child unnecessary discomfort or pain with procedures or interventions.

CNS Role and Responsibilities

CNS practice typically encompasses three broad areas or spheres of influence: (a) direct care with patients/clients and their families; (b) direct support of individual nurse practice and professional nursing practice as a whole; and (c) attention to systems/organizational issues affecting patient care (National CNS Competency Task Force, 2010). The CNS addresses these spheres through activities such as consultation, mentoring, project management, and program evaluation (Fulton, Lyon, & Goudreau, 2014). The development of thoughtful, respectful relationships with those one is engaging with is essential to the work at hand. Through collaborative, partnering relationships with patients and families and with the healthcare team members caring for them, CNSs are in a prime position to support the achievement and maintenance of healthy work environments (Disch, Walton, & Barnsteiner, 2001). CNSs can accomplish these functions, for example, by assisting staff with developing the needed competencies to safely and comfortably take care of children and their families, thereby reducing fears and anxieties generated by the unknown. GP strategies are ideally suited to accomplishing this goal.

Pediatric CNS practice in a community hospital setting involves effectively sharing specialized knowledge about children and families in order to position nurses and interdisciplinary colleagues to provide safe, timely, and developmentally sensitive care in ways they can feel good about (Blake, 1964b). This knowledge sharing also includes giving attention to assisting staff with identifying and developing the competencies— attitudes, behaviors, knowledge, and skills (Wright, 2005)—needed to consistently deliver appropriate care to children and families in keeping with professional practice standards and expectations. In turn, this attention supports efforts to offer care in truly family-centered ways (Blake, 1964a), a gold standard approach which has gained traction over the years yet remains a work in progress (Harrison, 2010).

GP PRACTICE IN ACTION

Using GP concepts and methods offers one way to address and reduce healthcare team member anxiety when confronted with caring for pediatric patients of all ages (newborns through age 17) with a range of common childhood medical and surgical diagnoses (e.g., pneumonia, asthma flare-ups, gastroenteritis, appendicitis, tonsillectomy, extremity fracture repair). GP practice as a CNS working with healthcare team members is often fluid and dynamic, reflective of and responsive to the nature of the relationships, internal working models of the issue at hand, and needs for competency development or support in the moment as care is being given (see Chapter 1). This section reviews GP competencies needed to success-fully address issues and reach goals, offers a clinical case example for consideration, then illustrates how GP processes can be used with health-care team members in parallel fashion to support the care of children and families. The content is presented linearly to assist with recognition and identification of concepts, not to imply that GP practice usually proceeds in this order.

Issue/Goal

An important goal of the pediatric CNS in a community hospital setting is to address the concerns and reduce the anxiety (issue) of the nursing staff (e.g., nurses, certified nursing assistants, health unit coordinators) and interdisci-plinary healthcare team members (e.g., respiratory therapists, pharmacists, physical therapists, medical imaging technologists, consulting services) car-ing for children and families, who on average have more experience with and knowledge about taking care of adult patients than pediatric patients. Facilitating competency development for caregiving of children and fam-ilies through the relationship-based teaching–learning approach of GP allows nurses and interdisciplinary healthcare team members to acquire the knowledge and skills needed to safely, effectively, and efficiently care for children and families. This in turn helps to decrease the discomfort and anx-iety healthcare team members may experience when taking care of pediatric patients—and may even result in staff who come to appreciate and look forward to caring for children and families.

Competencies

The premise is that through GP-directed interactions with the CNS (guide), healthcare team members (learners) will continue to develop their own competencies and, in turn, be able to engage as the guide with chil-dren and their families (learners) in similar ways—or even with cowork-ers. The guide makes use of demonstration, discussion, and the learner's lived experience of the process in developing GP competencies. Becoming skilled at the relationship competencies of "being with the other" and "knowing and relating to the other" requires a willingness of the guide to commit to and invest in the learner (Schroeder & Pridham, 2006). Skill with these two competencies are foundational for engaging in GP effectively.

Being With the Other

A guide's competency in "being with the other" may include (a) displaying and expressing a calm, open, nonjudgmental demeanor; (b) recognizing, acknowledging, and acting upon the learner's expressed or implied need for the guide's presence when learning about or taking the lead on doing the task; (c) expressing appreciation for and satisfaction with the role of being the learner's guide; and (d) expressing respect for and appreciation of the learner's unique story and qualities (Schroeder & Pridham, 2006). Being with can be (a) demonstrated (e.g., remaining with the learner), (b) discussed (e.g., "I learn so much from and with you when we have the chance to work together—Thank you!"), and (c) experienced (e.g., making a point of checking back in with the learner later in the shift to see how the day is going).

Knowing and Relating to the Other

A guide's competency in "knowing and relating to the other" may include (a) referring and responding to the learner as someone with specific preferences, needs, and learning styles; (b) intentionally investing in getting to know the learner; (c) reflecting back to the learner their understanding of the learner's situation and experience; and (d) taking time to figure out the learner's preferences, needs, and learning styles (Schroeder & Pridham, 2006). This approach makes explicit how to "individualize" a teaching–learning plan for helping staff develop needed caregiving competencies, which in turn may translate into skill at "individualizing" a plan of care for children and their families.

Communicating and Engaging

Becoming competent in methods for communicating and engaging with healthcare team members who (understandably) are focused on the "tasks" which comprise the work of taking care of their patients is essential. Both written (e.g., charting, notes in mailboxes, emails, texts) and verbal (e.g., wireless communication devices, paging systems, phone, in person) methods may be needed in order to efficiently and effectively communicate with healthcare team members. Knowing the usual flow of the day and best times to catch staff assists with this. A willingness and ability to be flexible regarding communication methods and timing is useful. Taking advantage of "teachable moments" applies just as much to staff learners as to the children and families being cared for. Learning how to clearly, concisely, and accurately convey concerns, questions, and observations is crucial for caregiving and GP practice that is coordinated across team members.

Doing the Task

There are numerous "tasks" or activities in taking care of patients, children, and families, which typically involve multiple steps or components. The guide can assist the learner with (a) identifying what the tasks are;

(b) prioritizing which to address in what order; (c) understanding the complexity and sequencing of a task; and (d) learning the outcomes that signal successful completion of the task. Often, when a healthcare team member is new to doing a task or is in the process of learning it, mental and physical energy is directed primarily toward accomplishing the concrete steps for completing the task. Being able to attend to other important aspects of the activity, like acknowledging family members, clarifying expectations and intentions for the task about to be undertaken, involving family members as desired, and briefly summarizing what will happen before starting may be challenging at first for the learner.

Problem Solving/Decision Making

Developing competency at problem solving or decision making is crucial to the process of transferring responsibility. This competency is evidence that the learner's internal working model for the activity at hand has grown to include an understanding of the "bigger picture" and what it takes not only to accomplish the activity under usual circumstances but to also effectively identify and manage any unexpected, unanticipated aspects. Wondering along with the learner about potential explanations for what is observed and experienced is an opportunity to brainstorm possibilities, confirm hunches, correct misunderstandings, and determine next steps as needed. Recognizing that one is approaching or has progressed to independent problem solving contributes to reducing anxiety, as the learner realizes that what was once new is now known.

Regulating Emotion

Being able to effectively regulate one's emotions is especially important when working with children, who often take their cues (verbal and nonverbal) from the adults with them on how to react and respond to emerging situations. If the adult expresses dread, fear, anxiety, and worry—for example, through frowning, a tight or higher pitched voice, avoiding eye contact, or quick, hurried body motions—the child is likely to respond in kind. The same can be said of anxious learners. The guide can assist learners with developing competency at regulating emotion by (a) demonstrating the use of a calm approach (lower-pitched voice, paying attention to slowing down motions); (b) sharing observations and wondering along with the learner in order to identify and name emotions (e.g., "I'm noticing that you are frowning and your voice is pitched higher; I wonder what might be going on for you right now?"); and (c) offering calming techniques for decreasing tension and anxiety in the moment (e.g., pausing before entering a patient room to let go of previous distractions and tune in to this child and family, slow deep breathing, counting to 10, or stepping out for a moment to regroup).

As you think about these competencies and then read the case example (names changed to protect privacy), see if you can identify GP competency development the CNS could support through engaging in GP processes in order to accomplish the goal of reducing a healthcare team member's observed or stated anxiety in caring for a child.

Case Example 18.1

Jack is a typically developing 18-month-old toddler admitted to the Medical/Surgical/Pediatrics unit for a community-acquired pneumonia (Stuckey-Schrock, Hayes, & George, 2012) requiring treatment with intravenous antibiotics due to worsening respiratory symptoms and fever. He lives in town at home with his mother (Tracy), father (Dave), maternal grandmother (Patrice), and 4-year-old sister (Susie). This is Jack's and his family's first experience with hospitalization other than when Jack and Susie were born. Jack is receiving 2 L of oxygen via nasal cannula to keep his oxygen saturation above 92%, has acetaminophen elixir ordered every 4 to 6 hours as needed for fever, and can eat a general diet as tolerated. Tracy is staying with Jack at the hospital, while Dave comes after work to visit and Patrice is at home caring for Susie. The cross-trained adult nurse (Polly), who has worked on this unit for 15 years and has two teenagers of her own, is assigned to care for Jack and can count on one hand how many pediatric patients she has taken care of in the last 5 months admitted for a respiratory condition.

Processes

Getting and Staying Connected

Relationship-building is at the heart of an effective CNS practice. Healthcare team members need to know they can count on the CNS to respond promptly, thoughtfully, and nonjudgmentally when called upon for help in caring for children and families. Sometimes the CNS may want to initiate contact with team members prior to a call for help, anticipating the potential need for assistance based on past experiences or knowledge of the learner. With Polly, knowing that she did not mind caring for children but did so infrequently due to her work schedule and felt a little "out of practice," I connected with her early in the shift—to let her know I was there, that I was interested in helping her day as well as Jack's and his family's day go as smoothly as possible, that I was available to assist as needed (e.g., with tasks, with problem solving, with staying calm).

Joining and Maintaining Attention

At Jack's bedside, his mother, Polly, and I reviewed the plan of care for Jack—for the current shift, for the day, and for his hospital stay. This helped us all think together about what to focus our attention on regarding the needs of Jack, his family, and Polly at this time. Tracy wanted Jack to have a bath at some point during the day. Polly wanted to review the components of a pediatric respiratory assessment. We (Tracy, Polly, and myself) agreed it made sense to do a baseline assessment of Jack's respiratory condition first, before undertaking a bath, to (a) help collect data to be used for comparison as the day progressed; (b) do the assessment while Jack was relatively quiet, before moving him around to accomplish a bath; and (c) offer the bath as something fun to look forward to after the "work" of the morning was completed. This especially pleased Jack's mother, as she shared, "Jack loves the water!"

Sharing Understanding

Reviewing Jack's plan of care (e.g., interventions to put his body in the best position possible to manage and heal from the pneumonia) was an avenue for learning how we each understood what the plan involved and what it would take to achieve it. It was an opportunity to create and/or refine a shared, common understanding of the plan, and to evaluate how the current plan was working by asking questions about what was not clear or what was missing. Potential misunderstandings or misconceptions could be identified and clarified. Questions such as "What are you hoping will happen today? What are you expecting will happen?" (see Chapter 11) provided information about each other's internal working model of the task at hand, thereby helping to reduce uncertainties (and thus anxiety) about what was involved and what to expect.

Bridging

A GP process often effective for decreasing anxiety about the unknown is to build bridges from the known to the new—such as, make explicit what the learner already knows and how it can be built upon to connect with what is new or currently not known as well. For Polly, her request to review a pediatric respiratory assessment was appropriate and understandable, given the reason for Jack's admission and how often Polly had the opportunity to actually perform a respiratory assessment on children. We started by reviewing what Polly already knew about respiratory assessment with adults in order to identify those components which are essentially the same regardless of the age of the patient (e.g., assessing respiratory effort; where to place the stethoscope for auscultation of breath sounds; if on oxygen, checking that all equipment and supplies are attached correctly and in good working order).

Structuring the Task/Learning

Through building on the foundation created by the relationship (getting and staying connected), identifying the task or goal to be worked on (joining and maintaining attention), making internal working models explicit to understand where each partner is coming from and to help create common expectations and goals (sharing understanding), and making connections from the known to the new (bridging), the CNS is then in a good position to structure the task or the learning at hand to be accomplished in ways that are likely to be experienced as respectful, nonthreatening, and helpful.

Structuring the learning might include helping the healthcare team member locate evidence-based, relevant sources of information regarding the task at hand, such as (a) textbooks in the hospital library; (b) online databases for journal articles; (c) hospital policies and procedures; (d) online skills reference tools; (e) online video resources; and/or (f) other colleagues (coworkers, leadership staff, staff on other units, specialists) to assist with review either in the moment or later. It may include demonstrating all or part of the task first, if appropriate. It may mean team member and CNS doing the task together and/or determining who will do which part(s). It may mean acknowledging that the guide is unsure about the answer to a question, pairing an "I don't know" statement with a "Here's what we'll do to find an answer" statement. Ideally, the CNS (guide) and the healthcare team member (learner) together determine how best to structure the learning that needs to happen based on what the learner already knows, what they need to know, and their preferred learning method.

For Polly, I started by reviewing a few key developmentally based assessment points (Pridham, Adelson, & Hansen, 1987) use with toddlers, including (a) gather what information you can before approaching/touching the toddler (e.g., respiratory rate and effort; color; alertness, responsiveness), which might cause distress and thus affect the assessment; (b) allow the toddler to stay in a position of comfort, such as on the family member's lap; (c) position yourself at the toddler's eye level when possible; (d) give the toddler something of their own to hold while you perform the assessment (e.g., a favorite or new toy, pillow, blanket); (e) choose the appropriate-sized stethoscope and warm it before placing it on the toddler's chest; (f) talk to the toddler about what you are doing, what will happen next, what it will feel/smell/sound/look like; and (g) wrap up with "All done!" when you are truly all done.

Polly preferred to have me talk her through what to do as she was doing it, with me directly next to her and my own stethoscope ready to listen if called upon—after having briefed Tracy on what we would be doing and how she could help. This approach respected the learning Polly had already incorporated into her practice and started at the point of requested assistance. Tracy held Jack on her lap throughout, comforting him and distracting him as needed. We completed the assessment by praising Jack for holding still, complimenting Tracy on her skill at keeping Jack distracted and comfortable throughout the assessment, and thanking them both for their part in achieving an accurate respiratory assessment. Pointing out what went well strengthens the foundation for the next time Polly needs to "do the task" and creates several satisfying moments between the guide (CNS) and the learner (staff nurse). Feeling more prepared and confident about "doing the task" contributes to achieving the larger goal of decreasing staff anxiety and discomfort.

Transferring Responsibility

"Readiness" is one evaluation criterion for determining when and how much to transfer responsibility for doing a task. Readiness may be determined in several ways. These include (a) asking learners if they feel ready to do the task; (b) hearing an affirmative response to "How about today if I start, then we work together, and finally you do the last step?"; or (c) "Remember the last time you took care of a child admitted with a respiratory condition, we talked about you doing [xxx] on your own the next time. Tell me how confident you feel about doing that today. I will be right beside you." Effective transferring of responsibility is a process which tends to happen through repeated experiences over time—it is not typically completely accomplished the first time through. This process can be challenging when staff have limited opportunities to practice and maintain the skills needed for the care of children and families. Under these circumstances, the process of transferring responsibility may move back and forth; expectations for achieving a full transfer may need to be adjusted.

OUTCOMES

While it is not possible at the moment to directly link nurse, interdisciplinary colleague, child, and family outcomes to the use of GP methods at the hospital I work at, it is not unreasonable to speculate that using GP methods has contributed to several positive outcomes. Anecdotally, staff have described one strategy for problem solving issues in the moment when I am not directly present as asking themselves or each other "What would the pediatric CNS say or do?" They relate that this helps them feel calmer when confronted with caring for children and families, which in turn helps them (a) call to mind what they already know, (b) think more clearly about locating resources and help as needed, and (c) "do the task" with more confidence. This implies that GP methods are accessible to the learner and can be acted upon even when the guide is not directly present—a variation on the idea of "being held in mind" (see Chapters 1 and 23).

My direct supervisor has shared her assessment that, in general, our emergency services staff are more attuned to developmental and family-centered support of children and families than they were prior to consistent CNS interaction with and support of staff in caring for pediatric patients and families. She attributes this in part to a CNS practice directed specifically to staff competency development in the context of a relationship-based teaching–learning approach. Our interdisciplinary healthcare team members have successfully cared for children and families throughout the hospital, striving to do what is best for each child and their family, making use of available resources to creatively and safely meet the needs in the moment. While there are always opportunities for improvement, there have been no sentinel events as defined by The Joint Commission (2017) related to pediatric care—a testament to the healthcare team's commitment to caring for children and families.

CONCLUSION

Making use of GP methods when working directly with nursing and inter-disciplinary colleagues is not only possible it is highly desirable and it is achievable. It provides a built-in opportunity for staff to experience directly what the children and families they work with could also experience if staff were to engage with them in this manner. Further, the CNS can identify that parallel process explicitly for staff, assisting them not only with developing competencies in the care of children and families—thereby lowering anxiety levels about taking care of children—but also in developing competencies in the practice of GP.

QUESTIONS FOR REFLECTION

- Can you see yourself trying out this approach—that is, applying the GP methods you might use with patients and families—when working with your healthcare team colleagues?
- What would you need in order to do this?
- What does it take to engage in GP processes with colleagues in the presence of patients and their families?
- What happens if the learner's assessment of what needs to be done differs from the guide's assessment? How can GP methods be used to address this situation?
- What kind of education and how much "practice" does one need in order to competently engage in GP as a guide?
- What would you recommend we stop doing, continue doing, and start doing to promote fuller achievement of developmentally sensitive, family-centered care of children and their families?

REFERENCES

American Hospital Association. (2017). Fast Facts on U.S. Hospitals. Retrieved from http://www.aha .org/research/rc/stat-studies/fast-facts.shtml

Blake, F. G. (1964a). *Family-centered pediatric nursing care*. Ross Roundtable on Maternal and Child Nursing, #1. Columbus, OH: Ross Laboratories.

Blake, F. G. (1964b). *The functions of the clinical nurse specialist in the hospital organization*. Madison, WI: University of Wisconsin–Madison.

Blake, F. G., Wright, F. H., & Waechter, E. H. (1970). *Nursing care of children* (8th ed.). Philadelphia, PA: J. B. Lippincott.

Children's Hospital Association. (n.d.). About Children's Hospitals. Retrieved from https://www .childrenshospitals.org/About-Us/About-Childrens-Hospitals

Disch, J., Walton, M., & Barnsteiner, J. (2001). The role of the clinical nurse specialist in creating a healthy work environment. *AACN Clinical Issues, 12*(3), 345–355.

Fulton, J., Lyons, B., & Goudreau, K. (Eds.). (2014). *Foundations of clinical nurse specialist practice* (2nd ed.). New York, NY: Springer Publishing.

Harrison, T. M. (2010). Family-centered pediatric nursing care: State of the science. *Journal of Pediatric Nursing, 25*(5), 335–343. doi:10.1016/j.pedn.2009.01.006

The Joint Commission. (2017). Sentinel event policy and procedures. Retrieved from https://www .jointcommission.org/sentinel_event_policy_and_procedures/

National CNS Competency Task Force. (2010). *Clinical nurse specialist core competencies: Executive summary 2006–2008.* Retrieved from http://nacns.org/wp-content/uploads/2016/11/ CNSCoreCompetenciesBroch.pdf

Pridham, K. F., Adelson, F., & Hansen, M. F. (1987). Helping children deal with procedures in a clinic setting: A developmental approach. *Journal of Pediatric Nursing, 2*(1), 13–22.

Schroeder, M., & Pridham, K. F. (2006). Development of relationship competencies through guided participation for mothers of preterm infants. *Journal of Obstetric, Gynecologic, & Neonatal Nursing, 35*(3), 358–368. doi:10.1111/J.1552-6909.2006.00049.x

Stuckey-Schrock, K., Hayes, B. L., & George, C. M. (2012). Community-acquired pneumonia in children. *American Family Physician, 86*(7), 661–667.

Wright, D. (2005). *The ultimate guide to competency assessment in health care* (3rd ed.). Minneapolis, MN: Creative Health Care Management.

19

A Mobile Application as a Tool for Guided Participation

Jena Tanem and Anne Chevalier McKechnie

The use and feasibility of a mobile application (app) for tracking many chronic health conditions, including cystic fibrosis and depression, has been demonstrated (Birkhoff & Smeltzer, 2017). An app for clinic and home-based care of children, however, has only recently become available. Parent or child use in the home or community of a health tracking app for managing common acute illness problems or for monitoring physiologic stability and health status related to a child's chronic illness could extend clinician monitoring of and interaction about care, promote child well-being, and prevent hospitalization and time lost from everyday activities of living.

We believe that an app could support and extend the capacity of clinicians, parents, and children to engage in guided participation (GP) for learning to manage acute and common health issues related to chronic illness. Some readers might conclude that mobile phone apps are inconsistent with some or much of what is central to GP, particularly the relationship of teacher and learner. The relationship is the vehicle of knowing the motivation, goals, expectations, and intentions of the learner and dynamically structuring needed learning with this knowledge in mind. This knowledge, some may think, is hard to come by with use of a mobile phone app, even with interactive features for reciprocal sharing of information structured into its use. Interpersonal relationship is at the core of GP, a feature that is not obviously central or important to mobile app use for obtaining information, tracking health status, problem solving, or getting connected with help for attention to personal problems. Interaction cannot be equated with relationship, which, although it may gain in its formation and maintenance from interaction, has substance and endurance beyond a back and forth exchange with one person and another (Hinde, 1979).

This chapter shows how an app that structures the monitoring of chronic illness, tracking of physiologic status, and communicating with clinicians about health data can provide a platform for and information to structure GP. The goals of GP flow through the information obtained with health monitoring and parameter tracking gained with the app. The potential result of integrating app use and GP is increased knowledge about the chronic illness in the life of the child and parents, strengthened sense of ability to manage or efficacy, and enabled participation with competencies for care responsibility. This chapter provides an example of a health tracking app, designed and implemented by nurses in the care of children with complex congenital heart disease. The app described in this chapter was designed to monitor the physiologic well-being and health at home of infants born with a single ventricle between the first and second stages of their palliative surgery. Monitoring of physiologic status and tracking of health data has become the standard of care worldwide for the population of infants born with a single ventricle. Questions to ask yourself as you read this chapter could include how are an app for tracking health data and GP mutually reinforcing? How does GP come into play as health data are tracked? How can clinicians assess how well the app and GP work together as a learning system for parents of an infant with a complex chronic disease? What are the components of a model for the structure and function of an app articulated with GP for clinical practice with children who have a complex, chronic health condition that requires monitoring at home?

HYPOPLASTIC LEFT HEART SYNDROME AND THE HOME MONITORING PROGRAM

Congenital heart disease affects approximately 40,000 infants per year in the United States (Hoffman & Kaplan, 2002). Hypoplastic left-heart syndrome (HLHS) accounts for 2% to 3% of all congenital heart disease (Reller, Strickland, Riehle-Colarusso, Mahle, & Correa, 2008). This diagnosis carried a poor prognosis prior to the development of the Norwood operation, adopted in the 1980s. At our center, current management of HLHS entails stage 1 palliation (S1P) with the Norwood operation (Children's Hospital of Wisconsin, 2017), followed by stage 2 palliation (S2P) with a bidirectional Glenn operation, generally by about the age of 6 months, and stage 3 palliation (S3P) known as the Fontan procedure, which generally is done in the child's second or third year. The timeframe between S1P and S2P is universally known as the interstage period. The national mortality rate of interstage patients was reported at 10% to 20% in the early 2000s. Despite improving hospital survival rates, infants with HLHS remain vulnerable to even mild changes in physiologic state following S1P.

HLHS is hypoplasia or underdevelopment of the left-sided heart structures (mitral valve, aortic valve, aortic arch, and left ventricle). In utero, blood is able to bypass the hypoplastic left-sided structures and is pumped to the body through the patent ductus arteriosus (PDA) and patent foramen ovale (PFO). Shortly after birth the PDA closes leaving little to no systemic blood flow. Within the first week of life, a temporary shunt (Blalock–Taussig shunt [refer to Figure 19.1] or a right ventricle-to-pulmonary artery [RV–PA] conduit) is created to provide pulmonary blood flow. Systemic blood flow is achieved by creating a "neoaorta" which consists of combining the native aorta and pulmonary artery into one outflow tract.

Adequate circulation is often difficult to achieve in these infants since it requires a careful balance of pulmonary and systemic blood flow. Numerous circumstances, such as gastroenteritis, fever, respiratory infections, shunt stenosis or obstruction, neoaortic arch obstruction, restriction of the atrial septal defect, or atrioventricular valve insufficiency, can change the balance of circulation. Consequences of illness or change in hemodynamics can cause hypovolemia, hypoxemia, increased systemic vascular resistance, inadequate pulmonary or systemic blood flow, or impaired myocardial performance. These in turn can lead to significant morbidity and mortality for infants during the interstage period.

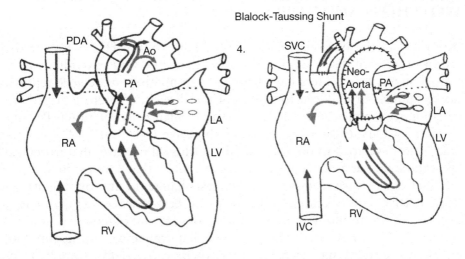

FIGURE 19.1 Anatomy and physiology of a hypoplastic left heart and its surgical modifications.

Ao, aorta; IVC, inferior vena cava; LA, left atrium; LV, left ventricle; PA, pulmonary artery; PDA, patent ductus arteriosus; RA, right atrium; RV, right ventricle; SVC, superior vena cava.

Source: May, L. E. (2012). *Pediatric heart surgery: A ready reference for professionals* (5th ed.). Minneapolis, MN: Cardiotext Publishing. Used with permission.

To combat the high mortality rate in this fragile population, the home monitoring program (HMP) was first implemented by Children's Hospital of Wisconsin in 2000. The program was developed on the hypothesis that detection of either decreased oxygen saturations or poor weight gain/acute weight loss may forecast the presence of serious intercurrent illness or physiologic compromise, and potentially allow for life-saving intervention to be implemented. Therefore, prior to S1P discharge, extensive parental education is implemented by a specialized medical team. Parents are provided with a home scale and pulse oximeter. Recordings of daily oxygen saturations, weight, and 24-hour enteral intake are followed. The family receives weekly phone calls from the HMP team and is seen at a minimum every other week in the interdisciplinary interstage clinic. Parents are instructed to contact the interstage team if SpO_2 is less than 75% or greater than 90%, there is weight loss of 30 g or failure to gain 20 g over 3 days, or enteral intake of less than 100 mL/kg/day.

At our institution, nurse practitioners (NPs) are vital to the interstage management of the infants. The NPs are responsible for daily rounding on hospitalized infants, educating parents, coordinating care related to discharge of patients, making weekly calls to families on the condition of infants now at home, facilitating interstage clinic visits, communicating consistently with referring clinicians, and being available via pager around the clock for medical questions.

QUALITY IMPROVEMENT IN THE CARE OF INFANTS WITH HLHS AND THEIR PARENTS

According to the National Institute of Health (NIH), HLHS fits the definition of a "rare disease," affecting less than 200,000 individuals in the United States. Few centers have large enough numbers to achieve representative samples of children for study of the disease. Therefore, a pediatric collaborative improvement network was formed titled National Pediatric Cardiology Quality Improvement Collaborative (NPC-QIC). The collaborative was developed to provide a multisite clinical network that fosters collaboration among practice-based teams at centers that care for infants with HLHS. Centers learn from one another, test changes to improve quality, and use collective data to understand and spread best practices. This collaboration in turn can result in improved quality of care and outcomes (Lannon & Peterson, 2013). For example, since the collaborative was formed in 2008, interstage mortality has decreased (per collaborative data) from 20% to a consistent 5%. This 15% decrease in mortality means hundreds of lives have been saved with the aid of collaboration.

The initial phase of NPC-QIC focused on interstage growth and mortality and relied heavily on chart review and collection of individual patient data. The second phase of the collaborative, currently in operation, expands the topics of phase I but also places an emphasis on optimization of family support. GP could provide a means of advancing this objective.

FAMILY INTEGRATED CARE

Family integrated care has become a topic of interest for our center, as well as for the NPC-QIC. This type of care is defined as an extension of family-centered care. Parents are not merely bystanders that are privy to information but partners in providing daily care for their child with education and guidance from knowledgeable medical staff. For example, parents are not only encouraged to participate in daily rounds and collaborate in decision making, but also to help lead daily cares (feedings, diaper changes, sleep schedules, bathing, medications, etc.) with support from bedside nurses. Preliminary studies for those participating in family integrated care demonstrate that infants grow faster and have increased rates of breastfeeding, parents have less stress/anxiety, and infants spend fewer total days in the intensive care unit (O'Brien et al, 2013; Örtenstrand et al, 2010).

Family integrated care is similar to that of GP. The NPs and bedside nurses help guide parents in performing socially meaningful activities of daily living for their infant with the overall goal to gain competence in caring for their baby and their complex medical needs at the time of discharge.

EVALUATION OF FAMILY INTEGRATED CARE DELIVERED THROUGH THE HMP

To gain insight regarding family integrated care delivered during the home interstage period from the parent's perspective, mothers and fathers were asked to complete a quality improvement survey at the conclusion of the HMP (the time of the infant's S2P). Survey topics ranged from feasibility of daily tasks, to use of the interstage binder in which the guidelines and records of health data were kept, to the overall experience in the HMP. Most parents reported favorable experiences in the program. A consistent theme concerning the burden of the binder record of data, however, was identified, as seen in the following comments:

> "It [the binder] was understandable and well made. It was a lot of writing. It would be much easier for parents if there was [sic] an electronic version online or with an app."

> "Dislike [in regard to binder]: bulky pages easily torn because using it every day."

"Binder got to be too bulky with the frequent in/out to doctor visits and hauling baby with meds, oxygen, car seat, bottles, etc."

"I liked that I had something to keep track of sats [oxygen saturations], heart rate and weight. I disliked bringing it [the binder] everywhere with us."

"It was great to know how closely we were followed and also how easy it was to contact the team if I had any concerns. A way to electronically send over daily logs with an app or webpage would make recording and giving the information to the team *much* easier on both ends. Other than that, I felt fully prepared and comfortable going home thanks to the awesome Interstage team that clearly worked hard on making this great program. THANK YOU!"

DEVELOPMENT OF THE INTERSTAGE MOBILE APP

To support parent satisfaction with participation in the HMP, and to develop and improve quality of care, ideas for developing the interstage app were proposed by the NPs. Ultimately, the app was created by NPs through a collaborative project funded by a philanthropic technology company, Red Arrow Labs, a Dohmen Company, aiming to reduce infant mortality. The goal of the project that the NPs shared with the company was to improve the experience of families participating in our HMP. We set out to accomplish this goal through the creation of an app that would do the following: (a) improve efficiency of data recording, (b) enhance safety, and (c) promote effective communication between parents and caregivers. To learn about parents' needs for monitoring, recording, and communicating their infant's physiologic and health status in the interstage period, members of the technology company spent time shadowing the healthcare team and held sessions with parents of infants who were previously home monitored to gain their perspectives on the use of an app. After investing over a year's time in app development, a "Journey Map" (refer to Figure 19.2) was created to inform design and content, and the interstage app prototype was born.

The interstage app is expected to be a valuable tool because it can offer both asynchronous and immediate access for communication, facilitate discussion that progresses over time, and can be useful for parents regardless of where parents live. Although the design was informed by parents' and healthcare clinicians' needs, the app—as well as other materials (e.g., HMP binder, journey board)—are provided by teachers to be used by learners. This app will remain a tool for GP because a parent cannot learn everything about an experience, what to expect, how to feel and think through a technological interface. Although the GP of the nurse cannot be replaced by this app, introducing this tool could shift the extent and timing of the nurse–parent relationship. The case below is intended to illustrate how the initial interstage app prototype can be used as a tool for GP.

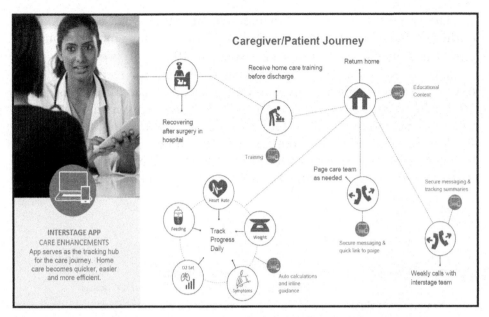

FIGURE 19.2 Journey map created to guide interstate app development.

Source: Copyrighted by Red Arrow Labs, a Dohmen Company.

THE INTERSTAGE APP AS A TOOL FOR GP WITH PARENTS OF AN INFANT WITH HLHS

Case Example 19.1

Parents Tina and Kyle anticipated that their infant, Tate, would be born with HLHS since he was diagnosed prenatally. Tate was born at 39 weeks, and immediately after delivery, he was assessed by the neonatal intensive care team. Tate was started on a prostaglandin infusion to maintain patency of his PDA and provide his lungs and body adequate blood flow and oxygenation. As typical for most infants with HLHS, he underwent his stage I Norwood operation within the first week of life. After approximately 1 week of intubation and sedation, Tate's breathing tube was removed and his parents held him for the first time.

While Tate was hospitalized, Tina and Kyle were eager to absorb any information and be involved in any special care that they could to speed up Tate's recovery. Shortly after Tate's extubation, an NP on the HMP care team introduced herself and initiated GP by getting connected with the parents as she described the program. Recognizing Tina and Kyle's eagerness, the NP sought to stay connected with an emphasis on the common goal of optimizing Tate's care and health outcomes. A copy of the HMP binder was introduced, and despite their fatigue, the couple was very interested in looking through the binder and other HMP materials.

The process of joining and maintaining attention was easily engaged in as the NP first focused on the HMP binder as a means for information gathering and daily data collection (refer to Figure 19.3).

The NP explained how the binder is used daily for recording weights, oxygen saturations, heart rates, and 24-hour enteral intake. Recording in the binder was discussed at length, and the teach-back method was used to assess the parents' understanding of the why, when, and how of using the binder. Next, the "Stepping Stones to Home" journey board (refer to Figure 19.4) was shared with Tina and Kyle. The NP explained that the journey board is used to improve communication between parents and all

Date: ___/___/___   **Date:** ___/___/___

Today's Weight: **Today's Weight:**
_____ 1bs/Kg/grams   _____ 1bs/Kg/grams

Yesterday's Weight: **Yesterday's Weight:**
_____ 1bs/Kg/grams   _____ 1bs/Kg/grams

Weight Change: **Weight Change:**
(Today–Yesterday):   (Today–Yesterday):
+/- _____ 1bs/Kg/grams   +/- _____ 1bs/Kg/grams

O$_2$ Saturation: _____%   **O$_2$ Saturation:** _____%
Heart Rate: _____Beats per minute   **Heart Rate:** _____Beats per minute

Feeds: **Time**   **Amount***   Feeds: **Time**   **Amount***
                    (cc/oz)   (cc/oz)

_____   _____   _____   _____
_____   _____   _____   _____
_____   _____   _____   _____
_____   _____   _____   _____
_____   _____   _____   _____
_____   _____   _____   _____
_____   _____   _____   _____
_____   _____   _____   _____
_____   _____   _____   _____

*If you breast feed, write bf under amount.   *If you breast feed, write bf under amount.

24 hour Feed Total: _____   24 hour Feed Total: _____

Comments _____   **Comments** _____
_____   _____
_____   _____
_____   _____

FIGURE 19.3 Binder record of infant physiologic and health data.

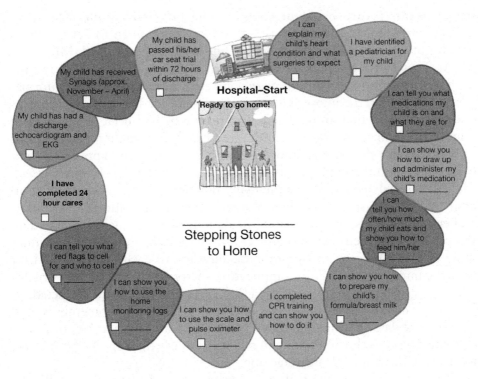

FIGURE 19.4 Journey board: "Stepping Stones to Home."

Source: Copyright © 2017 Children's Hospital of Wisconsin. CHW does not make any representation with respect to any sort of industry recognized standard of care for the particular subject matter of this form. Additionally, CHW form dcuments are subject to change, revision, alteration and/or revocation without notice.

care team members, ensuring that everyone is aware of tasks that still need to be completed prior to discharge home in the HMP.

The binder and journey board are examples of how to offer structure for learning by organizing larger tasks into manageable tasks.

Over the next few weeks in the hospital, Tina and Kyle helped to determine which tasks they were ready to complete using the journey board. The bedside nurses were assessing how the parents were holding up emotionally, and how they were doing with developing the new caregiving skills. The nurses also wanted to know how Tina and Kyle were thinking about how caregiving was going. To prepare Tina and Kyle to care for Tate at home, the nurses relied on their experience and knowledge to support their progress through joint problem solving and reflecting on what went well and what did not. As the tasks were accomplished and documented on the journey board, the NP met with the couple again and began bridging what the parents had learned with what might be new and would need to be applied in the home setting. They discussed HMP, identified common concerns, and considered scenarios that would require medical attention. Tina and Kyle were both very engaged in learning more about the real care experiences they had recently addressed with Tate as well as the hypothetical scenarios for future problem solving. The NP and couple shared an understanding that learning to assess and knowing when to act on Tate's health status after discharge was crucial and well-supported by HMP.

As Tina and Kyle became skilled with assessing Tate, identifying the health information needed, and were competent in recording daily information in the binder, the interstage app was introduced. The couple was introduced to the idea that an interstage app prototype had been designed to be a more streamlined means to record Tate's health information and could be viewed by both the parents and the healthcare team. The app was downloaded on their mobile phones as well as to a tablet that has Internet access. The NP showed Tina and Kyle the many functions of the app, including (a) easily identifiable spaces for daily weights, oxygen saturations, heart rates, and enteral feedings; (b) automatic calculations of weight gain/loss based on the previous day's entered weight; (c) automatic calculation of daily minimum enteral intake goal; (d) automatic addition of each recorded feed for visible cumulative total; (e) in-application alerts when a breach of criteria occurs, notifying the family that the HMP care team should be contacted; (f) sharing of data between numerous mobile devices of family members; and (g) real-time data sharing with Tate's healthcare team (refer to Figure 19.5).

Since this was the first family in the HMP to use the app, the binder was used as a backup to the interstage app.

Tina and Kyle became well-practiced at using the app along with the binder in the time leading up to Tate's discharge from the hospital. The NP and bedside nurses recognized that it was appropriate to focus on fully transferring responsibility of infant care to the parents. Tina and Kyle saw themselves

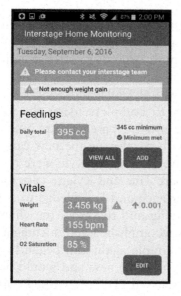
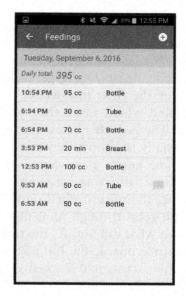

FIGURE 19.5 Interstage app screenshots of Tate's 1-day feeding and vital signs data.

Source: Copyrighted by Red Arrow Labs, a Dohmen Company.

as ready for the next step, which would be the 24-hour infant care periods, often referred to as "24-hour cares." The 24-hour cares take place in the safe environment of the hospital and allows for the parents to independently practice all care for the infant, including bathing, diaper changes, feedings, medication administration, and recording of HMP data. During this time, the bedside nurse is only available for parents' questions as needed. Tina and Kyle felt very successful, and the nurses agreed that the 24-hour cares went particularly well for the couple and their infant. The NP sat down with the parents and examined their use of the interstage app and binder. She pointed out specific competencies related to the infant's health status, and provided encouragement and support as they would soon be going home with Tate.

After 6 weeks of hospitalization, Tate and his parents were ready for discharge. As was customary HMP practice, weekly phone calls were made to the parents to assess Tate's enteral intake, growth, and oxygen saturations as well as overall well-being. With previous families who used only the binder, this phone call was rather tedious because the parent was asked to read out to the NP the bulk of the information they had recorded in the binder during the past week. The interstage app prototype, however, was partnered with the use of a secure website, known as the provider portal. In this portal, HMP team members have access to real-time data recorded by parents in the app. Data could be graphed to show patterns of weight, feeding, as well as physiologic data such as oxygen saturation over the period of a week (refer to Figure 19.6).

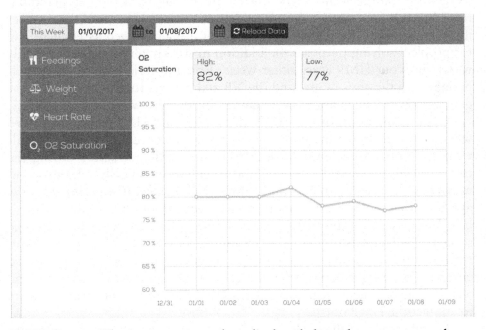

FIGURE 19.6 The interstage app data displayed through a secure portal as a clinician interface. Patterns of weight, feeding, and physiologic data are shown for a period of 1 week.

Source: Copyrighted by Red Arrow Labs, a Dohmen Company.

Now, prior to calling Tina and Kyle, the NP reviewed the data seen on the provider portal and confirmed with the parents that this information was correct. The ability to check the data in advance left the NP and parents more time for proactive use of the NP as a resource and for the NP to use clinical resources for problem solving. For example, if the NP logs onto the portal and sees that the infant has lost weight over the past few days, clinical discussions with other team members, such as dieticians, can take place prior to the call with the parents, therefore making the process more efficient.

The app data being available in real time was a tangible benefit to both the parents and the healthcare team, and a promising tool for GP. In addition to the clinician interface, Tina and Kyle could access app data on multiple mobile devices. Tina explained that she typically cared for Tate during the day, and when Kyle was away at work, he could log onto the app and see how Tate's day was going. The app data were reassuring, informative, and could be used to discuss concerns when needed. The app noticeably reduced the burden of data collection by the NP over the phone with parents. It is important to point out, however, that great emphasis is always placed on verbal communication with the parents as a valuable source of information that extends beyond the data displayed. The parents' time on the phone with the NP or other members of the healthcare team was focused on important health concerns and additional teaching and learning activities. For example, when a concern was identified regarding Tate's weight and oxygen saturation declines, the question came up with the parents about recording this information. An agreement was reached to record these values more frequently for the upcoming week for a finer grained assessment and for problem-solving purposes. In addition to weekly phone calls, the family was seen in our HMP every other week. Tina and Kyle both brought their phones with the apps in use, and the NP and parents together examined the data entries and calculations and planned for the next week.

Upon completion of the HMP, the family and HMP staff considered whether the goals for the interstage app were reached. The primary goals were to improve efficiency of data recording, enhance safety during the transition from hospital to home, and to enhance clinically relevant communication between parents and healthcare clinicians. It was clear that the app used as a tool for GP supported early recognition of a decline in Tate's health status and allowed the parents and healthcare team to intervene sooner. The couple saw the value in app alerts related to the health information entered at home that by design signaled a breach in preestablished criteria (e.g., weight below a set value). The app was not designed to send alerts to the healthcare team, but instead the alert for parents prompts them to contact the HMP nurse.

Despite reaching the goals, some limitations in the interstage app prototype were noted. From a healthcare clinician perspective, though the information was easily attainable, it did not directly connect to our electronic health record, which would improve efficiency even further. In addition, there were no educational resources embedded in the app prototype, whereas these resources were easily accessible in the binder. Similarly, there is no place to view a list of the breach in preestablished criteria, which forces parents to rely on the built-in alerts that appear only after data entry. From the parents' perspective, the main missing piece was a visual display of the weekly trends. Tina and Kyle also found it hard to follow the cumulative totals which were set to log from midnight to midnight for a 24-hour time frame. Both the healthcare clinician and parent user experiences were evaluated by the app development team. The current app prototype has been improved with visual displays for parent viewing and a cumulative feeding total that mimics that of the hospital setting (7 a.m.–7 p.m.). The interstage app development will be ongoing, with design and functionality modifications based on feedback from new families and the HMP healthcare team.

CONCLUSION

The nature of family integrated care and the educational process of the HMP fits well with GP methods and the interstage app as a tool for intervention. Specifically, teaching with the interstage app easily incorporates all GP processes. The nurses can employ the app to get and stay connected as the app can easily catch the parent's interest. The app is a tool for structuring data with displays of information for the nurse and family to join and maintain attention in order to identify health issues and work on competencies such as health assessment and problem solving. The nurse can use the process of bridging during discussions, reinforced with common experiences of other families and app data, for testing "what if" scenarios. With the transfer of responsibility of infant caregiving to parents, the app appears to be an effective tool as they manage the daily interstage tasks. Yet the app data display relies on their responsibility to accurately record information and ultimately make informed decisions if breach of preestablished criteria occurs.

As described in this chapter, the interstage app used for tracking health data is a resource for healthcare clinicians who aim to advance the competencies of parents and children in adapting to the challenges of complex chronic illness, including managing the intricate decisions of day-to-day care. While the interstage app has been created specifically for parents in the HMP, the easy-to-use design and real-time data for parents and healthcare clinicians have resulted in a valuable platform. For example, with modification of the app, additional or alternate data regarding tube feedings could be recorded. Similarly, the app platform lends itself to other cardiology populations, such as those needing blood pressure or blood sugar monitoring, or those requiring frequent blood work while titrating anticoagulation medications. It could also be possible to embed relevant functions of the insterstage app into other apps designed for parents preparing and caring for infants with a range of major, life-threatening conditions. Overall, access to this type of app creates efficiency for families and healthcare clinicians, and, most importantly, allows for high-quality tailoring of care through clear communication.

With approaching universal ownership of mobile phones, the use of mobile app methods of obtaining and presenting information potentially will strengthen the support GP offers parents and children in managing chronic health conditions.

REFERENCES

Birkhoff, S. D., & Smeltzer, S. C. (2017). Perceptions of smartphone user-centered mobile health tracking apps across various chronic illness populations: An integrative review. *Journal of Nursing Scholarship, 49*, 371–378. doi:10.1111/jnu.12298

Children's Hospital of Wisconsin. (2017). Norwood procedure for hypoplastic left heart syndrome. Retrieved from http://www.chw.org/medical-care/herma-heart-center/for-medical-professionals/pediatric-heart-surgery/norwood-procedure-for-hypoplastic-left-heart-syndrome/

Hinde, R. A. (1979). What do we mean by a relationship? In *Towards understanding Relationships* (Vol. 18, pp. 14–39). London, UK: Academic Press.

Hoffman, J. I., & Kaplan, S. (2002). The incidence of congenital heart disease. *Journal of the American College of Cardiology, 39*(12), 1890–1900. doi:10.1016/S0735-1097(02)01886-7

Lannon, C. M., & Peterson, L. E. (2013). Pediatric collaborative improvement networks: Background and overview. *Pediatrics, 131*(Suppl. 4), S189–S195. doi:10.1542/peds.2012-3786E

O'Brien, K., Bracht, M., Macdonell, K., McBride, T., Robson, K., O'Leary, L., . . . Lee, S. K. (2013). A pilot cohort analytic study of family integrated care in a Canadian neonatal intensive care unit. *BMC Pregnancy and Childbirth, 13*(1), S12. doi:10.1186/1471-2393-13-S1-S12

Örtenstrand, A., Westrup, B., Broström, E. B., Sarman, I., Åkerström, S., Brune, T., . . . Waldenström, U. (2010). The Stockholm neonatal family centered care study: Effects on length of stay and infant morbidity. *Pediatrics, 125*, e278–e285. doi:10.1542/peds.2009-1511

Reller, M. D., Strickland, M. J., Riehle-Colarusso, T., Mahle, W. T., & Correa, A. (2008). Prevalence of congenital heart defects in metropolitan Atlanta, 1998–2005. *The Journal of Pediatrics, 153*(6), 807–813. doi:10.1016/j.jpeds.2008.05.059

20

A Neonatologist's Guided Participation With Parents of an Infant With Trisomy 18

Steven Leuthner and Anne Chevalier McKechnie

When a chromosomal defect, such as Trisomy 13 or 18, is diagnosed prenatally, what parents need and want to know to get their bearings, anticipate what the future holds, and make critical, pressing decisions is sometimes beyond what clinicians have personally experienced. Parents may be grief stricken and overwhelmed with the anticipated infant's health problems, and highly likely to require a knowledgeable and compassionate guide through processes and transitions of care (McKechnie, Pridham, & Tluczek, 2015; Patterson et al., 2017).

As a neonatologist, I have worked with many parents expecting and delivering an infant with Trisomy 13 or 18 or another potentially terminal condition. A protocol for decision making with parents who have received a diagnosis of a fetal anomaly has limited usefulness because of the idiosyncratic features of the fetal diagnosis, every family's circumstances, and the ethical questions that are generally very personal. What I learn accrues as expectations of what parents and the clinical team will confront and as intentions for care develop. Moreover, what I know about the parents' needs in light of the infant's status and prognosis helps me to discern the ethical considerations. As a neonatologist in this context, I view myself as a guide and parents as apprentices in learning to become parents of an infant with a severely life-limiting condition. Unlike a typical apprenticeship, however, knowing what should be set out for parents to learn and the processes of learning depend on what the parents expect and intend and on the realities of the infant's condition (Pridham, 1993).

This is an account of one family and how my expectations and intentions for clinical practice and my learned knowledge of the parents' expectations and intentions intersected with concepts of guided participation (GP). This chapter crystallized through several conversations with my clinical and academic colleagues about how these concepts helped me to provide teaching and learning opportunities to parents expecting an infant with Trisomy 18 (T18), as well as work with other members of the healthcare team to assist the parents. Together with the second author, a conceptual diagram (refer to Figure 20.1) was generated to inform and organize the telling of this account.

The conceptual diagram specifies how GP is used by the physician—myself as a neonatologist—with parents and the healthcare team after a fetal diagnosis. The variables in relation to GP are illustrated in a conceptual diagram. The issues that the physician, parents, and members of the healthcare team are working on are the focus of the guided participation process. In the center as a guide, the physician engages with parents and members of the healthcare team to discuss clinically relevant issues that can have a substantial bearing on the health outcomes of the infant and the family. The issues for the physician as illustrated in this

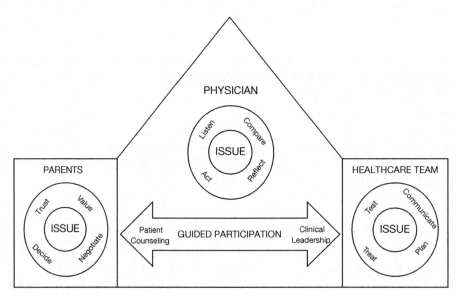

FIGURE 20.1 GP can be used by a physician through patient counseling with parents and through clinical leadership with members of the healthcare team. Clinical discussions focus on the issues that the physician, parents and healthcare team need to work on to achieve health outcomes. Related to each issue are contextual factors that inform the direction of mental work or behaviors.

GP, guided participation.

case involve (a) relating to parents and members of the healthcare team, (b) communicating medical information as well as the individualized approach to fetal/infant care to the parents, and (c) developing the healthcare team's support for the parents' goals. The contextual factors informing the physician's issues have to do with when and how one listens, compares new and prior experiences, reflects on the complexities, and ultimately acts to reach clinical outcomes.

The physician can use GP through patient counseling with consideration for the parents' hopes and goals for their infant's quality of life. The issues for the parents raised here include (a) managing a perceived adverse environment on behalf of their daughter, (b) making their voices, as parents, heard, and (c) preparing for and protecting the infant's physical and spiritual life. The contextual factors regarding each parent issue involve trust, what they value, and the need to negotiate and make decisions regarding maternal–fetal health management.

The physician can also use GP through clinical leadership to examine the ethics related to the medical condition and power dynamics inherent in the decision making of the healthcare team with the parents. The issues for the healthcare team that required attention include (a) considering before birth invasive procedures and blood transfusions to be used after birth, and (b) providing medical care for the infant during a short life expectancy. The issues faced by the healthcare team were shaped by contextual factors represented by their approaches to test for, communicate about, plan for, and finally treat the condition.

My aim is to tell the story of how the clinical care actually unfolded, including interactions with other members of the healthcare team, and, in the course of the telling, to identify major GP concepts as I drew on them in the following case. In the text that follows, my description is shown in regular font; my interpretation is shown in *italics*. The GP processes (see Chapter 1, Figure 1.1) are shown as headings. The issues of GP are shown in sidebars.

Case Example 14.1

A 35-year-old gravida 2, para 1 woman and her husband were referred from their obstetrician to a maternal–fetal medicine (MFM) specialist because of anatomic abnormalities consisting of growth restriction, a left-sided congenital diaphragmatic hernia (CDH), and a large perimembranous ventricular-septal defect (VSD) of the heart. These defects led to genetic counseling and testing that confirmed the fetus had T18 as the underlying condition. The family was referred for confirmation and counseling regarding decision making and management of the pregnancy and fetus. Prior to visiting our institution, the parents were connected, through social media, to a family who had a surviving infant with T18. This infant had been cared for at our center.

GETTING AND STAYING CONNECTED

At our center, the findings were confirmed by the MFM specialist. Meetings were arranged for the family with a fetal cardiologist, a neonatologist, and a pediatric surgeon. As the consulting neonatologist, I began the consultative process as I normally do. I introduced myself as one of our center's neonatologists whom the parents could consider to be their infant's pediatrician during the initial hospital stay. I shared that I knew they had heard about their infant's condition from other physicians or research reports. I asked them if they could share with me what they had been told, what their understanding was of their daughter's condition, and what goals they had thought about for their family.

This mother and father spoke with intensity in their voices, making their points with sharpness, while maintaining themselves just on the other side of anger. I could understand why many on the healthcare team saw them as both aggressive and defensive. They shared that they understood the infant they were expecting had birth defects that would require surgery. The one concern they had was whether we (physicians) would be honest with them about what options there were for any infant with these defects. The parents requested that we not discriminate in our care of their infant based on the genetic condition. They wanted to essentially take the T18 out of the picture and treat their infant as her own individual, as if she didn't have this genetic make-up. The father said, "Well, you know, we're not sophisticated enough to know what we don't know," acknowledging that he and his wife were not medical experts. He asked how he would know if we were telling him everything. The mother then shared that they were told by their social media friend that I, as the attending neonatologist, had personally refused to send an infant who had T18 home with a pulse oximeter, and that I had "kicked her (the social media friend) out of the NICU" when she considered herself as doing her best to be a parent advocate.

> Clearly, I had some trust building challenges on my hands here. The GP issue evident was that the parents wanted to nurture and protect their future infant from what they perhaps perceived as a nontruthful or hostile environment. I would need to figure out a way to relate to them. My goals were to build trust, allow them to feel empowered to nurture and protect their infant, and, at the same time, bring in considerations regarding quality of life for the infant, who had a significant genetic disorder that could not be ignored. I thought about how I would structure learning and bridge what the parents were thinking and believing (i.e., what was currently known to them) to what would be most facilitative of good medical care and quality of life for the infant (i.e., what was unknown or new to them) from the beginning of our interaction.

Parent Issue 1: Managing a perceived adverse environment on behalf of their daughter
Physician Issue 1: Relating to parents

As a guide, I had to develop trust through communicating medical information, understanding hopes, and assessing their goals for the quality of life and future of their infant. They recognized the power differential in knowledge between themselves and the physicians. Unlike the majority of families, the parents directly addressed the difference in power. I could now, hopefully, use this direct expression of power difference to break down barriers of us versus them and build trust.

I shared with the parents that my goal was to work with them to help them understand what medical and surgical interventions were available, that is, what we "could" do, and then help them decide what would be best for their infant, or what we "should" do. What "should" be done is based not only on their infant's individual needs but also on the parents' values, which would help determine their goals. In order to try and break down some barriers and build trust, I shared a few key pieces of information in an effort to amend their understanding of the situation the social media friend had reported about me in the NICU (described previously), trying not to sound defensive. First, it had been the insurance company that had refused the pulse oximeter because the infant had no respiratory distress, and so did not go home on supplemental oxygen. I did, however, send the infant home on an apnea-cardiac monitor. Second, I was not the physician who had "kicked" that mother out of the NICU, but a physician partner. That mother was asked to leave after she was loudly saying in public areas that we were not offering or doing tests on the infant in question. These tests, I explained, were not medically indicated for this infant. I suggested that this event actually demonstrated that we treat each infant as an individual. At our center, physicians address the medical needs of individual infants without assuming all infants with T18 have the same complications and need the same tests and interventions. I pointed out to the parents that demanding testing and treating of every infant with Trisomy 18 in the same manner was as discriminating as not testing or treating any infant because of the condition.

Parent Issue 2: Making their voices, as parents, heard

The issue became about how the parents could make their voices heard so that they and the physicians could work together for the best outcome. The goal was to establish trust and begin to establish a relationship, part of the process of "getting and staying connected." These parents were demonstrating the parental role of protecting their infant, as well as advocating for themselves as the decision-making authority for their infant. If I could not connect with these parents, there would be no way to help guide them. Their level of distrust is not typical in perinatal consultation, but, if present, must be recognized and dealt with. I realized my goal in this one hour I had with them was to develop a level of trust that would lead us to have further conversations. This was going to be a process.

TOWARD SHARED UNDERSTANDING: GETTING AND STAYING CONNECTED, JOINING, AND MAINTAINING ATTENTION

We needed to understand the meaning of each of the infant's health problems and to get and stay on the same page. As a goal towards that end, I wanted to learn what was on the parents' minds and to help them understand how, as a physician/neonatologist, I work with families. My larger goal was to support the parents in maintaining hope and having confidence in me as a guide. I wanted to have confidence in myself as a guide as well. Hoping and being confident are competencies for dealing with parenting and professional challenges. The guiding that I was doing was structured for the parents' learning about individualized care for the infant, the process of making treatment decisions, and the need to see how health events would unfold for the infant.

Building on the discussion of individualization of care, I suggested we begin to talk about some of the complex anomalies their infant had, with the understanding that we could take each condition, one at a time, to better understand typical management. This approach would hopefully build their trust by sharing what we "can do" medically and surgically for specific birth defects, yet always leaving open the idea that "can" does not automatically mean "should" in medicine.

Physician Issue 2: Communicating medical information as well as the individualized approach to fetal/infant care to the parents

I referred to experience in similar medical situations with families. This reference led to a discussion of how we manage a typical CDH, including problems of pulmonary hypoplasia and hypertension, and how we might assess and treat those processes. In this discussion, the idea of extra-corporeal membrane oxygenation (ECMO) came up, at which point the father shared that they were members of the Jehovah's Witnesses faith community, and as a consequence they would not want any blood given to their infant.

Through communication I now had new information. The parents' values could determine goals and contribute to outcomes. Therefore, knowledge of the Jehovah's Witnesses faith would have to be incorporated into decision making and development of a treatment plan. So I drew on my prior clinical experiences with families of similar faith communities to explain our approach to care for the infant.

Parent Issue 3: Preparing for and protecting the infant's physical and spiritual life
Healthcare Team Issue 1: Considering invasive procedures and blood transfusions

What these parents valued as Jehovah's Witnesses led us down an interesting path, a tangent from the usual discussion of what to expect with CDH. The parents understood that the ECMO circuit was filled with blood, and for an infant this was necessary because of the need to maintain blood volume. On the one hand, I shared that for an infant with severe CDH and pulmonary hypoplasia we typically recommend not doing ECMO. We consider ECMO optional for any infant with CDH, T18 or not, as we consider benefits and burdens and long-term outcomes. I also shared that our typical response to a parent who is a Jehovah's Witness is to do whatever we can to avoid transfusing blood into an infant, but in the end if we felt it was necessary as a life-saving measure, we typically go against parental wishes by getting a court order to transfuse blood products.

It has been suggested by some that seeking a court order is appreciated by some parents because it removes the moral responsibility aspect of decision making from them. I asked them their thoughts about this, and about whether their infant would be considered spiritually damaged if we gave blood. I suggested they think about whether a shorter, spiritually intact life was better or worse than a longer life after blood transfusion. I also shared that even if the infant did not need ECMO, it would be a rare case for an infant with CDH to not require a transfusion at some point in time. We left that conversation agreeing that ECMO would not be used. I also shared that if we got through the CDH repair, the issue of considering invasive procedures and blood transfusion would come up again for additional potential cardiac surgery. I shared that on one other occasion we refused to perform cardiac surgery on an infant with T18 and a VSD without blood consent. Five other centers around the country agreed with us and refused to take the infant for surgery. For the first time, the parents began to consider whether aggressive treatment was the right path. They wanted, however, to continue the conversation concerning aggressive care options.

TRANSFERRING RESPONSIBILITY

The parents needed to explore their faith and which goal might be more important—an infant who was spiritually intact or who had a longer life. The bridging and connection making I was guiding the parents in led them to confront their faith and the limitations it presented to them. They had to negotiate their own internal struggles with these limitations.

From the perspective of ethics, we had to explore whether we should factor typical Trisomy 18 (T18) outcomes, like the infant's death, into the decision about blood product administration. If we did not discriminate among the individual care needs of each infant and family, we would, by default, seek a court order to give blood products against the parents' wishes. The other ethical option was to support parental autonomy and not seek a court order. This option is based on the concept that, in the best interests of an infant with T18, infants would not undergo invasive procedures requiring blood transfusions. The medical team had some level of power to make the call on which way we would go.

After discussing the possible outcomes regarding CDH, I pointed out that I had not yet addressed the cardiac defect, partly because that would not typically be something to deal with in the first days to weeks of life. Neither had we discussed T18. Only after pointing this out did the parents appreciatively acknowledge it. They seemed to recognize that my not bringing up T18 meant I was not constraining the infant's medical care decisions by the fact the infant had T18. They also seemed to recognize that I was willing to meet them where they were in their view of their infant's needs. When I asked what they understood about infants with T18 and their outcomes, they acknowledged that they hadn't looked into that because they didn't want the infant's T18 to affect their decisions. I gently led them to a discussion about how T18 can potentially affect medical and surgical response to therapies and the implications of T18 for outcomes and quality of life should the infant survive a CDH repair (Andrews et al., 2016; Haug, Goldstein, Cummins, Fayard, & Merritt, 2017). The parents had by then shared that quality of life was important to them. I suggested they think about levels of quality of life worth pursuing that we could address in future meetings.

> It was clear to me that the parents needed to think about one condition at a time and were having trouble putting the many facets of their infant's medical condition together. As they needed to move on to meet with one of our pediatric surgeons, there was a consensus that this would really be the first of our meetings. We would continue to meet to discuss plans of care and answer their questions as we saw how the infant did throughout the pregnancy.

CONTINUING BRIDGING: BRINGING WHAT WAS FEARED INTO THE LIGHT OF WHAT IS KNOWN

Subsequent meetings with the parents focused on helping them know what to expect. Supporting the parents in regulating emotions occurred in these meetings. They had to wait and see what would happen, and through their waiting maintain hope and trust. I informed them of possibilities and kept out in front the understanding that they, the parents, wanted the doctors to assess things and then inform them of what they, the doctors, had learned. While the parents expressed not wanting to know too much about T18 outcomes, it was important to gently lead them to hear some outcome data and how the genetic condition would affect their infant. My responsibility was to help the parents know what kind of condition their infant had, what they could expect for her and themselves, and how they could participate in decision making in the context of the medical team's expertise and my guidance.

> Allowing the parents to reject information about T18 would not help them be the best decision makers they could be for their infant. To support their ethic of being autonomous parents, they had to be informed with the medical information that mattered for making decisions.

MAKING CONNECTIONS IN PROBLEM SOLVING, WEIGHING ALTERNATIVES, AND DECISION MAKING

My impressions were that the parents were moving from a relationship with me of not trusting to a relationship of trusting, and they were likely to not want palliative care, admittedly my preference for their infant. We had briefly reviewed a few of the positive features of palliative care if the infant's condition seemed to be even more concerning than we anticipated. My goal was for the parents to at least understand what that process might look like at some point in the infant's life.

After meeting with the surgeon, the parents were excited about being offered an MRI at 32 weeks gestation to assess fetal lung volume. Perhaps their excitement was based on the hope it gave them of the pregnancy lasting at least until 32 weeks, and on the hope that we would do everything diagnostically we generally recommend. I interpreted the parents' excitement as wanting us to proceed with the assessment of lung function. Privately with the healthcare team members, I acknowledged I was not happy that a fetal MRI was discussed and offered, because the ultrasound had already shown lung volumes were reasonable. The MRI is another expensive test with consequent findings that, in my opinion, were not likely to change the management strategy. The surgeon and the fetal nurse, however, thought that in the short time the parents had been alone while waiting for the surgery consult, they had reconsidered their expressed desire during the earlier conversation with me to decline palliative care. The surgeon and the nurse thought the parents were thinking palliative care could be the best option for their infant, and that a fetal MRI finding of poor lung volume could sway them to choose palliative care.

BRIDGING: TO NURTURE REALISTIC HOPE AND TO BRING IN THE EXPERTISE OF OTHERS

As a guide, offering tests that may provide information to help parents make a decision consistent with their goals is clearly valuable. Whether the fetal MRI was necessary for this decision was debatable. The next step for a guide would be to help the family interpret the fetal MRI results. These results, however, are not necessarily definitive in predicting physiologic processes and behavior after birth. The guide, as a consequence of limitations in the information provided by a test like a fetal MRI, must put the perimeters around the test for interpretation if the result is to help in decision making.

My next meeting with the parents came after the fetal MRI, which as expected revealed very good fetal lung volumes. The parents were ecstatic. I was concerned that the fetal MRI results gave the parents false hope. Knowing of their response, I had to meet them in the place of having hope, yet bring them back to a two-pronged reality—their infant still had the underlying T18 genetic disorder, and they would still not want to transfuse blood products. Together, these two realities made their hopes for long-term survival of their infant futile.

> I now had to help explain to the parents how the fetal MRI results were informative but limited in value. While initially the healthcare team set up the test to possibly help the parents move toward palliative care if the results showed poor fetal lung volumes, we now had to deal with "good" test results. I had to determine the parents' understanding of the results and whether the positive test had backfired in the messages we were trying to give them about their infant's likely death due to the T18.

I began my meeting with the parents by agreeing with them that while the fetal MRI findings were encouraging, I reiterated that we still had to see how their infant would respond to our medical therapies. I suggested it was time to acknowledge that the T18 could or could not negatively affect unfolding health events, and that the VSD could also affect the infant's response to therapies if there were significant pulmonary hypertension present. It was time to start to put all these things together. This led me to discuss again the cardiac condition, including outcomes with or without surgery. I began to guide them in thinking about things essentially backwards instead of forward.

The backwards walk, a way of structuring the learning, would begin with the fact that we (and five other centers we had conferred with) would not offer to nor perform cardiac surgery if the parents would not provide consent for blood products administration. Without surgical repair, their infant would die from congestive heart failure somewhere in the range of 4 to 12 months after birth. We discussed whether our surgeons and anesthesiologists would perform CDH surgery without consent for blood products. This would require the pediatric surgeons to agree to surgery without giving blood, which meant accepting the possibility they might bring her out of the operating room to die or accepting that the infant could die slowly of anemia in the NICU. The parents still agreed to forego ECMO. For the first time, they asked the question about whether they should start invasive treatments/surgery if, in the end, their infant would die without undergoing cardiac surgery. We reviewed what comfort care would look like from the beginning of their infant's life, prior to invasive procedures. Comfort care included parents having the opportunity to hold their infant, without having a sense of separation. There would be no painful procedures. All care usually provided to newborn infants would be given as the infant tolerated them until death occurred. Their infant could die in the hospital, or possibly go home with hospice, depending on the infant's physiologic status. We talked about spiritual support and memory making, which would be offered with whatever kind of care their infant received, including aggressive care.

TRANSFERRING RESPONSIBILITY TO PARENTS AND TO OTHER CLINICIANS

I wanted to support the parents' problem solving and decision making. The father recognized we were talking about packed red blood cell (PRBC) transfusions and asked me to explain what blood products we typically provide. He was starting to question and hope that perhaps other blood products were acceptable in his faith and only whole blood was unacceptable. While I knew the answer, I explained about PRBC, platelets, fresh frozen plasma, and cryoprecipitate. I then suggested he go to his religious leaders and ask if any of these were acceptable, while knowing the answer he would get.

Physician Issue 3: Developing the healthcare team's support for parents' goals

I knew that I needed to use GP through clinical leadership. To do this, I focused on keeping clinical goals in mind and reminding others on the healthcare team about these goals. During the parent–team meeting, I also assigned some homework to pediatric surgery and cardiology physicians prior to a third meeting with the parents. My intent was to learn if going to the operating room without blood consent was something any of the physicians would do or not do. I wanted to be able to give the parents a final answer. In the process, I was developing the healthcare team's support for the goals for the infant's care.

The connections the parents were making with what they knew about their infant's condition and needs for care and the knowledge of their spiritual leaders' interpretation of religious doctrine concerning blood products use forced the parents to confront their faith and the restrictions it presented to their infant's treatment. At the same time, I was transferring some of the responsibility for informing parents about treatment options to the parents' religious guides and to other members of the healthcare team. Transferring responsibility supported me in not being the person to tell the parents that no blood products at all were allowed, and that the healthcare team would not support undertaking surgery without consent to give blood.

Healthcare Team Issue 2: Providing medical care for the infant during a short life expectancy

I held the third and final prenatal meeting with the parents. This meeting included the mother's delivering obstetrician, pediatric surgeon, cardiologist, and fetal support nurse. I began the meeting by asking for the information I had requested to guide our decision making. The parents very sadly acknowledged that their religion precluded use of blood products of any kind for the infant or the mother. The pediatric surgeon reported that a few of his colleagues would be willing to do the CDH surgery without consent for blood, and all were in support of not using ECMO. The cardiologist reported that the team would not operate without consent for blood products. It was agreed that further exploration with other centers would not be necessary for their decision making, as this has been done before. The parents told the healthcare team their goal was to support the infant at birth with any medical interventions we could provide except ECMO. They would like their infant to have the CDH surgery and to be able to go home.

We addressed labor and delivery planning in detail. Options offered included labor with and without fetal monitoring, within the context of natural vaginal delivery and cesarean section (C/S) options. While the goal was to give vaginal delivery a trial, the obstetrician asked what the parents would want if fetal monitoring were used and fetal distress was observed. Would the mother want an emergent C/S without the possibility of being given blood? The delivery options were explored in the context of the parents' goal of possibly bringing the infant home.

The parents now understood that the healthcare team might recommend different options based on the parents' goals. The team members stated that they strongly recommended against the mother taking too much risk for an infant who, in the end, would die. The parents' response, however, was that the mother was willing to take on the risks of anything, even up to C/S without blood products for her, knowing there might be a high likelihood of dying. Whether the parents' response was due to an unrealistic, false hope or not eluded me.

> In the course of problem solving and making decisions, while keeping the parental and the clinical goals in mind—that is, the infant's viability, quality of life, spiritual well-being, and the implications for outcomes of their decisions—transferring responsibility became my focus with these parents.

FINAL DAYS AND TRANSFER OF RESPONSIBILITY

Their infant girl was born by spontaneous vaginal delivery without any need for blood products for the mother. The infant's initial response to our respiratory support was good. There was no pulmonary hypertension that would have required ECMO, or lethal pulmonary hypoplasia. On the second day of life, with parental support and agreement, the pediatric surgeon made the decision to take the infant to the operating room for open primary closure of the CDH. The infant returned to the NICU in reasonable shape. However, over the next 4 days, she became more significantly anemic and consequently metabolically acidotic. She required more supplemental oxygen, and was started on an intravenous dopamine and epinephrine medication drip for cardiac support. While the pediatric surgeons had agreed to be available to fix the CDH without administering blood, they struggled with refraining from challenging the parents' wishes to not give blood postoperatively once back in the NICU. This struggle intensified while watching the infant slowly die from worsening, untreated anemia. They raised the question about getting a court order, but in the end agreed to stay consistent in following parental wishes, even if that led to the infant's death. The main reason the healthcare team was comfortable supporting the parents' wishes was the fact that the infant had T18. No member of the healthcare team thought we should have gone as far as we had gone with active/invasive treatment for their daughter to begin with.

At this time, the parents were counseled that the only treatment that could turn things around clinically now for their infant would be a PRBC transfusion. We would not, however, override the decision they had made. We explained that if their infant should experience a cardiac arrest, we would not do chest compressions because airway and circulatory support were already in place. The parents decided to withdraw care on their infant's sixth day of life in the face of progressive decompensation.

CONCLUSION

This case is a powerful example of GP. The parents were brought over time into full participation in medical decision making. This mother and father engaged in parenting through a prenatal diagnosis, birth, and eventually a death they had hoped would not happen. The patient counseling practices, or pattern of activities that were routinely and repeatedly performed over the pregnancy and into the NICU, included addressing the parents' needs for protecting their daughter. GP occurred through the relationship built over time, from the moments of distrust to support, through the processes of getting and staying connected, maintaining attention, bridging, structuring learning and tasks of parenting, and transferring the responsibility to both parents and healthcare team participants. The more skilled or resourceful person, the guide, learned from and with the less skilled person, the learner, about what is relevant, meaningful, useful, manageable, and emotionally tolerable.

QUESTIONS FOR REFLECTION

Trust and a Working Relationship Expressed as Getting and Staying Connected

Dr. Leuthner comments on the distrust he felt the parents had in their earliest interactions and the crucial need for establishing a trusting relationship:

> If I could not connect with these parents, there would be no way to help guide them. . . . I realized my goal in this first hour I had with them was going to be developing a level of trust that would lead us to have further conversations. . . . The goal [was] a working relationship, which is part of the process of "getting and staying connected."

- Are you or are you not in agreement with Dr. Leuthner's claim that trust is essential for a working relationship through which getting and staying connected, the grounds for GP, can be established? Reflect on your own experience.

Establishing Trust

- Identify the means Dr. Leuthner used to develop trust, expressed through and beyond getting and staying connected.
  One of the means Dr. Leuthner used was reflecting with the parents about what they were expecting and intending and the goals and values that set a direction, oriented and corrected their actions, and shaped their perspectives. Reflecting with parents was implicit in the GP that Dr. Leuthner described himself as doing with parents:

  > They [the parents] were likely to not want palliative care, admittedly my preference for their infant. We had briefly reviewed a few of the positive features of palliative care if the infant's condition seemed to be even more concerning than we anticipated. My goal was for the parents to at least understand what that process might look like at some point in the infant's life.

- How would you reflect on the parents' values and goals, or encourage this type of reflection with parents?
  Here is how Dr. Rana Limbo has written about "wondering with" parents of an infant with abnormalities as a means of reflecting on distrust accompanied by feelings of anger that need to be regulated for connecting in a relationship and doing GP:

  > It must be so hard to have heard and read about those stories and now you are here in the same place with your own infant. I am wondering what I could do right now to help you feel more comfortable about being here with me.

  Dr. Limbo continues beyond reflecting in the active form of wondering to build trust by speaking directly to her principles of working with parents, for example:

  > I am careful to not speak about other patients and families so I cannot explain the situation you heard about. I of course offer that same level of privacy and confidentiality to you. I want you to trust me and hope we can start building that trust right now.

- What means do you use to build trust and how do you or would you structure it into GP practice?

The Problem of Hope: Nurturing and Maintaining Hope, But Preventing False Hope

Dr. Leuthner wrote in his case study:

> My next meeting came after the MRI, which as expected revealed very good fetal lung volumes. This now gave me concern of giving the family false hope as the parental response was ecstatic. Knowing of their response, I had to meet them in that place of having hope, yet bring them back to the reality that the infant still has the underlying genetic disorder, and that they still would not want to provide blood products, which together made their hopes for long-term survival futile.

One of Dr. Leuthner's goals for the GP was to nurture and maintain hope while countering false hope.

- Why, how, and when does hope surface in GP?
- What are the ethical issues associated with hope?
- When and how would you make issues of hope explicit in GP?

For clinicians, Feudtner and his colleagues (Hill & Feudtner, 2016; Rosenberg & Feudtner, 2016) stress two ideas concerning hope: (a) the importance of recognizing that hope influences the experience for parents whenever pediatric illness is serious; and (b) hope is not a singular concept in parents' thinking, but rather a set or range of issues, including not only length of life but opportunities and life experiences and quality of life from various perspectives.

- How would you apply these ideas in your GP if and when you work with parents who are anticipating or currently caring for an infant with a serious illness?

Power and Its Articulation With GP

Dr. Leuthner referred to power in his case in two senses, the first in regard to empowering parents as follows:

> I would need to figure out a way to relate, building trust and allowing them to feel empowered to nurture and protect their infant, and at the same time bring in quality of life issues for the infant who had a significant genetic disorder that cannot be ignored.

The second reference is to his own power as perceived by the parents:

> As a guide I had to develop trust through communication of facts, understanding of hopes, and assessing their quality of life goals for their future infant. They recognized the power differential in knowledge and addressed that directly,

which a majority of families never do. I could now hopefully use this to break down barriers and build bridges of trust.

- How does the decision-making power parents have make a difference in how you do or could practice GP in your setting?
- What would inform you that your own power was hindering the effectiveness of your GP practice?
- What would or could you do to regulate power issues between yourself and the person(s) you were providing guidance to?

REFERENCES

Andrews, S. E., Downey, A. G., Showalter, D. S., Fitzgerald, H., Showalter, V. P., Carey, J. C., & Hulac, P. (2016). Shared decision making and the pathways approach in the prenatal and postnatal management of the trisomy 13 and trisomy 18 syndromes. *American Journal of Medical Genetics Part C: Seminars in Medical Genetics, 172,* 257–263.

Haug, S., Goldstein, M., Cummins, D., Fayard, E., & Merritt, T. A. (2017). Using patient-centered care after a prenatal diagnosis of trisomy 18 or trisomy 13: A review. *JAMA Pediatrics, 171*(4), 382–387.

Hill, D., & Feudtner, C. (2016). Hope, hopefulness, and pediatric palliative care. In B. P. Black, P. M. Wright, & R. Limbo (Eds.), *Perinatal and pediatric bereavement in nursing and other health professions* (pp. 223–247). New York, NY: Springer.

McKechnie, A. C., Pridham, K. F., & Tluczek, A. (2015). Preparing heart and mind for becoming a parent following a diagnosis of fetal anomaly. *Qualitative Health Research, 25,* 1182–1198. doi:10.1177/1049732314553852

Patterson, J., Taylor, G., Smith, M., Dotters-Katz, K. P., Davis, A. M., & Price, W. (2017, March 16). Transitions in care for infants with trisomy 13 or 18. *American Journal of Perinatology, 34,* 887–894. doi: 10.1055/s-0037-1600912

Pridham, K. F. (1993). Anticipatory guidance of parents of new infants: Potential contribution of the internal working model construct. *Image–The Journal of Nursing Scholarship, 25*(1), 49–56.

Rosenberg, A. R., & Feudtner, C. (2016). What else are you hoping for? Fostering hope in paediatric serious illness. *Acta Paediatrica, 105,* 1004–1005.

21

Guided Participation: The Role of the Speech– Language Pathologist

Katherine Frontier

When I was studying to become a speech–language pathologist (SLP), I was taught guided participation (GP) practice early in my graduate coursework. The focus was on facilitating language development in young children. As an SLP, the process of guiding a toddler's meaningful use of language was very rewarding. Although my career and clinical practice shifted to the care of infants over 20 years ago, the focus on communication and guidance of meaningful learning is still something I practice every day.

The aim of this chapter is to introduce how GP can be practiced by an SLP to support parents in feeding their premature or medically compromised infant as the parent/infant dyad together develop feeding skills. The SLP uses professional expertise acquired in part through work with numerous infants to assess an individual infant's ability to communicate cues of hunger and satiety, communicate readiness to feed (e.g., awake enough), physically engage in effective feeding (e.g., suck, swallow, and breathe coordination, oral and overall body muscle tone and strength), communicate cues of distress, manage swallowing difficulties, and effectively respond to the parent's feeding behavior. The SLP uses this information to guide the parent (e.g., through processes of sharing understanding, bridging, and structuring the task of feeding) in successfully doing the feeding task (e.g., developing competency in interpreting the infant's responses and actions during feeding), and thus gain confidence as a feeder.

In effect, the SLP creates a learning environment which invites and supports the parents to become competent feeders of a compromised infant.

Simultaneously, the process of developing feeding competencies also offers the opportunity to be with and get to know the infant as a person—that is, to develop a relationship with the infant (Schroeder & Pridham, 2006). As parents gain confidence in their feeding competencies and those of the infant, they are able to coregulate the feeding experience. This forges a bond between the compromised infant and caregiver. The SLP transfers her knowledge of feeding, swallowing, and breathing and the responsibility of feeding the infant to the parents over the course of assessment and treatment sessions.

LEARNING THE INFANT'S LANGUAGE: A COMPETENCE TO BE DEVELOPED

My role in the NICU is the assessment and treatment of infants with a primary focus on the acquisition of the skills for safe and efficient oral feeding. Parents are often surprised when they hear that "Speech" is coming to evaluate their baby. Many think of the role of the SLP as primarily to assess and treat communication disorders. Although the objective is successful oral feeding, and infants do not speak in the truest sense of the word, they communicate throughout feeding. The infant may exhibit shifts in their respiratory pattern, subtle sounds can be heard during swallowing, changes in facial expression, shifts in muscle tone as well as other autonomic and or physiologic cues—this absolutely is communication. "Engagement—important for learning a new skill—requires an awake state, sufficient energy, robustness, and focused attention" (Rogoff, 2003). Teaching parents to recognize their infant's cues can lead to more effective, positive, and nurturing feeding experiences. Premature infants begin to show readiness cues for oral feeding at 32 to 33 weeks postconceptual age. Nurses are trained to see these cues and are able to respond to the infant to help introduce oral feeding practice. This introduction begins with nonnutritive oral input with mouth cares of swabs of the mother's breast milk and progresses to the initiation of oral feeding.

GP ISSUES, PROCESSES, AND COMPETENCIES

I take my role in the patient's treatment team very seriously. Parents of hospitalized newborns have to entrust the care of their infant to others and I approach my care of their child as a responsibility and with gratitude. Pamela Dodrill, PhD CCC-SLP, at Brigham and Women's Hospital in Boston, described feeding preterm infants as a responsibility requiring competencies acquired through learning processes. In her words, "There is no other time that a human is more vulnerable" (Dodrill, 2015). The infant is wholly dependent on the caregiver for all nutrition and hydration. A preterm infant is learning new skills as they mature to complete the complex task of sucking, swallowing, and breathing. Newborns feed at minimum eight times per day. If the caregiver is unable to read signs of feeding readiness, to respond to the infant's responses during feeding, and to recognize completion cues, there is risk that the infant will fail and be readmitted to hospital. Through teaching, reciprocal interactions, and transfer of knowledge through the course of being guided by an SLP, parents become the experts in guiding the infant to eat safely and efficiently.

As an SLP, when called to consult on an infant's development of feeding competencies, I provide assessment of oral motor skills, oral reflexes, oral sensorimotor skills, the infant's feeding pattern, respiratory pattern, as well as timing and safety of swallowing. After my initial assessment, I follow the infant and partner with the family, the nurses, and the other team members, including lactation consultants, clinical dietitians, and physical and occupational therapists. Together, we are able to teach the parents how their infant reacts to the environment and responds to stimuli. A plan of care for oral feeding (refer to Figure 21.1) is developed to be followed by caregivers and nurses.

The feeding plan includes when to feed, what feeding readiness cues to look for, what bottle/nipple to use, positioning guidelines, indications of stress during feeding, factors that influence respiratory function, and strategies to promote the infant's stability during feeding. These strategies could include breathing breaks, pacing, and limiting the duration of feeding. Feeding plans are continually modified and updated as the infant gains resilience and advances to the ultimate goal of total oral feeding. Stress cues (refer to Figure 21.2) in the infant's subsystems (state, respiratory, motor, and swallowing) are acknowledged and acted on to facilitate feeding success.

GP with parents for the development of competence in feeding the infant starts as opportunities for caregivers to observe as I describe the infant's behaviors and reactions during feeding. Parent partners are guided to recognize and respond to these stress signs to support their infant. As the infant becomes more competent during feeding, my role as the person feeding the infant changes to that of a guide or coach as the parent learns to recognize infant cues in the process of feeding the infant.

An aim of guiding parents to become the expert in feeding their infants is to teach coregulated feeding, a process in which the caregiver and infant take cues from each other. Goals in guiding parents in learning to feed the infant in a coregulated manner are to both improve the feeding experience and to have safe and effective feeding (Horner et al., 2014; Ross & Browne, 2002, 2013; Ross & Philbin, 2011; Shaker, 2013, 2017a, 2017b); Thoyre, Holditch-Davis, Schwartz, Melendez Roman, & Nix, 2012). The concept of coregulation fosters the principle that the infant and the parent respond to each other during bottle or breastfeeding for safe and successful feeding experiences. The transfer of knowledge for coregulated feeding practice from the SLP to parents supports them in developing competence for understanding and communicating with others to ensure their infant's success in feeding.

Every infant being discharged from the hospital must be able to be fed in some way. The infant must tolerate feeds and demonstrate appropriate weight gain and growth before consideration of discharge. Attainment of oral feeding is often what prolongs hospital length of stay. The ideal route for feeding is through oral feeding and may include total breastfeeding, total bottle-feeding, or a combination of breast and bottle-feeding. However, there are many infants

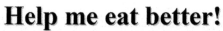

Help me eat better!

Right now, I am working on practice and pleasurable oral feeding times. Please focus on the quality of feeding experiences not necessarily the amount of volume taken.

- ONLY orally feed me if I am awake, showing readiness cues and am able to suck on my pacifier at my feeding time.
- Use the slow-flow nipple.
- Hold me in a cradled position for feeds. I need to be swaddled to help me stay organized and to conserve my energy.
- Give me breathing breaks at the beginning of the feeding, usually every 5-6 sucks.
- I may need my pacifier again if my sucking becomes disorganized or I am biting the nipple.
- Limit feeds to 15 minutes to help me conserve my energy.

Thanks!
Baby H. and Family

Please page Katherine if I'm having oral feeding problems.
3/3/2017

FIGURE 21.1 Plan of care—oral feeding.

who are unable to take necessary volume by oral means. In these situations, there are thoughtful discussions with the medical team and the family to determine the best and safest route for feeding. Alternative feeding methods may include nasogastric feeds, gastrostomy, or jejunal tube placement. Surgically placed

Examples of Stress Cues Observed During Infant Feeding

State Stress Cues

Diffuse sleep or wake states
Eye floating/eyebrow lift
Staring
Gaze aversion
Panicked or worried look
Glassy-eyes
Frenzy or inconsolability

Respiratory Stress Cues

Tachypnea
Gasping
Head bobbing
Nasal flaring
Stridor
Congestion
Retractions

Motor Stress Cues

Gagging
Grimacing
Arching/turning away
Shifts in muscle tone
Raised hand ("Stop sign")

Swallowing Stress Cues

Gulping
Gurgling/pharyngeal pooling
Drooling
Choking
Coughing

FIGURE 21.2 Examples of stress cues observed during infant feeding.

feeding tubes are used for various medical causes, and may also be used in cases when an infant is not safe to be fed orally and/or oral feeding intake is limited for some reason. These limitations could include aspiration, poor endurance to complete feeds, altered oral motor skills, or other causes.

Feeding preterm infants is not the same as feeding healthy, term infants and requires a different set of parental skills. For an infant to be discharged from the neonatal or cardiac ICU, the parents must know how to feed the infant and the infant must be able to feed and grow as expected. All parents must be guided in reading infant behaviors relevant to oral feeding. This guidance gives parents the skills to independently feed their infant at hospital discharge (Reyna, Pickler, & Thompson, 2006). No matter the family situation, my SLP role must be to facilitate positive feeding experiences for the infant and the parents by guiding them to understand their infant's behavioral language. Parent teaching within a GP framework is constantly adapted for the learner in an informed and compassionate way.

THE EMOTIONAL COMPONENT OF GP

The SLP needs to be prepared to guide parents in understanding the meaning of the feeding experience and the emotions they experience, along with the infant's learning to feed. Reflecting on the experience of caregiving, I asked myself: What do we do as caregivers of an infant? We feed them, diaper them, and make sure they are comfortable. Imagine if feeding your baby was a challenge. Parents of NICU graduates often say that the waiting for their infant to learn to feed was the most challenging part of the NICU stay. It is also the most difficult for friends and family members outside of the day-to-day NICU experience to understand. A mother recently told me that her brother asked her why her 4-month-old premature infant, born at 25 weeks postmenstrual age, was still in the hospital. He had told his sister that the baby was past the expected due date, so why wasn't the baby home? When she told him that her son was still working on feeding, his reply was, "Infants eat. Aren't you taking good care of him?"

This question was emotionally heartbreaking for the mother. She was at the bedside every day, helping her infant learn to eat, but he was still having stress cues and falling asleep, unable to take full bottles. I guided her to recognize the small steps he had made over the past weeks of feeding practice as he built endurance and became more successful every day. This infant was succeeding, as was his mother. By guiding the mother in building a mental bridge between how things had been with feeding for both her baby and herself and how they were now, I was helping her to regulate her feelings of distress, experience confidence in her and her infant's capacity to learn to feed competently, maintain her optimism, and to have hope that she could communicate effectively to others, like her brother.

Case Example 21.1

Baby Elliott was born at 28 weeks gestation via caesarean section due to maternal preeclampsia. Elliott required resuscitation at delivery and was intubated. He was extubated by 32 weeks gestation and by 34 weeks had transitioned to simple nasal cannula. Nursing staff and his mother provided opportunities for nonnutritive sucking with pacifier and mouth cares with breast milk. Oral feeding was started at 33 6/7 weeks with Elliott's display of feeding readiness cues with waking for feeds, rooting, and accepting his pacifier. A speech consult was placed when Elliott was 35 weeks because he was only taking 25% of the required volume by mouth. Nursing documentation reported that Elliott would wake and show hunger cues, but would fall asleep after feeding for 8 to 12 minutes. He showed stress cues of tachypnea, drooling, and occasional choking and coughing. It was also reported that the mother did not want to feed him because she was afraid that he would choke.

At the time of my initial assessment, at 35 weeks, Elliott demonstrated rooting and had rhythmical sucking with his pacifier. Prior to feeding, I gave him tastes of breast milk on the pacifier. He was fed with a newborn-flow nipple, but showed immediate stress cues including head bobbing, gulping with swallowing, and drooling. During the assessment, his feeding position was changed from cradled to side-lying and the nipple was changed to one that was slower flowing. With these changes, he had less drooling and was no longer gulping with swallowing.

I fed Elliott for the next three sessions with his mother observing. I was able to point out his competencies, including coordinated nonnutritive sucking, rooting to the nipple, and timely swallowing when given breaks. I was able to describe Elliott's breathing pattern to his mother and help her see his cues of rapid breathing without needing to look at his cardiorespiratory monitor. We discussed how pacing gave Elliott breaks to breathe and increased his endurance at feeding.

At the fourth feeding session, Elliot's mother wanted to feed her son. I helped her with the new positioning so she felt comfortable with him in her arms. She told me that we should start with the pacifier to "help him get organized." This was something we had discussed at earlier sessions. She had joined attention with me and understanding was shared between us. She asked me to get him started with eating, but after just a few minutes of my initiation of the feeding, she was holding the bottle with me as I showed her the rhythm of pacing Elliott by tilting the bottle down so the contents of the bottle could not flow into Elliott's mouth and he could take a breath. Soon, she was feeding him independently. At the end of that feeding, Elliot's mother proudly remarked that he "took half of his bottle for me!"

Over the next 2 weeks, Elliot progressed to take full feeds by mouth. I continued to follow his progress and partner with his mother. When she fed her son, she would talk to him with phrases that I had used when teaching her. I heard her say "let's take a break with your pacifier to put you back together." She recognized feeding cues and asked the nurse to get the bottle ready early because "I can tell he's getting hungry, he's going to his hands." Prior to discharge, she was showing Elliott's father how to swaddle him before feeding "so he keeps his body together."

In just a few weeks, Elliott's mother had gone from being fearful of holding and feeding her son to directing the behavior of others to assure his feeding success.

CONCLUSION

GP is constantly present in my clinical practice. Through observation, demonstration, and description of infant behaviors, my attention and knowledge is shared with the parents and young infants needing guidance in feeding practice and leads to successful relationships. These reciprocal interactions create shared understanding of the processes. This understanding is transferred to parents and the infants and from them to me as all become expert in feeding with the infant. Taking Vygotsky's (1978) concept of the zone of proximal development, we have extended understanding and competence all the way around. In the process, parents are not only competent in feeding their infant but also advocates for the infant as well. The advocacy is marked by the parents' skills in describing their infant's competencies and needs for support and the contributions the parents are making to the infant's support.

Through my observations as an SLP and reflection with parents on the progress of their infant's feeding, I have opportunities for in-depth learning about variations in parental and infant learning. This learning extends my competencies as an SLP who provides GP. Through SLP practice grounded in GP, I am able to integrate the best available evidence for supportive feeding of vulnerable infants, develop my clinical expertise, and discern the preferences of parents and infants for feeding that functions well for them in the context of their families (Taylor, Priefer, & Alt-White, 2016; Turkanis, Bartlett, & Rogoff, 2001).

QUESTIONS FOR REFLECTION

This chapter contributes a number of significant ideas about GP practice. One of these ideas is that the ways of being with others, learning, and living out one's chosen vocation and life responsibilities are likely to be permeated with ways of thinking, knowing, behaving, and enacting roles that are consistent with the practice of guided participation. Another distinctive idea is that guided participation may be carried out simultaneously on several levels, including a clinician guide with a parent concerning the parent's guidance, in a manner consistent with GP practice, of a young child and even a very young infant who is compromised in capacity to learn to feed because of prematurity or medical condition.

A third significant idea is that the same concepts of GP of clinician (e.g., SLP) and infant or parents and infant are applicable to the practice as is the case for clinicians and parents with an older child. Attention must be shared, even though the infant or young child may not be aware of focusing on the same thing as the guide. The language of the other needs to be understood and shared in respect to its meaning. Bridging, in the form of sensorimotor associations, needs to occur, and transfer of responsibility of a guide for pacing the process of sequential sucking, swallowing, and breathing gradually advances to the parents. The SLP in the case example demonstrates a keen sense of an infant's language and a finely tuned skill in helping parents to make sense of that language as parents learn to feed a premature or medically challenged infant—and in the process, help the infant learn to feed.

In respect to your own practice, whether, clinical, educational, or research focused, consider the types of "languages" you engage with in your functions as a guide. These "languages" could take several forms, ranging from behavior to the expressions of a toddler or to the newly forming language of a school child, adolescent, or adult parent or grandparent who is an immigrant in a new country.

- How do you or would you learn language that is adequate to be a guide in the process of GP for the person?
- How would or could you use another person, for example, a parent, in communicating so that you share attention and understanding with the person you have taken on the responsibility of guiding?

Think of yourself working with a team that (clinical, educational, or research focused) includes members engaged in GP for various goals.

- What are some of the paths you, as a team, might take and strategies you might use to integrate your work, keep it from conflicting, and coordinate it?
- What kind of verbal and written reporting would be indicated among your group and even necessary to make the GP practices of all team members beneficial to recipients and guides?
- If you have a clinical practice, does it lend itself to structuring or laying out a plan for GP? Why or why not?

REFERENCES

Dodrill, P. (2015, October). *Feeding Difficulties in the NICU.* Lecture presented at the Innovative Care in Pediatric Feeding and Swallowing: Bringing It All Together Conference, Boston, MA.

Horner, S., Simonelli, A. M., Schmidt, H., Cichowski, K., Hancko, M., Zhang, G., & Ross, E. S. (2014). Setting the stage for successful oral feeding: The impact of implementing the SOFFI feeding program with medically fragile NICU infants. *Journal of Perinatal and Neonatal Nursing, 28*(1), 59–68.

Reyna, B. A., Pickler, R. H., & Thompson, A. (2006). A descriptive study of mothers' experiences feeding their preterm infants after discharge. *Advances in Neonatal Care, 6,* 333–340.

Rogoff, B. (2003). Learning through guided participation in cultural endeavors. In *The cultural nature of human development* (pp. 282–326). Oxford, UK: Oxford University Press.

Ross, E. S., & Browne, J. V. (2002). Developmental progression of feeding skills: An approach to supporting feeding in preterm infants. *Seminars in Neonatology, 7,* 469–475.

Ross, E. S., & Browne, J. V. (2013). Feeding outcomes in preterm infants after discharge from the neonatal intensive care unit (NICU): A systematic review. *Newborn & Infant Nursing Reviews, 13*(2), 87–93.

Ross, E. S., & Philbin, M. K. (2011). Supporting oral feeding in fragile infants: An evidence-based method for quality bottle-feedings of preterm, ill, and fragile infants. *Journal of Perinatal and Neonatal Nursing, 25*(4), 349–357; quiz 358–349. doi:10.1097/JPN.0b013e318234ac7a

Schroeder, M., & Pridham, K. F. (2006). Development of relationship competencies through guided participation for mothers of preterm infants. *Journal of Obstetric, Gynecologic, & Neonatal Nursing, 35*, 358–368.

Shaker, C. S. (2013). Cue-based feeding in the NICU: Using the infant's communication as a guide. *Neonatal Network, 32*(6), 404–408. doi:10.1891/0730-0832.32.6.404

Shaker, C. S. (2017a). Infant-guided, co-regulated feeding in the neonatal intensive care unit. Part I: Theoretical underpinnings for neuroprotection and safety. *Seminars in Speech and Language, 38*(2), 96–105. doi:10.1055/s-0037-1599107

Shaker, C. S. (2017b). Infant-guided, co-regulated feeding in the neonatal intensive care unit. Part II: Interventions to promote neuroprotection and safety. *Seminars in Speech and Language, 38*(2), 106–115. doi:10.1055/s-0037-1599108

Taylor, M. V., Priefer, B. A., & Alt-White, A. C. (2016). Evidence-based practice: Embracing integration. *Nursing Outlook, 64*, 575–582. doi:10.1016/j.outlook.2016.04.004

Thoyre, S. M., Hubbard, C., Park, J., Pridham, K. F., & McKechnie, A. (2016). Implementing co-regulated feeding with mothers of preterm infants. *MCN: The American Journal of Maternal Child Nursing, 41*(4), 204–211. doi:10.1097/nmc.0000000000000245

Turkanis, C. G., Bartlett, L., & Rogoff, B. (2001). Never-ending learning. In B. Rogoff, C. G. Turkanis, & L. Bartlett (Eds.). *Learning together: Children and adults in a school community* (pp. 225–244). New York, NY: Oxford University Press.

Vygotsky, L. S. (1978). *Mind in society: The development of higher psychological processes.* Cambridge, MA: Harvard University Press.

22

Using Principles of Guided Participation to Develop and Maintain a Bereavement Program

Mary Beth Hensel and Rana Limbo

Healthcare professionals who support a woman and her loved ones facing perinatal death know the acute emotional, physical, and psychosocial suffering that surrounds such an experience (Capitulo, 2005; Chan, Chan, & Day, 2003; Gold, 2007; Smart & Smith, 2013). How those healthcare professionals are educated and trained to deal with these situations either carries and empowers them, or defeats and impairs their ability to administer appropriate support to their patients, and to sustain themselves and coworkers during these devastating life events.

This chapter provides two perspectives on the development of an internationally recognized training program for healthcare clinicians (primarily nurses) who care for those who are grieving the death of someone close to them. The first segment traces the historical roots of the program Resolve Through Sharing® (RTS) from its 1980 planning committee to the present. Although guided participation (GP) practice was unknown to program leaders during the first approximately 20 years of the program, one can identify elements of GP that were incorporated into building the infrastructure and content (see Figure 1.1). The second half of the chapter examines results of contemporary training success, specifically measuring associations between pre- and posttraining surveys of change in participants' learning.

THE BEGINNING OF A PROGRAM THAT WOULD BECOME INTERNATIONALLY KNOWN

RTS began in 1981 as a healthcare program for providing excellent care to families when their baby died at any point during the pregnancy, during labor, or in the newborn and early infant periods. As is often the case with innovation, one person had an idea. A labor and delivery nurse, during her certification course for becoming a maternal nurse practitioner, saw ways that perinatal bereavement care at La Crosse Lutheran Hospital (now Gundersen Health System) could improve. After enlisting the help of her nursing colleague, they went to their department's nursing director, asking for improvements in the way families were cared for. Specifically, they desired an interprofessional team approach, grounded in a strong educational component and standardized through policies and checklists to ensure safety, quality, and continuity.

DETERMINING KEY LEADERS

Fortunately, the director listened to their concerns and agreed (i.e., they developed joint attention) that the process should begin with an interprofessional planning committee. The three carefully chose the members to include bereaved parents, bedside and senior leadership in nursing, social workers, a chaplain, hospital administrators, a project manager, and two physicians (neonatologist and maternal–fetal medicine specialist [MFM]). After meeting together for approximately 8 months, this group came to know each other (i.e., getting and staying connected), forming a strong base of support for introducing the innovation (a system-wide perinatal bereavement program). The term "buy in" is often used in business practices in which the ongoing support of diverse disciplines is needed to make change successful. Once a coordinator was selected (see next section), she invited all planning committee members to a small party at which recognition certificates were given to each committee member. This ritual signaled the end of formal planning, passing the baton for program development and education (i.e., transferring responsibility) to a coordinator who was recently hired. The committee's charge to the coordinator was to implement RTS on all units where perinatal losses occurred, educate all staff about RTS, and most important, train a cohort of RTS support persons (a 16-hour training) who would be bereavement specialists and leaders in the areas in which they worked. The first educational program in fall 1981 was taught by the two maternal nurse practitioners, both of whom were recognized as having the greatest expertise in this area. After that, the coordinator was in charge of scheduling and conducting education via both formal (the 16-hour training to create experts) and less formal learning opportunities (e.g., staff meetings, written materials for staff conference rooms).

CHOOSING A COORDINATOR

The person who became coordinator was suggested by one of the planning committee members. A small group of planning members (including bereaved parents) interviewed the coordinator candidate and made the final selection. The person chosen was experienced as a bedside nurse in mother/baby care, had studied grief and loss in depth during her master's in nursing program, and was highly motivated to serve in this capacity. She had speaking and writing experience, both helpful to those who are in charge of innovation, which requires skill in motivating through face-to-face interaction and written communication.

Many members of the planning committee moved into an advisory committee role, a group that met quarterly initially. Those trained as support persons met monthly to discuss concerns, issues, and successes, creating cohesiveness among the group while developing the competencies of knowing and relating to each other as persons, communicating, and doing the task (that included problem solving).

After several months of working to coordinate and expand RTS, the coordinator recognized the need for patient care coordinators (the nurse manager role) to meet. Their importance in "spreading the word" and offering strong support for the bereavement standard of care became clear as the weeks and months progressed. Their meetings served several purposes. One was that although they knew each other, coming together to discuss a singular program or specific patient care services was an opportunity they rarely had. They used the time to develop competencies important to GP, including problem solving, communicating, and getting to know each other. The time together also allowed those who were farther along in development of integrating bereavement care into the daily practice of bedside nurses to serve as role models and mentors for others.

Joining and maintaining attention (which could be described as "being on the same page") can be more challenging with some professionals than with others. In this case, the coordinator identified the need to work with the MFM to bring the obstetricians and gynecologists into joint attention. They provided the medical care for most of the patients with perinatal loss, and their support of the standardized protocols and regard for the experts providing bedside care was critical. A turning point for this group came about after summaries of clinical care evaluations were sent to families whose baby died or pregnancy ended during the past year. Using bar graphs and other visuals, the coordinator demonstrated the overwhelming satisfaction patients expressed with bereavement care, both quantitatively and qualitatively. The group of physicians seemed especially moved when a sample of comments were projected on the screen. In fairness, these included both positive and negative (of which there were very few). One mother whose baby died in the NICU wrote, "This was the worst thing that has ever happened to us. But I know now that I could get through it again if I had [my nurse] with me." Documenting the relational nature of family-centered care proved to be the cornerstone of the program, with all materials and trainings focused on relationship. In fact, the booklet for parents, still offered and used today, is named from a quotation received from a parent in that very first evaluation: ". . . it means so much to know that someone cares."

Another significant department that needed to embed perinatal bereavement care was the pathology laboratory. Fortunately, the laboratory supervisor worked closely with the coordinator and those providing bereavement care, gaining and maintaining joint attention to create respectful ways of treating the remains after miscarriage (defined as less than 20 weeks gestation). Patients whose pregnancy ended were aided in making decisions about whether they preferred private burial or hospital disposition, which by the late 1980s included a hospital-sponsored annual burial service and a grave marker. A mother, whose baby died early in pregnancy, called the coordinator at some point after her loss, asking, "Where is my baby?" Like nearly all hospitals and laboratories, the tissue from a miscarriage or ectopic pregnancy went to a landfill. With the laboratory supervisor's help, this mother's wish to create a special place for all babies was created and continues today. Laboratory personnel store the remains, marked with the patient's name, and prepare caskets for a select place in a local cemetery.

DEVELOPING RELATIONSHIP-BASED MATERIALS

During the early to mid-1980s, the need grew quickly for reading materials for parents and training materials for staff. Three occurrences gave a strong impetus to design and create the materials: (a) requests from nurses and others to "have something to give to patients," (b) high interest in the program expressed from participants at two national conferences, and (c) the decision to do research, a step toward making the program more evidence based and to answer questions raised by several nurses caring for women during and/ or after miscarriage. These decisions used the process of bridging the current status to something new, thereby structuring the task and promoting learning.

HAVING SOMETHING TO GIVE TO PATIENTS

Given the newness of RTS at our organization, we needed to start from the beginning to develop materials that would supplement the quality care we were learning to provide. Bedside nurses were asking for things such as information on stillbirth, a brochure about miscarriage, or what to do for grandparents. Numerous members of the interprofessional team contributed their writing and clinical skills to develop these and other materials, all of which grew from the relationships between and among professionals and parents; the coordinator and her supervisor, a clinical nurse specialist (CNS); and the coordinator and RTS-trained support persons. Examples of brochure topics included miscarriage, stillbirth, newborn death, grief of grandparents, helping children, and subsequent pregnancy. The need for keepsakes following miscarriage led the spiritual care team to design a "Remembrance of Blessing" card that could be framed or saved as a precious memory after a baby's death.

NATIONAL INTEREST

After the coordinator and CNS spoke at a large national nursing conference, the interest was so high in wanting to replicate our program that our advisory committee recommended that we create a manual using current policies, protocols, and teaching materials, which we did. We also decided that because our program was committed to providing compassionate care for patients and resources for professionals that we would write a book using the already existing brochures and material from the manual. Titled *When a Baby Dies: A Handbook for Healing and Helping*, it was a uniquely presented piece at the time, combining compelling stories from parents with useful information for hospital professionals, community clergy, funeral directors, parent support group leaders, and others.

THE DECISION TO DO RESEARCH

In listening to bedside nurses who cared for those who experienced miscarriage, the CNS and coordinator opted to design a mixed methods research proposal, which was funded by the Wisconsin Nurses Foundation (Limbo & Wheeler, 1986). We followed more than 70 women at the time of loss and over the next year. The most significant finding was that approximately 75% of the women felt the emotional loss of a pregnancy or baby and the concomitant grief; the other 25% regarded their miscarriage or ectopic pregnancy as a "life event" and did not feel sad. This was some of the early research done on miscarriage. The data from several research studies conducted after this one demonstrated consistent results. This left clinicians with the need to carefully assess the *meaning of the miscarriage* for every patient they cared for, establishing a connection and joint attention between patient and clinician. The results guided clinical care and brochure updates, and let others know of the program's scholarly endeavors, an important element of innovation in healthcare.

INTRODUCING THE PROGRAM TO OTHER SITES

Formal and informal education continued at our organization. Nurses posted "What to say and what not to say when someone has a miscarriage" in bathrooms, a strategy we called "potty talk." A mother whose baby was born healthy shared with the coordinator (also an on-call bedside nurse) that "I have been crying all day ever since the person who drew my blood was rough." The coordinator immediately recognized that a bereaved mother who experienced the same thing could or would feel even more wounded. More and more we learned that parent and professional stories would provide the underpinning for our program training and that every training would include a parent panel.

Once the manual was written, we were invited to a large medical center in the southern part of the United States to train their staff. The training was highly successful. It was the first of hundreds of trainings we have done internationally to bring the message of relationship, compassion, empathy, and evidence to a continually more diverse audience of professionals (e.g., child life specialists, ultrasonographers, genetic counselors, support group leaders, managers, perinatal palliative caregivers, and others). At that training, the coordinator and CNS were forever transformed by the father on the parent panel, reminding them once again of the significance of hearing a parent tell their own story. Two things made an amazing impact. Part of his story was that he himself, someone with limited education, having never spoken in front of a large group previously, was able to powerfully talk about his premature twin sons: "These were the boys I was going to take fishing one day and now I'm holding them in the palms of my hands." He also related a story that rings true for many experiencing grief. Yet the way he relayed his story led to tears in the eyes of everyone present. The long day was ended, his boys were dead, and he was on his way home. He understood how much his life had changed. This is how he described it: "I was standing at the stoplight waiting to cross [the main street in front of the hospital]. Traffic was quickly passing. I slumped to the curb, sobbing, with my head in my hands. When I looked up, I saw the cars continuing to whiz down the street. I wondered how everyone could just go on with their lives when mine had ended that day."

In 1985, we created and presented the first Resolve Through Sharing Coordinator Training. This train-the-trainer model had been used successfully in numerous businesses, and after 2 years of doing the 2-day training, we came to realize that to round out our educational offerings we should provide the content that a coordinator would need to start a program, gaining joint attention with a whole host of those who were in some way connected to the desire for a gold standard method of caring for bereaved families. The initial coordinator training featured numerous protocols and policies that had been developed; identified groups who needed to be brought along on the journey; and gave practical advice on how to effectively teach a course on grief (e.g., we always use the team-teaching method with two faculty as one of our relationship-based educational components (Limbo, 2008–2013, 2017). Go to **www.springerpub.com/pridham**, Chapter 22, for supplemental material on the RTS Bereavement Education Model Position Paper. We introduced "talking points," videotaped participants answering questions potentially asked by the media (e.g., local television or radio station), and provided scenarios that led to complex discussions of problem solving difficult situations.

Perhaps the most unexpected outcome of these trainings was the personal and professional growth and transformation the participants described. "That course changed my life" continues to be the single most common statement we hear from participants who took the training in the 1980s, in the 2010s, or anywhere in between. GP includes an element called *parallel process*. In the beginning, we did not know that term, but nonetheless, we were making use of the way it functions. The faculty work with training participants in the way that they hope participants will work with families (i.e., a parallel process). This may include demonstrating and developing competencies such as being with another (e.g., if a participant shares a particularly painful story with a faculty member in private); doing the task (a participant describes what she did and said when she was with a patient whose partner was angry); or achieving joint attention by showing and discussing a videotape in which the father (an actor) is disengaged until the nurse makes small but effective efforts to bring him into the conversation.

USING GP TO ESTABLISH RELATIONSHIP-BASED EDUCATION

For a practice such as GP to be effective, it must be integrated into the content and process of education. It can be seen in many places: within parents' stories; within professionals' explanations; the description of policies, protocols, and standard operating procedures; within talks for large or small audiences; within how an individual shows personal growth and transformation; and within a research protocol, to name a few. Yet it does not need to be named in order to be effective. GP works most effectively when it is integrated into one's usual way of interacting. One strategy that is particularly useful enhances the reflective processes that are incorporated into GP. The strategy is "wondering."

Case Example 22.1

The second author attended a noon conference about 2 years ago. The speaker was a physician, internationally known for her work in pediatric palliative care. She wanted to do a short role play and needed someone to be the mother of a very ill young child with little hope of survival. If one were to name this role play, it could be titled "Hope and Miracles," two concepts that are mentioned frequently in all aspects of palliative care. Another palliative care physician played the role of the child's mother, and the only preparation she had was that they were going to talk about her son who was (hypothetically) critically ill. They sat together on the stage, each in a folding chair at a 45° angle to each other. After some discussion that got each centered on the topic at hand, which was "What shall we do to help your son?" Dr. A. said to the mother, "I wonder what you are hoping for." [short pause] "Well," the mother responded, "we're hoping for a miracle, that he will get better." "So am I," acknowledged Dr. A. At this point, the pause is a long one. The two sit together, not moving, and with no signal from Dr. A. that she wanted or planned to intervene. She "wondered," which sets the stage for another to reflect (or pause and think), and Dr. A. joined the mother in her hope by saying "So am I." In GP language, we would say that the two had joint attention. There was no need at that point to judge the comment as being "denial" or "outrageous" or "impossible." Who wouldn't want a miracle? Dr. A. was simply stating the obvious. But at the end of this pause something amazing happened. The mother said, "But that's [a miracle] probably not going to happen, not when he's this sick." Dr. A. then interjected, "Well, what else might you be hoping for?"

The guide, in this case the physician, had been in these situations many times previously, so she would be considered the expert. This is the mother's first experience, so she is a learner at knowing what to expect or what to do. However, she is resourceful and she knows her child better than anyone else. This demonstration of a guided rather than directive or prescriptive approach lets the mother reflect on multiple options, more than one decision, and what she herself is thinking. She was not robbed of being a mother or forced to make a choice that did not feel right. And the two of them did all of this within a few minutes, coming together in a moment to make a connection, to be in relationship. That was the end of the role play, but we can imagine how this may have played out in real life. The elements are few: hope, miracles, reflecting, wondering, learner and guide, resourcefulness, and relationship. That is how GP is taught, demonstrated, and used and how it becomes central to an educational training on caring for the bereaved.

While GP principles were part of the organic process of program development in the early 1980s and a critical part of the education model, it was not until 2008 that the practice was intentionally added as a framework to the training itself. GP practices were incorporated in three ways: (a) inclusion into the 2-day training manual and PowerPoint; (b) creation and distribution of a pocket card outlining the elements of GP practice and would later become an infographic; and (c) creation of a full-length video (see https://www.youtube.com/watch?v=t3ptAGfg6EE&feature=youtu.be) with clinician and patient scenarios demonstrating how to use GP processes and competencies around issues specific to perinatal bereavement circumstances. The video would later become part of the RTS Coordinator Starter Kit. Go to **www.springerpub.com/pridham**, Chapter 22, for supplemental material on the GP Pocket Card and Caregiving Theory and GP Infographic. GP practice remains foundational as one of the tenets of the RTS program, setting it apart from all other bereavement education offerings currently available.

PROGRAM TRAINING EFFECTIVENESS EVALUATION

As an evidence-based program, RTS has been evaluated since it began with a local audience in 1981 and continued through expansion to national audiences in 1983. The evaluation process served two main purposes: (a) to provide continuing education credits to participants and (b) to collect participant feedback for continuous program development and improvement. Since 2012, RTS has increased its scope of measurement to include a pre- and postsurvey aimed specifically at understanding the impact of the training on participants' comfort level, knowledge, and skills in providing care to bereaved families. The method of data collection and measurement scale for the survey went through several iterations before settling on its final version—a 5-point Likert scale with pre- and post-items and participant responses on the same page. As part of a master's thesis project, the first author analyzed survey results over a 12-event span to measure three areas (comfort level, knowledge, and skills). GP practice itself is incorporated in RTS training content and relates to what RTS measures in the pre- and post-survey in a number of ways (see Table 22.1).

The RTS team wanted to determine how the standardized training with GP competencies was associated with pre- and posttraining change in how participants viewed their professional practice. Given that RTS trainings include a plethora of disciplines, the survey is brief and applicable to any participant's care of bereaved families. The seven domains evaluated in the survey correlate to GP elements explained in the results and discussion sections of the thesis summary that follows.

Literature Review for Program Evaluation

Definition of Perinatal Pereavement

No death comes without loss, but certainly those occurring during a pregnancy, intended or otherwise, merit special consideration. Perinatal death is defined as the unintended ending of a pregnancy before or during birth, or death of a newborn in the first month after birth (Limbo & Kobler, 2010). It touches thousands of lives each year in the United States alone. Using 2013 statistics, MacDorman and Gregory (2015) estimated that perinatal deaths, including miscarriage, were close to 750,000 annually. Because perinatal death occurs at such a significant rate, the likelihood that all nurses and many other healthcare professionals, even those outside of clinical maternal/child settings, will encounter and care for a woman who has experienced the death of a baby is high, and further demonstrates the need to prepare them to deliver quality bereavement care (Limbo & Kobler, 2010).

TABLE 22.1 RTS Survey Items Related to GP Principles

RTS Survey Item	GP Issues	GP Processes	GP Competencies
A. I am comfortable caring for bereaved families.		Getting and staying connected	Being with, knowing and relating, communicating and engaging, regulating emotion
B. I have enough knowledge to create a relationship with a bereaved family.		Getting and staying connected, joining and maintaining attention	Being with, knowing and relating, communicating and engaging
C. I have the skills to effectively communicate with a bereaved family.	Relating and guiding	Getting and staying connected, joining and maintaining attention, bridging	Communicating and engaging, problem solving, regulating emotion
D. I am able to guide a family with end-of-life decision making.	Nurturing and protecting, maintaining life quality	Bridging, structuring the task/learning, transferring responsibility	Doing the task, problem solving
E. I understand how to use interdisciplinary care for bereaved families.	Helping others understand family needs	Communicating, transferring	Communicating and engaging, joining attention
F. I have the knowledge to help create meaningful keepsakes with families.	Nurturing and protecting, relating and guiding	Structuring the task/learning, transferring responsibility	Doing the task
G. I have the skills to help myself and coworkers with our own grief.	Issues: relating and guiding, maintaining life quality		Being with, knowing and relating, communicating and engaging, regulating emotion

GP, guided participation; RTS, Resolve Through Sharing.

Perinatal bereavement—including when life-limiting diagnosis are present prior to birth—is the time surrounding perinatal death (Wool, 2016). Healthcare professionals who plan and provide support to women and families during this time need to be aware of the psychosocial and cultural needs that accompany the complex nature of this particular grief (Capitulo, 2005; DiMarco, Renker, Medas, Bertosa, & Goranitis, 2002; Fenstermacher & Hupcey, 2013).

Knowledge and Comfort Levels

How healthcare professionals perceive their ability to provide sufficient care and support to those experiencing perinatal death and bereavement, coupled with the actual work they do, affects their own personal experience. We have learned this over the years from the results of our pre- and postsurvey measuring RTS training effectiveness in the domains of comfort levels, skills, and knowledge. A number of studies spanning over a decade show that the vast majority of nurses recognize a need for specialized training to care for and support bereaved parents, and that those who received it held more positive attitudes about their level of competency (Chan et al., 2003; Chan, Lou, & Arthur, 2010). Knowledge, experience, communication skills, management of personal feelings, and support from team members topped the list of education and training objectives (Steen, 2015).

Supporting families experiencing perinatal death can cause a broad range of emotional responses for healthcare clinicians, from discomfort to feelings of being overwhelmed (Limbo & Kobler, 2010; Roehrs, Masterson, Alles, Witt, & Rutt, 2008). Lack of perinatal death-specific knowledge and skills is the primary cause for clinicians' discomfort and can actually cause them to avoid this patient population in the healthcare setting, or mistake their own level of competency in providing beneficial care (Capitulo, 2005; Limbo & Kobler, 2010; Steen, 2015). Under these conditions, negative encounters with tactless, ill-equipped, or uncaring practitioners have a lifetime impact and can compromise the course of bereavement for parents for years to come (Browning & Solomon, 2006; Gold, 2007).

Need for Competency Development and Training

It follows that using a standardized approach to perinatal bereavement care throughout an organization has been found to be effective in increasing confidence and skill levels. A standardized approach benefits patients, families, and staff (Smart & Smith, 2013). A literature review of hospital-based bereavement intervention studies found families and professionals agree that a standardized approach should be incorporated within a formal model of care that is theory and evidence based. However, a lack of a clear evidence base from which healthcare providers set the standard for bereavement care and support continues to hold back best practice (Donovan, Wakefield,

Russell, & Cohn, 2015). Though the altruistic focus of nursing practice is meeting patient desires and needs, it must be guided by standards and protocol, increasing the probability that professionals will be able to provide consistent, quality care (Limbo & Kobler, 2010; Steen, 2015).

Data from research establish a continued need to increase standards and consistency when delivering perinatal bereavement care around the world (Steen, 2015). While RTS has trained approximately 50,000 persons since its inception, the need for effective, high-quality bereavement education still exists. Smart and Smith (2013), who used the RTS model for their organization's perinatal program, reported a lack of programs among numerous healthcare organizations in the southeastern United States, showing a paucity of standardized bereavement care regardless of gestational age or point of entry into the hospital system. Considering the extensive body of evidence in favor of standardized approaches to perinatal bereavement care, it follows that their 1-year study at their own independent regional tertiary care center, after adopting the RTS model of bereavement support and education, found their nurses had a significant increase in their confidence level when caring for women suffering pregnancy loss (Smart & Smith, 2013). By creating a proven, standardized bereavement program throughout a healthcare system, end-of-life care—provided in any unit—ensures patient-centered, relationship- and evidence-based, interprofessional, and meaningful care for all those experiencing the loss of a loved one (Wilke, 2014).

To conclude the background information for program evaluation data, evidence-based and standardized bereavement training and education are critical to the future of supporting the holistic needs of grieving individuals and families. Healthcare professionals require and desire standardized, evidence-based training and education to build their comfort levels, skills, and knowledge. Providing programming to ensure excellence in caring for the bereaved in professional settings worldwide has been the mission of RTS for more than 35 years. While RTS has been the leader in gold-standard bereavement education since 1981, its long-term effects and sustainability have not been entirely measured. To fully understand the value of end-of-life/bereavement education on comfort levels and skills of healthcare professionals, additional studies are needed with larger provider populations (Zhang & Lane, 2013).

Methods

To ensure a reliable and representative sample size for the evaluation of the RTS training effectiveness, 471 total participant responses from 12 training events (average = 39 registrants per event) spanning a 1-year period were examined. RTS promotes interprofessional care as a core component of its framework and offers training to enhance multidisciplinary skills and extend professional growth. Therefore, for the period surveyed, we were able to include responses from nurses, social workers, chaplains, physicians, genetic counselors, and those from other disciplines who provide perinatal bereavement care, in our assessment.

RTS faculty designed the survey tool to measure the effects of the standardized RTS training on participants' comfort level, knowledge, and skills when delivering perinatal bereavement care. Pre- and postsurveys consisting of one demographic and seven assessment items using a 5-point Likert scale (see full list of items in the Results section) were administered routinely at the beginning and again at the end of the 2-day training during the course of the 12 events. The surveys contained no participant identification. Pre- and post-survey items and responses were included on the same page so that the change for each individual could be verified. After each training event, the surveys were returned to the national RTS office where the data were compiled.

The intervention tested in the study was the Resolve Through Sharing Bereavement Training: Perinatal Death. The standardized training is evidence based and follows the RTS practice handbook (manual) now in its 9th edition (Walter, Limbo, & Wilke, 1984–2012, 2017). Since its inception, RTS has incorporated relevant theories, research, and more than 35 years' experience into its classroom and patient education materials. Critical components of RTS education include emphasis on interprofessional collaboration, honoring cultural practices, integration of the GP framework, and coordination of care through documentation, education, and the utilization of RTS coordinators to ensure quality and sustainability. The training is built on a relationship-based education model. The RTS Bereavement Education Model Position Paper may be accessed through **www.springerpub.com/ pridham**, Chapter 22.

All of the survey data analyzed are historical data and none of the respondents who participated in the training can be identified by name, employer, address, age, gender, or discipline. The study was conducted with permission from Resolve Through Sharing, a program of Gundersen Medical Foundation.

Results

Descriptive Satistics Analysis

The RTS pre- and posttraining survey measured responses to the following items.

A. I am comfortable caring for bereaved families.
B. I have enough knowledge to create a relationship with a bereaved family.
C. I have the skills to effectively communicate with a bereaved family.
D. I am able to guide a family with end-of-life decision making.
E. I understand how to use interdisciplinary care for bereaved families.
F. I have the knowledge to help create meaningful keepsakes with families.
G. I have the skills to help myself and coworkers with our own grief.

The survey items are rooted in the three GP elements: issues, processes, and competencies (see Table 22.1).

After the responses were appropriately grouped, SPSS was used to perform statistical analysis. Following are four selected tables from the study characterizing the information most relevant to the GP discussion.

Out of 471 possible respondents, rates for all of the pretraining survey items were very high, ranging from 469 to 471, as shown in Table 22.2. The group mean response scores on presurvey items ranged from 3.09 to 3.75 (Hensel, 2015). Respondent rates for the posttraining survey items ranged from 463 to 468, as shown in Table 22.3. The group mean response scores on postsurvey items ranged from 4.27 to 4.63 (Hensel, 2015).

Table 22.4 shows participant responses indicating change in comfort level, skills, and knowledge from prior to taking the RTS training to completing it. Change was measured using only data pairs that included a participant response for both the presurvey and corresponding postsurvey items. The highest level of change occurred for item D (I am able to guide a family with end-of-life decision making), with a group mean change score of 1.17. The lowest level of change occurred for item A (I am comfortable caring for bereaved families), with a group mean change score of 0.68 (Hensel, 2015).

TABLE 22.2 Pretest Comfort Level, Skills, and Knowledge Responses Group Mean

Items	N	Mean	Standard Deviation
A. I am comfortable caring for bereaved families.	471	3.75	1.011
B. I have enough knowledge to create a relationship with a bereaved family.	471	3.58	0.988
F. I have the knowledge to help create meaningful keepsakes with families.	469	3.58	1.056
C. I have the skills to effectively communicate with a bereaved family.	469	3.52	0.955
E. I understand how to use interdisciplinary care for bereaved families.	470	3.42	1.002
G. I have the skills to help myself and coworkers with our own grief.	470	3.41	0.950
D. I am able to guide a family with end-of-life decision making.	471	3.09	1.051

TABLE 22.3 Posttest Comfort Level, Skills, and Knowledge Responses Group Mean

Items	N	Mean	Standard Deviation
F. I have the knowledge to help create meaningful keepsakes with families.	465	4.63	0.702
B. I have enough knowledge to create a relationship with a bereaved family.	467	4.56	0.728
E. I understand how to use interdisciplinary care for bereaved families.	464	4.53	0.740
C. I have the skills to effectively communicate with a bereaved family.	467	4.49	0.733
G. I have the skills to help myself and coworkers with our own grief.	463	4.45	0.722
A. I am comfortable caring for bereaved families.	468	4.43	0.752
D. I am able to guide a family with end-of-life decision making.	465	4.27	0.770

TABLE 22.4 Change in Comfort Level, Skills, and Knowledge Group Mean

Items	N	Mean	Standard Deviation
D. I am able to guide a family with end-of-life decision making.	464	1.17	0.981
E. I understand how to use interdisciplinary care for bereaved families.	462	1.11	1.058
F. I have the knowledge to help create meaningful keepsakes with families.	462	1.06	1.049
G. I have the skills to help myself and coworkers with our own grief.	461	1.04	0.927
B. I have enough knowledge to create a relationship with a bereaved family.	466	0.97	0.935
C. I have the skills to effectively communicate with a bereaved family.	464	0.97	0.903
A. I am comfortable caring for bereaved families.	467	0.68	0.819

Inferential Statistics Analysis

Table 22.5 shows that changes reported for all seven survey responses were statistically significant at the 0.05 level (Hensel, 2015).

1. Participants having no previous RTS perinatal bereavement training showed a greater change (p = .000, t = 4.451) in being comfortable caring for bereaved families.
2. Participants having no previous RTS perinatal bereavement training showed a greater change (p = .008, t = 2.644) in having enough knowledge to create a relationship with bereaved families.
3. Participants having no previous RTS perinatal bereavement training showed a greater change (p = .006, t = 2.743) in having the skills to effectively communicate with bereaved families.
4. Participants having no previous RTS perinatal bereavement training showed a greater change (p = .000, t = 3.854) in having the ability to guide a family with end-of-life decision making.
5. Participants having no previous RTS perinatal bereavement training showed a greater change (p = .001, t = 3.495) in understanding how to use interdisciplinary care for bereaved families.
6. Participants having no previous RTS perinatal bereavement training showed a greater change (p = .001, t = 3.409) in having the knowledge to help create meaningful keepsakes with bereaved families.
7. Participants having no previous RTS perinatal bereavement training showed a greater change (p = .011, t = 2.564) in having the skills to help themselves and their coworkers with their own grief.

TABLE 22.5 Paired t Test of Change from Pre- to Posttest for Respondents Having No Previous RTS Perinatal Bereavement Training

Items	N	t	df	Sig. (2-tailed)
A. I am comfortable caring for bereaved families.	428	4.451	53.638	0.000
B. I have enough knowledge to create a relationship with a bereaved family.	427	2.644	459	0.008
C. I have the skills to effectively communicate with a bereaved family.	425	2.743	457	0.006
D. I am able to guide a family with end-of-life decision making.	425	3.854	48.000	0.000
E. I understand how to use interdisciplinary care for bereaved families.	423	3.495	455	0.001

(continued)

TABLE 22.5 Paired *t* Test of Change from Pre- to Post-test for Respondents Having no Previous RTS Perinatal Bereavement Training (*continued*)

Items	N	t	df	Sig. (2-tailed)
F. I have the knowledge to help create meaningful keepsakes with families.	423	3.409	455	0.001
G. I have the skills to help myself and coworkers with our own grief.	422	2.564	454	0.011

RTS, Resolve Through Sharing.

Discussion

Because the research strongly demonstrates the need for specialized care and understanding of those experiencing perinatal loss, RTS engaged in full examination of change levels in the areas of comfort level, knowledge, and skills of interprofessional healthcare providers from across the United States after taking part in its perinatal bereavement training. The standard pre- and postsurvey areas (being comfortable with providing care, having enough knowledge to create meaningful relationships, effective communication skills, the ability to guide end-of-life decision making, the understanding of how to use interdisciplinary care, the knowledge to create meaningful keepsakes, and the skills to help themselves and their coworkers deal with their own grief when caring for families experiencing perinatal death) were measured. A number of demographics relevant to what might affect RTS training outcomes were analyzed. One conclusion stood out above the others: the impact of the training on how healthcare professionals view their competencies using GP language—being with, knowing and relating, doing the task (to include problem solving), communicating, and regulating emotion (self and those cared for) —is clearly evidenced in the results (see Table 22.1 for the list of RTS survey items and corresponding GP principles).

Data support statistical change levels for 100% of the survey items for first-time RTS-trained respondents. The RTS training offers an overwhelming opportunity to address the issues faced by professionals caring for those experiencing perinatal loss as outlined in the literature review section of this chapter. As shown by the survey and the results, RTS training, with its relationship-based education model, GP principles incorporation, and approach to perinatal bereavement care, positively impacts participants' levels of comfort, knowledge, and skills in learning and delivering consistent care standards to those who lose babies to perinatal death.

The survey did not ask participants whether they had any other form of bereavement training previously, only if they had received RTS training in the past. However, since all items showed statistically positive change levels for all who had not had previous exposure to RTS training, it could be presumed that if respondents had previous non-RTS bereavement education, it was not effective in the areas specifically measured by this study. The study showed sustainability of the learned RTS principles and practice guidelines by the correlation of the assessment results for participants who had previously taken the RTS training (Hensel, 2015).

Future Research

Because pre- and postcourse participant surveys scores were paired, we identified certain descriptive information that would not be available if the pre- and postsurvey were administered in another fashion. In some instances, participants altered their answers on the presurvey items. In all of those cases, the pretraining assessment answers were changed to indicate lower levels than initially marked. One hypothesis for interpreting these data is that participants learned more in these areas than they expected to, thereby creating a condition for lowering of pretraining scores. A simple qualitative question to accompany the survey could be, "If you changed any of your pretest scores at any point during the training, in what direction did the score(s) change? Please provide an explanation for the change."

This study provided foundational research data on a standardized educational program. The next step in a program of research designed to validate and extend the RTS program is to continue gathering quantitative data similar to the Likert design used in the present study combined with qualitative data from the same participants. This triangulated approach will create more robust findings that help curriculum designers extend the current standardized educational program.

Future studies should also measure program sustainability in organizations posttraining where RTS-trained individuals, especially coordinators, are present. This would support the research done by Smart and Smith (2013). Using a different evaluation tool, RTS has collected additional participant information specific to RTS training learning objectives and application to participants' work from the same training events where the pre- and postsurveys are conducted. This could provide further information if analyzed to compare post-RTS training learning with pre-RTS training learning. Currently, RTS has three principal training programs. Each has GP method embedded within teaching and learning content and methods. To further assess disciplines in addition to nursing, RTS works to reach greater numbers of professionals outside the nursing discipline. RTS has surveyed participants from its other relatively new core trainings (Neonatal and Pediatric Death and Pediatric and Adult Death), but statistical analysis has not been completed.

Conclusion—Training Effectiveness Evaluation

For those taking the training for the first time, the standardized Resolve Through Sharing Bereavement Training: Perinatal Death has a statistically significant impact on participants' levels of comfort, knowledge, and skills. The evidence- and relationship-based model, which incorporates GP practice, can be seen as one solution to increase confidence and competence for those healthcare professionals who support this special group of parents whose babies died.

Clinical and Educational Implications: Principles for a Perinatal Bereavement Program

The following clinical and educational implications briefly summarize some key points from the historical and evaluative summaries of a perinatal bereavement program.

- Education in perinatal bereavement is necessary for all disciplines caring for the bereaved.
- Critical domains of learning include the GP competencies of:
  - Being with
  - Knowing and relating to the other as a person
  - Communicating
  - Doing the task, including problem solving
  - Emotion regulation
- The competencies are centered around relationship. Faculty may use relational training through positive responses to participants' questions or comments, telling stories that demonstrate how relationship supports compassion among professionals and patients and between parents and their baby, to name a few.
- The incorporation of in-person narratives from parents provide maximum value in education. This training method increases empathy and compassion, and substantiates what parents want and need. Brief video clips of parents, their families, and professionals also add richness to the training.
- Parallel process is central to guide and learner. The term refers to how teaching and learning occur with the guide relating to the learner in a way that demonstrates how parents could ideally react to their baby, how professionals show compassion and sensitivity toward patients or coworkers, or the way an expert avoids judgmental or prescriptive responses in helping someone learn.

CONCLUSION

The clinical and educational implications of RTS provide a summary format highlighting the richness of integrating a teaching–learning practice into a bereavement program. By learning through RTS training, using processes and competencies, and taking on issues of greater or lesser magnitude (i.e., GP), clinicians engage in what many refer to as a "life-changing experience." In a world in which death is often feared and grief misunderstood, the RTS training, integrated with GP practice, become one with the other. The social worker from midtown, the nurse who lives on an Iowa farm, and the chaplain who spends every weekend kayaking face the world of loss with competence. They know how to make a difference because education has touched their souls.

ADDITIONAL READING

Ballantine, A., & Feudtner, C. (2010). The 10 R's of clinician education: A checklist. *Archives of Pediatrics & Adolescent Medicine, 164*(4), 389–390. doi:10.1001/archpediatrics.2010.33

Engler, A. J., Cusson, R. M., Brockett, R. T., Cannon-Heinrich, C., Goldberg, M. A., West, M. G., & Petow, W. (2004). Neonatal staff and advanced practice nurses' perceptions of bereavement/end-of-life care of families of critically ill and/or dying infants. *American Journal of Critical Care, 13*(6), 489–498.

Limbo, R., & Kobler, K. (2013). *Meaningful moments: Ritual and reflection when a child dies.* La Crosse, WI: Gundersen Medical Foundation.

Limbo, R. K., & Wheeler, S. R. (1986–2003). *When a baby dies. A handbook for healing and helping.* La Crosse, WI: Gundersen Lutheran Medical Foundation.

Londa, S. (2010). Consoling Rachel: A bereavement program for perinatal loss. *Chaplaincy Today, 26*(1), 27–31.

Raddi, S. A., Samson, S., & Kharde, S. N. (2009). Knowledge and attitude regarding 'perinatal bereavement care' among nurses working in the maternity unit and neonatal intensive care unit. *South Asian Federation of Obstetrics and Gynecology, 1*(3), 81–84.

Thieleman, K., & Cacciatore, J. (2013). When a child dies: A critical analysis of grief-related controversies in DSM-5. *Research on Social Work Practice, 24*(1), 114–122. doi:10.1177/1049731512474695

REFERENCES

Browning, D. M., & Solomon, M. Z. (2006). Relational learning in pediatric palliative care: Transformative education and the culture of medicine. *Child and Adolescent Psychiatric Clinics of North America, 15*(3), 795–815. doi:10.1016/j.chc.2006.03.002

Capitulo, K. L. (2005). Evidence for healing interventions with perinatal bereavement. *MCN: The American Journal of Maternal Child Nursing, 30*(6), 389–396.

Chan, M. F., Chan, S. H., & Day, M. C. (2003). Nurses' attitudes towards perinatal bereavement support in Hong Kong: A pilot study. *Journal of Clinical Nursing, 12*(4), 536–543.

Chan, M. F., Lou, F. L., & Arthur, D. G. (2010). A survey comparing the attitudes toward perinatal bereavement care of nurses from three Asian cities. *Evaluation & the Health Professions, 33*(4), 514–533. doi:10.117/0163278710381092

DiMarco, M., Renker, P., Medas, J., Bertosa, H., & Goranitis, J. L. (2002). Effects of an educational bereavement program on health care professionals' perceptions of perinatal loss. *Journal of Continuing Education in Nursing, 33*(4), 180–186.

Donovan, L. A., Wakefield, C. E., Russell, V., & Cohn, R. J. (2015). Hospital-based bereavement services following the death of a child: A mixed study review. *Palliative Medicine, 29*(3), 193–210. doi:10.1177/0269216314556851

Fenstermacher, K., & Hupcey, J. E. (2013). Perinatal bereavement: A principle-based concept analysis. *Journal of Advanced Nursing, 69*(11), 2389–2400. doi:10.1111/jan.12119

Gold, K. J. (2007). Navigating care after a baby dies: A systematic review of parent experiences with health providers. *Journal of Perinatology, 27*(4), 230–237.

Hensel, M. B. (2015). Exploring change in comfort level, knowledge, and skills of health care professionals after a standardized training in perinatal death. Unpublished manuscript. Department of Business Administration, Viterbo University, La Crosse, WI.

Limbo, R. (2008–2013, 2017). *Resolve through sharing: Bereavement education model position paper.* La Crosse, WI: Gundersen Lutheran Medical Foundation.

Limbo, R., & Kobler, K. (2010). The tie that binds: Relationships in perinatal bereavement. *MCN: The American Journal of Maternal Child Nursing, 35*(6), 316–321. doi:10.1097/NMC.0b013e318f0eef8

Limbo, R., & Wheeler, S. R. (1986). Women's response to the loss of their pregnancy through miscarriage: A longitudinal study. *Association for Death Education and Counseling Forum Newsletter, 10*(4), 4–6.

MacDorman, M. F., & Gregory, E. C. W. (2015). Fetal and perinatal mortality: United States, 2013. *National Vital Statistics Reports: From the Centers for Disease Control and Prevention, National Center for Health Statistics, National Vital Statistics System, 64*(8), 1–23.

Roehrs, C., Masterson, A., Alles, R., Witt, C., & Rutt, P. (2008). Caring for families coping with perinatal loss. *Journal of Obstetric, Gynecologic, and Neonatal Nursing, 37*(6), 631–639.

Smart, C. J., & Smith, B. L. (2013). A transdisciplinary team approach to perinatal loss. *MCN: The American Journal of Maternal Child Nursing, 38*(2), 110–114. doi:10.1097/NMC.0b013e318270db45

Steen, S. E. (2015). Perinatal death: Bereavement interventions used by U.S. and Spanish nurses and midwives. *International Journal of Palliative Nursing, 21*(2), 79–86. doi:10.12968/ijpn.2015.21.2.79

Walter, M., Limbo, R., & Wilke, J. (Eds.). (1984–2012, 2017). *Resolve Through Sharing, bereavement training: Perinatal death, practice handbook* (9th ed.). La Crosse, WI: Gundersen Lutheran Medical Foundation.

Wilke, J. (2014). *Investing in resolve through sharing creates a culture of compassion, enhances quality, improves patient and staff experience, and suppoRTS national standard benchmarks*. La Crosse, WI: Gundersen Lutheran Medical Foundation.

Wool, C., Black, B. P., & Woods, A. B. (2016). Quality indicators and parental satisfaction with perinatal palliative care in the intrapartum setting after diagnosis of a life-limiting fetal condition. *Advances in Nursing Science, 39*(4), 346–357.

Zhang, W., & Lane, B. S. (2013). Promoting neonatal staff nurses' comfort and involvement in end of life and bereavement care. *Nursing Research and Practice, 2013*, 1–5. doi:10.1155/2013/365329

23

Case Examples: Using "Holding in Mind" and "Joining Attention" as Relational Strategies

Rana Limbo

I was a guided participation (GP) intervention nurse for Dr. Karen Pridham's Feeding Support Project (FSP) during my doctoral studies. My role was to test GP with families of preterm infants during hospitalization in the NICU and in the first year after discharge. The study design focused on the infant's feeding and growth. Nurses worked closely with the family and other health-care team members, using videotape playback of feedings, monitoring intake and growth, and emphasizing that the mother/infant relationship could positively influence the feeding experience itself and the amount of intake.

This chapter illustrates two case examples that highlight aspects of GP. The first, "Holding in Mind," describes how the nurse and mother came to know each other over time. The second, "Joining Attention," demonstrates for the reader how the nurse and the mother were able to discuss a difficult subject (the mother's depression), ultimately leading to a vastly improved feeding experience for both mother and infant.

Case Example 23.1

This is a story of 19-year-old LeeAnn, the single mother of 2-year-old Bobby and baby Priscilla. I began seeing her while her baby Priscilla, born very prematurely, was still in the hospital. LeeAnn was only 19, her older son 2, and her baby approximately term (age adjusted for prematurity). I visited LeeAnn first in the hospital's NICU and then in a small rented home, where she lived with her children. Sometimes she was home, sometimes she was not when I arrived for our scheduled home visit. I felt discouraged that I was not able to establish a connection with her, one in which she felt satisfied and even eager to see me. My role with the project was supporting feeding and growth in very preterm babies and relationship between mother and baby. After all, I brought my large (but very accurate) weight scale, a length measuring board, a growth chart, a diet log for little Priscilla, and numerous ideas for how LeeAnn could help her daughter eat healthily and grow. I consistently scheduled our visits and left a friendly note for her when she was not at home. The idea of holding someone in mind (i.e., remembering an appointment) seemed especially poignant during these times that LeeAnn and I were working to build a relationship.

One day my ears perked up when LeeAnn told me how much her birthday meant to her. She said it was the best day of the year and (fortunately for me) was coming up in about a month. The day closest to her birthday on which I had a visit scheduled, I gave her a birthday card. The card remained, displayed on the shelves where she kept special things, for as long as I continued visiting her. Thus began a personal understanding of what it meant to hold someone in mind (LeeAnn) and to be held in mind (me).

Into the next year, when Priscilla was about 8 months adjusted age, I arrived for an afternoon visit and there was a note on the door. I knew instantly when I saw the note that this was what it meant to be held in mind. LeeAnn could not keep our visit and had left me a note to explain why. It has been 20 years since that day and I still have her note in my desk. In fact, that day was a turning point. From then, we had a mutual sense of each other— we valued our visits, occasionally opting to have phone calls instead, and were committed to finishing out our year together, aware of the other and the value of our relationship. One of the last moments I remember of LeeAnn was the evening we had arranged a videotaping of her discussing how she made healthcare decisions for Priscilla. LeeAnn preferred that we schedule the filming in the evening. As Dr. Pridham and I drove toward LeeAnn's mother's house, there was LeeAnn, wildly waving to us so we would be certain to see the house. The meaning of this step was profound. She had agreed for us to videotape her talking about how she cared for her daughter, specifically about how she recognized and attended to symptoms of illness. She had now moved to holding others in mind through her willingness to create a videotape that other parents and professionals could watch and learn from her.

The questions that follow this brief case example may assist you as a reader apply the principle of "Holding in Mind" in developing relationship competencies for the client and for you. I first read about the concept of "Holding in Mind" (or "being held in mind") in Dr. Jeree Pawl's 1995 article that described her work with a mother and her young daughter. The mother praised Dr. Pawl for giving her daughter a doll, a doll that literally changed the little girl's life. The doll represented to this little girl and her mother that Dr. Pawl was holding them in mind in their absence, understanding how the dynamics of their relationship could change if therapist and family created a special connection. Dr. Pawl wrote, "It seems to me that one of life's greatest privileges is just that—the experience of being held in someone's mind. Possibly, though, there is one exception—and that is the privilege of holding another in one's own" (Pawl, 1995, p. 5).

DISCUSSION QUESTIONS AND STRATEGIES

1. What examples can you identify in your professional and/or personal life that resonate with the idea of holding someone in mind (thinking of them in their absence) or being held in mind (knowing you were being thought about in your absence)?
2. Why do you think this is a powerful way of making a connection with another?
3. Some examples of how "Holding in Mind" could be worded are "I remember what you told me," "You said I should . . .," "I've been thinking about that problem you talked to me about and I have some ideas for you," "I know you love painted rocks and when I saw this one, it reminded me of you."
4. Some examples of "being held in mind" might be "When I wonder about a decision, I think about what you might do" and "I remembered what you told me and it helped a lot."

You may want to purchase a special notebook (small size) that you call your "Holding in Mind" book. Use it to keep track of examples of this special concept. Perhaps you will find that dividing the notebook into two sections, "Holding in Mind" and "Being Held in Mind," will be the better way for you to take notes. Or your style may be more narrative, meaning you write a story about each encounter involving this powerful way of knowing and relating to others.

Case Example 23.2

Giving birth to a baby born at 23 weeks gestation who survives may sound like a miracle to some. At the same time, what it takes to keep that precious baby healthy, growing, and connected to others is a challenge that few understand. The following field notes from the Smith family's FSP intervention nurse highlight how the GP process of "joining attention" affects the baby and her family. The first note is a summary of a visit in December. Sarah was 2 months old, age adjusted for prematurity. She had been in the NICU from her birth in May until her original due date in mid-September. On her due date in September, she came home. Her mother Anne and father Jerry, who worked full time, cared for her without additional assistance. I have included several graphs in the online materials that demonstrate how, in four areas (family psychosocial events, illnesses, feeding, and medications), this family was constantly counting milliliters of intake consumed, feeding, monitoring, problem solving, worrying, seeking medical and nursing care, and treating illnesses. At times, Sarah's parents simply did not know what to do. The illness graphs included as Figures 23.1 and 23.2 provide a window into the challenges they faced in one area of Sarah's life. The complete timeline for Sarah's first year may be accessed through this link: **www.springerpub.com/pridham,** Chapter 23.

This family, as evidenced by the graphs, experienced numerous contextual factors that served as an underpinning for Anne's depression. Anne struggled with fatigue and irritability. The caregiving demands, parenting challenges, Sarah's illnesses, and physical condition (i.e., breastfeeding a very preterm baby with gastroesophageal reflux) were wearing. Sarah also needed extra calories, which often meant that her mother pumped breast milk until letdown (to reach the hindmilk, higher in calories), nursed Sarah, and then supplemented with high-caloric-density formula. A feeding could easily take 1 hour. The following excerpt is from a field note from an audio-recorded visit in December:

Nurse: [What] we've been experiencing, it can be overwhelming and terribly discouraging in the best of circumstances. But when one is depressed, the discouragement can feel like hopelessness.

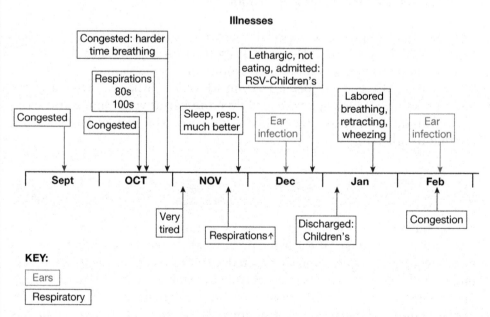

FIGURE 23.1 The illnesses of a prematurely born infant, Sarah, in the first half of her first year.

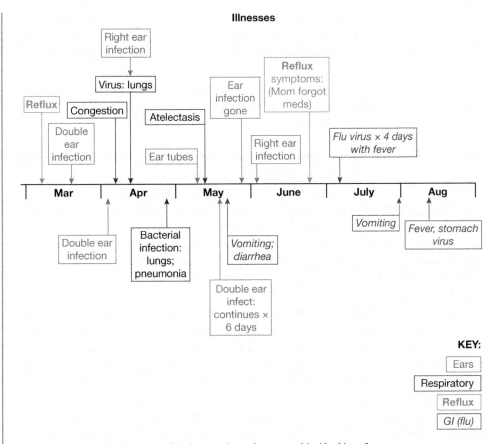

FIGURE 23.2 The illnesses of baby Sarah in the second half of her first year.
GI, gastrointestinal.

Mom: But for the first time that we've been meeting [about 5 months], I heard myself in the car say to Jerry, "Rana's comin' Thursday. Sarah hasn't gained weight. She's [the nurse] going to wanna know why. And what am I gonna tell her? (All of these sentences were clipped off, spoken abruptly, hopelessly.) Before it was, you know, I always knew that we get ideas, we're gonna work, and now I'm just like 'I don't, I don't know.'"

Nurse: "Is there a spiritual component to this as well?" Is there a thing like if your faith were better you wouldn't feel this way? Do you have that sort of belief?" She didn't think so. She feels she has "strayed" from her personal prayer life because she is so busy with the children.

The most significant part of this conversation took place on the curb with mom standing alongside the car as I was getting ready to leave. I told her there was a time in my life when I was depressed and I learned that I didn't have to feel quite as awful as I felt [This represents a careful use of self-disclosure as a strategy for relationship development. Its effectiveness can be evaluated immediately by determining if the focus of the communication remains with the mother and not with the nurse's story—it did]. I said something like "I don't have any doubt that you're doing your best for everyone else and that they may not be affected so much by this. But I'm concerned what the price is for you personally and how much you are suffering. I wonder if it has to be this bad." She immediately began to cry, and as I walked toward her I asked, "Am I on the mark?" She nodded her head vigorously. I put my arms around her and we just stood there on the curb for quite a long time. She made no effort to move.

It can be difficult to know whether the guide and parent have joint attention around something of importance, in this case Anne's mood and possible depression. One way of checking for joint attention is listening for change, or perhaps what one might call "surprise outcomes." A field note approximately 2 weeks after the one above contained this description of a change in healthcare practice: "She [Anne] has now gone to see her own physician and they have discussed the possibility of her thyroid medication needing to be increased, that doing so may reverse the symptoms of depression."

When one has an extremely premature baby with multiple medical conditions, the demands of parenting reach new heights. We invite you to look at all eight pages of the graphs, titled "Family Timelines for Baby Sarah" (access to this supplemental material can be found at **www.springerpub.com/pridham**, Chapter 23). Attempt to grasp the reality of caring for a child while considering multiple, potentially life-threatening conditions. Sarah experienced some of the usual complications of immaturity: lung problems, susceptibility to acute illness, respiratory difficulties, hospitalizations, difficulty sleeping, gastroesophageal reflux, need for continuous oxygen, and what was probably most difficult for her mother, trying to maintain calories and adequate feedings.

The beginning of joint attention between the intervention nurse and Anne regarding the possibility she had a major depression that needed treatment began in December (or before). A video recording of two feedings (at 4 and 8 months, respectively, age adjusted for prematurity) is accessible through this link: **www.springerpub.com/pridham**, Chapter 23. These videos demonstrate the effect of joint attention on treatment of an identified issue concerning the infant's feeding behavior. Ultimately, Anne and Jerry sought counseling; Anne had her thyroid medication adjusted, and her physician prescribed a low-dose antidepressant. These changes had occurred at the time of the 8-month feeding.

ASSESSING THE ONLINE VIDEO RECORDING

1. What do you see in the first video when Sarah tried to eat?
2. Have you heard the term "gastroesophageal reflux"? This is what Sarah had and was taking medication for.
3. What positioning do you notice? Anne held her upright to compensate for the pain from food getting into her esophagus.

4. How does the feeding end?
5. Consider the changes Anne and Jerry made to help with their relationship and Anne's depression.
6. Now study the 8-month feeding (in which Anne is holding a bowl and spoon, kneeling in front of Sarah, who is in a swing). Discuss the competencies of being with and knowing, comparing what Anne was capable of at 4 months and the changes evident at 8 months.

In summary, joint attention around complex issues frequently develops over time. Providing information is a beginning, but is rarely sufficient. The guide's skill in monitoring and noting small changes and wondering ("I wonder if it has to be this bad") can be components of joint attention. Another is getting the other's ideas about possible solutions to the problem ("What might be going on?"), which is how the past thyroid condition emerged and what led to Anne independently setting up an appointment with her medical provider. This paragraph briefly summarized how the process of joining attention led to transferring responsibility. At the same time, Anne developed expanded competencies in problem solving, communicating, and most of all, regulating emotion.

Study Guide: Examples for Initiating or Maintaining Joint Attention

In conclusion, here are some key assessment questions that could be used for the scenario above. You may wish to think through them yourself, take notes, and/or use them in a professional setting to introduce your colleagues to "joint attention."

1. What are you hoping for regarding feeding?
2. What if those hopes are not realized?
3. What else could we try?
4. How do you calm yourself when all three children have needs at the same time?
5. What does depression mean to you?
6. If it does, how does depression affect a new mother?
7. How would you decide if it was time to reach out to a professional for advice or even treatment?

Use of GP is shown in three video scenarios, A, B, and C: **www.springerpub .com/pridham**, Chapter 23. These scenarios center on discharge instructions for a couple after a stillbirth. Scenario A shows the nurse and couple interacting without engaging in GP, B demonstrates the use of GP among the three, and C is a discussion between two nurses of the meaning of scenarios A and B. Taken together, these three scenarios will help the reader differentiate how a focus on processes and competencies lead to relationship development and, in this case, prepare a couple in shock for what they will likely face in the immediate hours and days to come.

CONCLUSION

The content in this chapter features ways that GP was central to working through situations common to those who provide healthcare. Working to form a trusting relationship, discussing a mental health issue, and preparing to explain a very painful loss provide examples of how each can be addressed in ways that foster being with and knowing another, communicating respectfully, problem solving together, and regulating emotions. These ways of providing GP could be used with the discussion questions and questions about preparation to provide staff education, orient new staff, or create challenging real-life situations for a monthly team meeting.

REFERENCES

Feudtner, C. (2009). The breadth of hopes. *New England Journal of Medicine, 361*(24), 2306–2307.

Pawl, J. H. (1995). The therapeutic relationship as human connectedness: Being held in another's mind. *Zero to Three, 15*(4), 1–5.

24

Guided Participation Now and in the Future

Karen Pridham

THE VISION AND AIM OF THE BOOK

Our overarching vision in writing this book was to make guided participation (GP) as a practice of teaching and learning accessible, useful, and available to others to critique and develop. Our intent in making this vision a reality was to encompass aspects of GP in description of its structure, function, and use that we had come to know in pediatric nursing practice. The authors we chose to help us describe GP and to make clear what it could contribute to pediatric nursing practice substantially advanced the richness and the depth of our understanding. The chapters were written by clinicians and academicians who had a mind-set (or internal working model) for pediatric care and who were engaged in GP or thinking about it with some conception of the practice. Our ultimate aim is to develop concepts and practices of GP with parents, children, and clinicians which will support teaching and learning through developmental changes and across populations with the gamut of care responsibilities, a project that surpasses the limits of this book. The book, however, is a major step toward our aim.

The first section of this chapter is a discussion of what we learned about GP through the chapters our contributors wrote. The second section sketches next steps and questions for accomplishment of our aim. The care responsibilities, constructed in the context of the family's environment and the resources and competencies of family members, include managing chronic and acute illness, preventing illness, and promoting health. In many respects, the contributors to this book were guides to the book's editors in bringing out and making plain the kind of teaching–learning we had experienced or anticipated through GP.

Perspectives

In the process of the authors' discussions of GP from their multifaceted perspectives, the GP they were doing or designing was specified, described, reflected on, questioned, and further developed as a practice and a theory. We expected, as editors, that the boundaries of our assumptions and the limits of our understanding of GP and its implications for parents, children, clinicians, and academicians would be stretched and expanded to new zones of proximal development (Vygotsky, 1978) of pediatric nursing practice, along with education, research, and scholarship—its praxis. Now we know a great deal more about GP and have a clearer understanding of our assumptions and knowledge of our claims. Clearly, much development of theory and many research investigations are needed to determine the contribution to outcomes of GP as a teaching–learning practice in clinical settings.

WHAT WE HAVE LEARNED THROUGH THE CREATION OF THIS BOOK

The authors actively collaborated with us in structuring the chapters of this book. Assessment of what we have learned in this process reveals a broad scope of understandings and questions about GP in pediatric nursing practice.

- GP is grounded in the experience of real problems to be grappled with in the context of illness and health, and, within this experience, participation in the teaching–learning of socially important activities for acquiring the competencies that enable responsibility, whether full, partial, or collaborative.
- The premise that a relationship with a person who has the knowledge, skill, and commitment to understanding the motivation, goals, expectations, and intentions of the parent and child facilitates participation in learning was advanced by several authors.
- The nature of GP is revealed in authors' description of their work directly with children and parents or through academic study. GP goes beyond simply using open-ended assessments or interventions in which a choice is given. GP is distinct from merely involving parents and child in their care. This teaching–learning approach is oriented and directed to competent, responsible participation in the community that views the activity as important to be engaged in safely, effectively, and with satisfaction on the part of all participants, guide included.

- The relationship at the core of GP is not incidental, to be taken for granted, or to be treated like a black box that cannot be understood when doing GP. The relationship may need to be brought to the center of attention and focused on for the purpose of developing, strengthening, or maintaining it. When GP for teaching–learning is being practiced, the relationship is nurtured so that sharing attention on matters to be learned, making connections, and transferring responsibility can effectively and efficiently proceed.

- A culture is involved in GP from which the operative motivation, goals, expectations, and intentions (i.e., internal working model) are drawn or shaped. When GP is underway, culture and relationships are kept in mind by the guiding person(s). Communication with others involved in the GP contributes to understanding of the history and anticipated future of the person(s) being guided.

- The goals that direct or evolve with GP processes may have many sources or influences, including the population of families and children, condition and stage of the child, clinical setting, specialty of clinical care, mental status of the parents, and the internal working model of child or parent.

- Across cases of GP, a major source of variation surfaced. The goals that are giving direction to the GP populate, structure, and give a quality to the issues that specify the activity. Goals also determine processes of addressing issues and highlight competencies to be developed or strengthened to increase the odds of successful outcomes.

- GP processes can incorporate traditional strategies or techniques of education or adopt developing technologies, for example, a mobile application, without losing its distinctive features and contribution to development of experience through experience and participation.

- Clinicians have been and are learning to do GP in many settings where pediatric care is offered. Although initially developed with pediatric nurses in mind, GP is shown by authors of this book to be used in discipline-specific ways by dietitians, physicians, speech and language pathologists, and by pastors or spiritual guides.

- GP is for the most part nascent, incorporated into practice with commitment by clinicians who may be practicing it on their own volition, perhaps with the acquiescence of the clinical agency but not necessarily with fully expressed or formal support. Yet, there is at least one case of an agency, Resolve Through Sharing®, that has adopted GP as the standard of teaching–learning, relationship-based care.

GP for clinical practice in pediatric nursing has promise, but is undeveloped from theoretical, research, and health systems perspectives. We conclude, on the basis of our own experience and that of authors of this book, that GP is feasible, useful, and highly acceptable to parents, children, and clinicians. We have not yet located what we have learned about

GP within a theoretical framework that has concepts and relationships among them for context, conditions, sources, and outcomes. Our application of the internal working model construct (Bretherton & Munholland, 2008, 2016), including concepts of motivation, goals, expectations, intentions, competencies, and activities, is consistent with the construct of positive development, which attends to self-efficacy, competencies, and agency, among other concepts (Lerner, 2017). We are looking toward trends in developmental, educational, nursing, and healthcare science (Leman, Petersen, Smith, & SRCD Ethnic-Racial Issues and International Committees, 2017) to clarify what GP is about. Writing this book developed our understanding of GP as a construct of concepts and a practice from multiple perspectives. These perspectives are described in the next section.

GP FOR THE FUTURE

GP, with its goal of developing competencies for health-relevant responsibilities and tasks of children and parents, is consistent with current healthcare system directions. These directions, among them the Quadruple Aim, are toward improved health of populations, patient experience, and the work life of clinicians and staff, as well as reduced cost of care (Berwick, Nolan, & Whittington, 2008; Bodenheimer & Sinsky, 2014). These aims support participation of individuals and families in healthcare for development of competencies in its management. In writing this book, we recognized the consistency of GP, in its various forms of practice, with these healthcare aims. We also recognized, however, that much needs to be learned about how GP could effectively fit into and stimulate new healthcare system models of management of acute health problems, long-term chronic care, prevention of health problems, and promotion of health.

An initial step to learning what GP as a teaching–learning practice could contribute to the healthcare of various populations is to plumb the depths of what the GP in operation is about, that is, (a) its primary aims; (b) its orientation to prevention, day-to-day chronic illness care, and to relationship development and maintenance for the benefit of child, parents, family member, and healthcare team; (c) its methods or processes; and (d) its outcomes, both positive and negative. What may assist in sensitively and adequately characterizing the GP practice in operation is to have types of GP available to reference and to specify the kind of teaching and learning that is underway or intended. Several types of GP are revealed in this book. One type varies on formality, ranging from prestructured programs for children with the same or similar diagnosis to highly unstructured teaching and learning, as GP for a family with a prematurely born, extremely low-birth-weight baby might be. The dimensions of description and characterization of GP, if defined, could advance the testing of the effectiveness of GP.

Metaphors of GP as experience could be identified, among them, as a game metaphor (see Dewey, 1963; Fingarette, 1965, for metaphors of experience as learning in the form of a game). We could discern music composition as another type of metaphor for GP. Like a game, music composition has rules that distinguish types of composition, and when played, singly or with others, expectations of performance. This book illustrates improvisation as a feature of music composition and performance types that GP practice. GP may resemble a jazz group improvising the performance, displaying rules that operate to determine who performs next and with what style, but always with freedom and uncertainty about where the music is heading in terms of its aims and its strategies or processes. In contrast, GP may more closely resemble a classically constructed sonata in three-part form, with a phase of getting acquainted through assessment of issues, followed by a phase of wondering about the issue determined to be most pressing, and then making connections from the issue's sources to the present and future conditions or from what has worked in the past to what might work in the future, to a phase of explicitly transferring responsibility to the learners who are ready to accept it.

Other GP types of practice are distinguished by attention given to development or maintenance of health or relationship in an open-ended long-term condition, in contrast to the kind of rapid-response attention that is given when there is a crisis or psychological damage needs to be prevented or contained. Between these two extremes of GP implementation is the short-term, time-limited type associated with an acute illness, condition, or procedure.

A type of GP practice described in this book concerns competency development for care of a child with a complex chronic condition, whose development is uncertain and for whom feeding is a problem and growth is a challenge. This type of GP deliberately occurs over sessions not only for follow-up of the previous session but also for refining and developing competencies needed for conditions and issues that change as the child grows and develops. The GP best implemented has a complexity that may parallel that of the child's health condition. Issues for GP may become less complex and require less urgency of parental response as the child grows older, becomes more robust and competent in managing feeding and sleeping, and demonstrates expected developmental accomplishments.

The need for more intense GP, however, may resurface with transference of responsibility to a nurse or other clinician for decision making or managing caregiving. A higher level of GP may be called for at times of scheduled or emergent medical procedures, acute health problems, or developmental or healthcare transitions. The trajectory of GP sessions may become an increased number of closely spaced sessions, sometimes with reconstruction of what occurred in previous contacts, and sometimes with longer sessions that deal with more issues within a session, another basis of typing GP practice. Trajectories of GP may be discerned in longitudinal case studies included in this book.

The time GP requires to make some difference for learning is an important question for study from the perspective of clinical practicalities and the cost of implementing the practice. GP may be opportunistically engaged in on the fly without preparation or forethought and still have a powerful effect due to its strategic offering. GP that is a continuing process with a family when a child has a chronic condition is likely to evolve in structure and content as the child grows older and the parents become more experienced in caring for the child and the child more skilled in self-care tasks.

Identification of types of GP and description of conditions in which a specific type is offered are important for determining the impact or effect of GP on outcomes. Variables that characterize types of GP practice may make a difference for outcomes important for health (e.g., caregiving competencies; physiologic, behavioral, and emotional regulation; sensitivity and responsiveness of interaction; quality of life) and warrant identification. Among these variables are the issues addressed, what is delivered in brief encounters, what distinguishes the evolution of competence and responsibility in ongoing GP, and the time spent in GP and family member involvement.

QUESTIONS FOR STUDY OF GP IN PEDIATRIC CARE

The questions raised in this section bring attention to what needs study for GP in pediatric nursing care.

The Practice of Clinical Care

To practice GP clinically, data are needed to answer these questions:

- What characteristics of behavior and perspective are needed to do GP? Who is suited to this kind of practice? Can anyone be a guide for GP with children and their parents when healthcare issues are present? What kind of training prepares for GP practice? Should GP be taught in nursing school? What is needed for teaching and preparing others for practicing GP?
- How is continuity of GP planned for and maintained? Dewey (1963) emphasized the importance of continuity in making experience educationally beneficial.
- How can GP practice be tracked or recorded in an electronic healthcare record? Could the language of issues, processes, and competencies be used to keep track of GP in easily retrievable electronic form for purposes of accruing a history of GP for children and their parents and for making plans for future teaching–learning experiences or sessions?
- What clinical and family resources and policies are required for GP practice? How is reflection structured into the practice of GP?

The Substance, Process, and Quality of GP in Pediatric Care

Other questions concern the quality, substance, process, and outcomes of GP:

- How is the quality of GP assessed?
- How can the validity of specific GP sessions be determined? Has a session addressed adequately or at all what a child or parents are working on? Has the GP interaction been faithful to the reality children and parents experience?
- How can children and parents who would gain from GP best be identified? What criteria could be used for implementing GP sessions or experience? Who are GP resources best offered to?
- When should GP be initiated relative to identification of a health-related issue?
- How is GP explained to children and their parents in a way that supports and encourages participation?
- What criteria might be used to terminate GP sessions? How is termination of GP best implemented? When is follow-up desirable?

GP Issues: Subject Matter for Study

Another set of questions identify subject matter for further study:

- GP is a practice tailored to individual children and parents. As a consequence, it is highly variable in the issues involved, the processes included or emphasized, and the competencies that are the focus of attention. GP also varies within sessions and across time for any one child or parent. How can GP best be explored, described, and examined in ways that maintain the integrity of GP, keeping it recognizable as a practice with distinctive and recognizable principles? We have used methods of description including structured field notes and dimensional or matrix displays (Bowers & Schatzman, 2009; Miles, Huberman, & Moldano, 2014; Schatzman, 1991) to explore GP. These kinds of descriptions, we propose, could support identification and specification of types of GP practice.
- What contextual variables—conditions, environment, and resources—go into a theoretical framework for study of how GP proceeds and affects outcomes? Dewey (1963), in his book *Experience and Education*, stated the importance of being attuned to the conditions and sources of participation in experience as a basis of learning. He went on to claim that practitioners of teaching–learning through experience (or GP) have to know what social and physical conditions, resources, and histories are conducive to growth or development of competencies. Various types of GP are likely to require different resources, conditions of practice, training for leadership and expertise in practice, and methods of study.

Questions About Learning

We have much to learn about guided GP as a practice and its relevance and effectiveness for the learning of children and their parents about caring for their health. Questions that concern learning listed here are a suggestion of what future study might address.

- What is being learned, in the process of GP experience, about the self, others, and the relationship and the difference it makes for what is being learned?
- What is learning like when the child or parents are distressed, depressed, anxious, or experiencing trauma?
- How do parents and child learn together when perspectives of the situation differ?
- What difference does the parents' quality of coparenting make for their own and the child's learning?

GP Outcomes

The outcomes of GP we need to focus on now include short-range effects, for example, increased evidence of reflective thinking, problem solving, emotion regulation, and pleasure in being with the other person, parent, or child. Longer range outcomes of guided participation as a relationship-based teaching–learning practice include the child's social, emotional, cognitive, and physical development; the parents' competence in supporting the child's health and development and in coparenting; and the quality of life and life satisfaction of parent and child.

GP Research: Description, Feasibility, and Pilot Study of Effectiveness

Descriptive studies have enlarged our understanding of what parents are working on in relation to the loss of an infant, feeding an infant born very prematurely and with very low birth weight, or preparing and caring for an infant born with complex congenital heart disease. The studies we have done to date describe aspects of GP and support the feasibility and effectiveness of GP practice (Brown, Griffin, Reyna, & Lewis, 2013; Brown & Pickler, 2013; Brown, Thoyre, Pridham, & Schubert, 2009; Limbo & Pridham, 2007; McKechnie & Pridham, 2012; McKechnie, Pridham, & Tluczek, 2015a, 2015b; McKechnie, Rogstad, Martin, & Pridham, 2017; Pridham et al., 2005, 2006, 2010, 2017; Schroeder & Pridham, 2006; Thoyre, Hubbard, Park, Pridham, & McKechnie, 2016). Our current research concerning cocreation of GP practice with clinicians and the coparenting relationship of parents takes descriptive, correlational, and pilot clinical trial forms.

Beyond in-depth awareness of and attentiveness to types of GP in operation, creative approaches to research design for study of GP practice, located on the continua of various types, are needed. The research designs we are using are suited to rich description of small populations available for study that, however, may be difficult to recruit to studies because of the intensity of the care they are engaged in. Single cases, replicative or multiple cases, and longitudinal studies that can reveal patterns or trajectories over time are included in the designs we have used and intend to use. Graphical description for these purposes is aided by ongoing development and rediscovery of useful computer software.

CONCLUSION

What we have learned and need to learn about GP directs us to attend to how it functions, how it contributes to healthcare outcomes, and the conditions required for effectiveness. We need to learn more about the potential articulation of GP with healthcare system developments and trends and how GP practice could evolve for maximal use. Critical examination of the types of GP that we have observed and that could be created are needed to tailor it to the characteristics of the pediatric healthcare system and the conditions that are opportunities for development of GP practice.

Opportunities for GP activity abound in many environments and settings of life, providing inspiration and strategies for its practice. As I wrote this chapter, I recalled a serendipitous occasion for learning that occurred years ago on a family vacation. We were happy that we could park our car and have an easy walk to Chinatown in San Francisco. After several hours of our visit there, we returned to find our car gone. We walked up the hill, beyond where we had parked, and saw a sign that a tree had hidden from our view earlier. The sign read, "Tow away zone after 4 p.m." Our 6-year-old daughter was devastated by the loss of the car, and wept out of fear. Her 9-year-old brother, attempting to calm and reassure her, said with a memorable expression of confidence, "We can learn something from this." His comforting words were effective, and his saying about learning from experience, even frightening ones, became a family mantra, called on at times of challenge.

REFERENCES

Berwick, D. M., Nolan, T. W., & Whittington, J. (2008). The triple aim: Care, health, and cost. *Health Affairs (Millwood)*, 27, 759–769. doi:10.1377/hlthaff.27.3.759

Bodenheimer, T., & Sinsky, C. (2014). From triple to quadruple aim: Care of the patient requires care of the provider. *Annals of Family Medicine*, 12, 573–576. doi:10.1370/afm.1713

Bowers, B., & Schatzman, L. (2009). Dimensional analysis. In J. M. Morse, P. N. Stern, J. Corbin, B. Bowers, K. Charmaz, & A. E. Clarke (Eds.), *Developing grounded theory: The second generation* (pp. 86–106). Walnut Creek, OR: Left Coast Press.

Bretherton, I., & Munholland, K. A. (2008). Internal working models in attachment relationships: Elaborating a central construct in attachment theory. In J. Cassidy & P. R. Shaver (Eds.), *Handbook of attachment: Theory, research and clinical applications* (2nd ed., pp. 102–127). New York, NY: Guilford Press.

Bretherton, I., & Munholland, K. A. (2016). The internal working model construct in light of contemporary neuroimaging research. In J. Cassidy & P. R. Shaver (Eds.), *Handbook of attachment: Theory, research and clinical applications* (3rd ed., pp. 63–88). New York, NY: Guilford Press.

Brown, L. F., Griffin, J., Reyna, B., & Lewis, M. (2013). The development of a mother's internal working model of feeding. *Journal of Specialists in Pediatric Nursing, 18,* 54–64. doi:10.1111/jspn.12011

Brown, L. F., & Pickler, R. (2013). A guided feeding intervention for mothers of preterm infants: Two case studies. *Journal of Specialists in Pediatric Nursing, 18,* 98–108. doi:10.1111/jspn.12020. Epub 2013 Mar 24

Brown, L. F., Thoyre, S., Pridham, K. F., & Schubert, C. (2009). The mother-infant feeding tool. *Journal of Obstetric, Gynecologic, & Neonatal Nursing, 38,* 491–503. doi:10.1111/j.1552-6909.2009.01047.x

Dewey, J. (1963). *Experience and education.* New York, NY: Collier Books.

Fingarette, H. (1965). *The self in transformation: Psychoanalysis, philosophy and the life of the spirit.* New York, NY: Harper Torchbooks.

Leman, P. J., Smith, E. P., & Petersen, A. C., SRCD Ethnic-Racial Issues and International Committees. (2017). Introduction to the special section of *Child Development* on positive youth development in diverse and global contexts. *Child Development, 88,* 1039–1044. doi:10.1111/cdev.12860

Lerner, R. M. (2017). Commentary: Studying and testing the positive youth development model: A tale of two approaches. *Child Development, 88,* 1183–1185. doi:10.1111/cdev.12875

Limbo, R., & Pridham, K. F. (2007). Mothers' understanding of their infants in the context of an internal working model of caregiving. *ANS: Advances in Nursing Science, 30,* 139–150. doi:10.1097/01. ANS.0000271104.34420.b6

McKechnie, A. C., & Pridham, K. F. (2012). Preparing heart and mind following prenatal diagnosis of complex congenital heart defect. *Qualitative Health Research, 22*(12), 1694–1706. doi:1049732312458371 [pii] 10.1177/1049732312458371 [doi]

McKechnie, A. C., Pridham, K. F., & Tluczek, A. (2015a). Preparing heart and mind for becoming a parent following a diagnosis of fetal anomaly. *Qualitative Health Research, 25,* 1182–1198. doi:1049732314553852

McKechnie, A. C., Pridham, K. F., & Tluczek, A. (2015b). Walking the "emotional tightrope" from pregnancy to parenthood: Understanding parental motivation to manage health care and distress after a fetal diagnosis of complex congenital heart disease. *Journal of Family Nursing.* doi:1074840715616603

McKechnie, A. C., Rogstad, J., Martin, K. M., Pridham, K. F. (2017). An exploration of co-parenting in the context of caring for a child prenatally diagnosed and born with a complex health condition. *Journal of Advanced Nursing,* accepted manuscript online, August 9, 2017. doi:10.1111/jan.13415

Miles, M. B., Huberman, A. M., & Saldana, J. (2014). *Qualitative data analysis* (3rd ed.). Thousand Oaks, CA: Sage.

Pridham, K. F., Brown, R., Clark, R., Limbo, R. K., Schroeder, M., Henriques, J., & Bohne, E. (2005). Effect of guided participation on feeding competencies of mothers and their premature infants. *Research in Nursing & Health, 28,* 252–267. doi:10.1002/nur.20073

Pridham, K. F., Harrison, T., Krolikowski, M., Bathum, M. E., Ayres, L., & Winters, J. (2010). Internal working models of parenting: Motivations of parents of infants with a congenital heart defect. *ANS: Advances in Nursing Science, 33*(4), E1–E16. doi:10.1097/ANS.0b013e3181fc016e

Pridham, K. F., Harrison, T. M., McKechnie, A. C., & Brown, R. (2017). Motivations and features of co-parenting an infant with complex congenital heart disease. *Western Journal of Nursing Research,* Epublication ahead of print, June 1, 193945917712693. doi:10.1177/0193945917712693

Pridham, K. F., Krolikowski, M., Limbo, R. K., Paradowski, J., Rudd, N., Meurer, J. R., & Henriques, J. B. (2006). Guiding mothers' management of very low birth-weight infants. *Public Health Nursing, 23,* 205–215. doi:10.1111/j.1525-1446.2006.230302.x

Schroeder, M., & Pridham, K. F. (2006). Development of relationship competencies through guided participation for mothers of preterm infants. *Journal of Obstetric, Gynecologic, & Neonatal Nursing, 35,* 358–368. doi:10.1111/j.1552-6909.2006.00049.x

Thoyre, S. M., Hubbard, C., Park, J., Pridham, K. F., & McKechnie, A. (2016). Implementing co-regulated feeding with mothers of preterm infants. *MCN: American Journal of Maternal Child Nursing, 41,* 204–211. doi:10.1097/NMC.0000000000000245

Vygotsky, L. S. (1978). *Mind in society: The development of higher psychological processes.* Cambridge, MA: Harvard University Press.

Index